Inpatient Cardiovascular Medicine

Hospital Medicine: Current Concepts

Scott A. Flanders and Sanjay Saint, Series Editors

Inpatient Cardiovascular Medicine

Edited by

Brahmajee K. Nallamothu, MD, MPH
Associate Professor of Internal Medicine
University of Michigan
Ann Arbor, MI
USA

Timir S. Baman, MD
Clinical Assistant Professor of Medicine
University of Illinois College of Medicine at Peoria
Peoria, IL
USA

Series Editors

Scott A. Flanders, MD, MHM
Sanjay Saint, MD, MPH, FHM

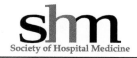

Society of Hospital Medicine

Hospitalists. Transforming Healthcare.
Revolutionizing Patient Care.

WILEY Blackwell

Published by John Wiley & Sons, Inc., Hoboken, New Jersey
Published simultaneously in Canada

For general information on our other products and services or for technical support, please contact our Customer Care Department within the United States at (800) 762-2974, outside the United States at (317) 572-3993 or fax (317) 572-4002.

Wiley also publishes its books in a variety of electronic formats. Some content that appears in print may not be available in electronic formats. For more information about Wiley products, visit our web site at www.wiley.com.

Library of Congress Cataloging-in-Publication Data:

Inpatient cardiovascular medicine / edited by Brahmajee K. Nallamothu, Timir S. Baman.
    p. ; cm. – (Hospital medicine : current concepts ; 6)
  Includes bibliographical references and index.
    ISBN 978-0-470-61000-8 (pbk. : alk. paper) – ISBN 978-1-118-48473-9 (Mobi) –
ISBN 978-1-118-48478-4 – ISBN 978-1-118-48481-4 (ePub) – ISBN 978-1-118-48482-1 (ePdf)
    I. Nallamothu, Brahmajee K., editor of compilation. II. Baman, Timir S., editor of compilation.
III. Series: Hospital medicine, current concepts ; 6.
  [DNLM: 1. Cardiovascular Diseases. 2. Inpatients. WG 120]
  RC674
  616.1′0231–dc23

2013017943

Cover image: Top left hand image – iStock file #3643872, middle left hand image – iStock file #10486652, bottom left hand image – iStock file #17324827

Printed in the United States of America

10 9 8 7 6 5 4 3 2 1

Contents

PART 5   Special Topics for the Inpatient Practitioner

Color plate section facing p. 212

Contributors

Keith Aaronson, MD, MS, Professor of Internal Medicine, Medical Director, Heart Transplant Program and Center for Circulatory Support, University of Michigan, Ann Arbor, MI, USA

Craig T. Alguire, MD, Assistant Professor, Michigan State University *and* Spectrum Health, Grand Rapids, MI, USA

William F. Armstrong, MD, Franklin Davis Johnston Collegiate Professor of Cardiovascular Medicine, Director, Echocardiography Laboratory, University of Michigan, Ann Arbor, MI, USA

David S. Bach, MD, Park W. Willis III Collegiate Professor of Cardiovascular Medicine, University of Michigan, Ann Arbor, MI, USA

Auroa Badin, MD, Assistant Professor of Clinical Medicine, University of Illinois College of Medicine at Peoria, Peoria, IL, USA

Timir S. Baman, MD, Assistant Professor of Medicine, University of Illinois College of Medicine at Peoria, Peoria, IL, USA

Anna M. Booher, MD, Assistant Professor of Internal Medicine, Division of Cardiovascular Medicine, University of Michigan, Ann Arbor, MI, USA

Sanders H. Chae, MD, Assistant Professor of Medicine, University of South Florida, Tampa, FL, USA

Stanley J. Chetcuti, MD, FACC, Associate Professor, Eric J. Topol Collegiate Professor of Cardiovascular Medicine, Director, Cardiac Catheterization Laboratory, University of Michigan, Ann Arbor, MI, USA

Jennifer A. Cowger, MD, MS, Assistant Professor, Medical Director Mechanical Circulatory Support Program, Cardiovascular Center, University of Michigan, Ann Arbor, MI, USA

Thomas C. Crawford, MD, Assistant Professor of Medicine, The University of Michigan, Ann Arbor, MI, USA

Melinda B. Davis, MD, Lecturer, Division of Cardiovascular Medicine, University of Michigan, Ann Arbor, MI, USA

Sharlene Day, MD, Assistant Professor of Internal Medicine, University of Michigan, Ann Arbor, MI, USA

Kim A. Eagle, MD, Albion Walter Hewlett Professor of Internal Medicine, and Director, Cardiovascular Center, University of Michigan, Ann Arbor, MI, USA

Dana P. Edelson, MD, MS, FAHA, FHM, Assistant Professor, University of Chicago Medical Center, Chicago, Illinois, USA

Anubhav Garg, MD, Lecturer, Department of Internal Medicine, University of Michigan, Ann Arbor, MI, USA

Zachary D. Goldberger, MD, MS, Assistant Professor of Medicine, Division of Cardiology, University of Washington School of Medicine/Harborview Medical Center, Seattle, Washington, USA

Sascha N. Goonewardena, Lecturer, Department of Internal Medicine, University of Michigan, Ann Arbor, MI, USA

P. Michael Grossman, MD, FACC, Associate Professor, Director, VA Ann Arbor Cardiac Catheterization Laboratory, University of Michigan, Ann Arbor, MI, USA

Sanjaya Gupta, MD, Assistant Professor of Internal Medicine, University of Missouri-Kansas City, *and* St. Luke's Hospital, Kansas City, MI, USA

Hitinder S. Gurm, MBBS, Associate Professor of Internal Medicine, University of Michigan, Ann Arbor, MI, USA

Peter G. Hagan, MB, Assistant Professor, Director, Cardiovascular Disease Fellowship Program, University of Michigan, Ann Arbor, MI, USA

Shea E. Hogan, MD, Cardiology Fellow, University of Michigan, Ann Arbor, MI, USA

Scott L. Hummel, MD, MS, Assistant Professor of Internal Medicine, Division of Cardiovascular Medicine, University of Michigan *and* Staff Cardiologist, Ann Arbor Veterans Affairs Health System, Ann Arbor, MI, USA

Karl J. Ilg, MD, Cardiac Electrophysiologist, Genesys Heart Institute, Grand Blanc, MI, USA

Renuka Jain, MD, Assistant Professor, University of Minnesota, Minneapolis, MN USA

Yogendra M. Kanthi, MD, Fellow, Cardiology and Vascular Medicine, University of Michigan, Ann Arbor, MI, USA

Christos Kasapis, MD, Interventional Cardiology Fellow, University of Michigan, Ann Arbor, MI, USA

Fareed U. Khaja, MD, Professor of Internal Medicine, University of Michigan, Ann Arbor, MI, USA

Gerald C. Koenig, MD, PhD, Assistant Professor of Medicine, Wayne State University and Henry Ford Hospital, Detroit, MI, USA

David C. Lange, MD, Fellow, Division of Cardiovascular Medicine, Cedars Sinai Medical Center, Los Angeles, CA, USA

Preeti N. Malani, MD, MSJ, Associate Professor of Internal Medicine, Divisions of Infectious Diseases and Geriatric Medicine, University of Michigan *and* Veterans Affairs Ann Arbor Healthcare System, Geriatric Research Education and Clinical Center (GRECC), Ann Arbor, MI, USA

Vallerie V. McLaughlin, MD, Professor of Medicine, Division of Cardiovascular Medicine, Director, Pulmonary Hypertension Program, University of Michigan, Ann Arbor, MI, USA

Brahmajee K. Nallamothu, MD, MPH, Associate Professor of Internal Medicine, University of Michigan, Ann Arbor, MI, USA

Hakan Oral, MD, Frederick G. L. Huetwell Professor of Cardiovascular Medicine, Director, Cardiac Arrhythmia Service, University of Michigan, Ann Arbor, MI, USA

Francis D. Pagani, MD, PhD, Otto Gago, M.D. Professor in Cardiac Surgery, Cardiovascular Center, University of Michigan, Ann Arbor, MI, USA

Amir B. Rabbani, MD, Cardiovascular Institute, DMC Harper University Hospital, Detroit, MI, USA

Michael C. Reed, MD, Interventional Cardiology, St. Patrick's Hospital, Missoula, MT, *and* University of Washington Affiliate, Seattle, WA, USA

Adam M. Rogers, MD, Kaiser Permanente Walnut Creek Medical Center, Walnut Creek, CA, USA

Sara Saberi, MD, Lecturer, University of Michigan, Ann Arbor, MI, USA

Michael J. Shea, MD, Professor of Internal Medicine, Section Head, Cardiovascular Medicine Outpatient Service and Clinical Education, Co-Director, Aortic Valve Clinic, University of Michigan, Ann Arbor, MI, USA

Nicklaus K. Slocum, MD, Traverse Heart & Vascular, Traverse City, MI, USA

Njeri Thande, MD, Assistant Professor of Cardiology, Albert Einstein Medical School, Montefiore Hospital, Bronx, NY, USA

Michael P. Thomas, MD, Lecturer, Division of Cardiovascular Medicine, University of Michigan, Ann Arbor, MI, USA

Thomas T. Tsai, MD, MSc, Director, Interventional Cardiology, Denver VA Medical Center *and* Assistant Professor, University of Colorado Denver *and* Investigator, Colorado Cardiovascular Outcomes Research (CCOR) Group, Denver, CO, USA

Scott H. Visovatti, MD, Lecturer, Division of Cardiovascular Medicine, University of Michigan, Ann Arbor, MI, USA

Preface

In the United States, the number of hospital admissions in which cardiovascular diseases play a significant role is increasing due to an aging population. The care for these patients also is becoming more complex with an ever-increasing amount of novel drugs and devices being introduced that target or impact on the heart. At the same time, many patients with cardiovascular diseases are now being managed by non-cardiovascular physicians in the inpatient setting when they are admitted for other diseases. As a result, hospitalists and other inpatient practitioners are increasingly exposed to these patients but faced with anxiety and uncertainty when contemplating their proper management. Current texts may discuss various cardiovascular diseases in detail, but less often convey to the reader how to best incorporate this information most effectively into everyday clinical practice. They also rarely discuss the secondary role of cardiovascular diseases during a hospitalization, when conditions like pneumonia or peptic ulcer disease can be strongly influenced by the presence of coronary artery disease or heart failure. This book focuses on cardiovascular medicine from the perspective of the busy inpatient practitioners. It is highly practical and algorithmic in nature, and our hope is that the reader will be able to care for his or her patient directly using contemporary evidence.

We have provided a format that we believe can be easily integrated into the daily practice of a broad range of non-cardiovascular physicians (e.g., hospitalists, internal medicine residents, nurse practitioners). We have divided the book into five major sections: 1) General Principles and Conditions in Cardiovascular Medicine; 2) Ischemic Heart and Vascular Disease; 3) Heart Failure and Cardiomyopathy; 4) Syncope and Arrhythmias; and 5) Special Topics for the Inpatient Practitioner. These sections serve as broad categories so that the reader can search for their specific topic of interest. Within each section, chapters are integrated with one another. We hope this flow is apparent and useful for readers utilizing the book. We have intentionally limited the text in the chapters as much as possible. We understand the busy nature of clinical practice and tried to place a special emphasis on the integration of charts, diagrams, and algorithms to make the book more user-friendly and applicable to daily patient care. We believe this approach also allows inpatient practitioners to immediately relay information back to the patient. Finally, we highlight several important points throughout the book, reflecting the informal but critical nature of a "Take Home Point" that is so familiar to clinicians everywhere.

Of course, we hope you will find our work interesting to read, but mostly that you find it useful for your patients.

Chapter 1

Cardiovascular History and Physical Examination

Melinda B. Davis and Michael J. Shea

Despite enormous technological advances in cardiovascular medicine, optimal care of patients with heart disease begins with a focused and thorough history and physical examination. Such an approach is needed not only to diagnose conditions but to relate findings obtained from additional testing into appropriate clinical context. A successful history and physical examination also establishes a foundation for a strong patient–physician relationship, which can greatly assist in complex discussions regarding therapeutic options.

1.1 HISTORY

Cardiac disease can masquerade in many different forms but classic symptoms include chest discomfort, fatigue, edema, weight gain, dyspnea, palpitations, syncope, cough, hemoptysis, and cyanosis. Symptoms of vascular disease include claudication, limb pain, edema, and skin discoloration. Patients' descriptions of symptoms yield a great deal of information and should never be discounted (Table 1.1). Basic elements of the history include the symptom onset, the nature and severity, duration, frequency, precipitating and relieving factors, impact on daily life and employment, and similarity to prior episodes. Major risk factors for coronary artery disease include age, male gender, family history, tobacco use, hyperlipidemia, hypertension, sedentary lifestyle, obesity, and diabetes mellitus.

Inpatient Cardiovascular Medicine, First Edition. Edited by Brahmajee K. Nallamothu and Timir S. Baman.

Table 1.1   Cardiovascular Symptoms and Conditions. Patients should be questioned about the following common cardiovascular symptoms. Different features in the history can provide valuable diagnostic information.

Symptoms and conditions	Patient descriptions
Paroxysmal nocturnal dyspnea	Occurs 2–4 hours after falling asleep, causes the patient to sit upright or stand, and resolves over several minutes
Palpitations	Fluttering, skipping, pounding heartbeat; differentiate between fast and sustained versus isolated beats
Orthopnea	Shortness of breath when lying flat, typically measured by the number of pillows needed to sleep
Sleep apnea	Loud snoring, or periods of interrupted breathing
Pulmonary embolism	Usually acute onset of dyspnea
Cardiac syncope	Sudden onset with quick restoration of consciousness
Neurocardiogenic syncope	Warning signs of nausea, yawning, diaphoresis, ashen skin, slower resolution of symptoms, without evidence of seizure or post-ictal state

Table 1.2   Comparison of the New York Heart Association Functional Classification with the AHA/ACC Heart Failure Stages Classification. Note that these are two different classification systems and that the different levels are not interchangeable.

Class	New York Heart Association Heart Failure Classification	Stage	AHA/ACC Heart Failure Stages
I (Mild)	No limitation in physical activities. No symptoms of fatigue, dyspnea, palpitations, angina	A	High risk for developing heart failure
II (Moderate)	Slight limitation in physical activity. Comfortable at rest, but ordinary physical activities cause symptoms	B	Damage to the heart, but never had symptoms of heart failure, e.g. after myocardial infarction
III (Moderate)	Marked limitation in physical activity. Less than ordinary activities cause symptoms	C	Heart failure symptoms from cardiac dysfunction. e.g. dyspnea, fatigue, exercise intolerance
IV (Severe)	Cannot carry out any physical activity without symptoms, and may have symptoms at rest	D	Advanced heart failure with severe symptoms

Chest discomfort is a common symptom and specific factors will increase or decrease the likelihood of acute coronary syndrome (ACS). Noncardiac chest discomfort is usually described as stabbing, pleuritic, positional, reproducible with palpation, or occurring *after* exertion (rather than during activity). If the pain is depicted as radiating to one or both shoulders or brought on by exertion or mental stress, a cardiac origin consistent with angina must be highly suspected.

Clinicians must be aware that, in some patients, chest discomfort due to angina may resolve with further activity due to recruitment of collaterals. So-called "anginal equivalents" include indigestion, belching, and dyspnea. Pain that is immediately relieved by sublingual nitroglycerin may be due to cardiac ischemia or esophageal spasm.

Patients with heart failure should be assigned to a New York Heart Association (NYHA) Functional Class based on their reported symptoms. Patients can also be classified based on the stage of disease progression using the AHA/ACC Heart Failure Stages (Table 1.2).

1.2 PHYSICAL EXAMINATION

Many cardiovascular diseases have commonly associated physical exam findings (Table 1.3). An adequate physical examination can streamline the use of additional diagnostic testing, such as laboratory studies and advanced imaging, and improve patient outcomes.

Table 1.3   Physical Exam Findings and Associated Cardiovascular Disease Pathology. Note that this is not an exhaustive differential diagnosis of each finding.

Physical exam Findings	Associated conditions
Carotid bruit	Carotid artery stenosis or transmitted heart murmur (e.g. aortic stenosis)
Femoral bruit	Arteriovenous fistula, peripheral arterial disease
Abdominal bruit	Celiac artery stenosis, transmitted heart murmur, renal artery stenosis, transplanted kidney
Cyanosis	Pulmonary hypertension
Cyanosis that affects the lower extremities	Patent ductus arteriosus
Large protruding tongue with parotid enlargement	Amyloid
Edema	Heart failure, medications, low albumin
Medial ulcers, hyperpigmentation, varicosities	Chronic venous insufficiency
Muscular atrophy, absent hair in extremity	Chronic arterial insufficiency
Anterior cutaneous venous collaterals	Superior vena cava (SVC) obstruction (or subclavian vein)
Kyphosis, lumbar/hip/knee flexion	Ankylosing spondylitis (look for aortic regurgitation)
Enlarged tender liver	Heart failure (right-sided)
Systolic hepatic pulsations	Severe tricuspid regurgitation
Ascites	Right heart failure, constrictive pericarditis, hepatic cirrhosis
Palpable abdominal mass	Possible abdominal aortic aneurysm

1.2.1 Blood Pressure

Proper blood pressure measurement is critical for patient care. A major source of error is using an incorrectly sized cuff, i.e. a cuff that is too small will read an artificially elevated blood pressure, and vice versa. Patients should be at rest for 5–10 minutes prior to measurement, seated with their arms at heart level. If a patient is supine, the arm should be raised on a pillow to the level of the mid-right atrium. The first Korotkoff sound is the systolic pressure and the final sound (when the Korotkoff sounds disappear) is the diastolic pressure.

If there is an *auscultatory gap* (the Korotkoff sounds disappear soon after the first sound), this first sound still denotes the systolic blood pressure. This is more common in hypertensive, elderly patients, with poor arterial flow in the upper extremities.

Pulsus paradoxus is an accentuated decrease (greater than 10 mm Hg) in systolic pressure with inspiration. The peripheral pulse may also disappear. This finding may indicate pericardial tamponade, severe airway obstruction, COPD, or superior vena cava obstruction. To test for pulsus paradoxus, the blood pressure cuff is inflated above systolic pressure. The cuff is deflated slowly (approximately 2–3 mm Hg per second). The pressure at which the first Korotkoff sound occurs should be noted. Initially, the sounds will be irregular as they vary with respiration (i.e. disappear with inspiration). The pressure at which the sounds become regular should be subtracted from the pressure of the first sound, and if the difference is >10 mm Hg, a pulsus paradoxus is present.

TAKE HOME POINT #1

Pulsus paradoxus is defined as greater than 10 mm Hg and is measured with a manual cuff. The pressure at which the sounds become regular and no longer vary with respiration should be substracted from the pressure of the first Korotkoff sound.

Intra-arterial measurement is generally higher than auscultatory measurement. Blood pressure taken distally at the wrist measures higher systolic pressure and lower diastolic pressure, but there is little change to the mean pressure.

Blood pressure should be measured in both arms; a difference of greater than 10 mm Hg is abnormal (Table 1.4). Blood pressure measured in the legs that is greater than 20 mm Hg higher than arm pressures may indicate peripheral arterial disease (PAD) or severe aortic regurgitation (Hill sign).

Table 1.4   Difference of more than 10 mm Hg of Pressure between the Arms.

Differential diagnosis if blood pressure between arms is greater than 10mm Hg
Normal variant (20% of normal subjects)
Subclavian artery disease (atherosclerosis or inflammation)
Supravalvular aortic stenosis
Aortic coarctation
Aortic dissection

1.2.2   Jugular Venous Pressure

Volume status can be assessed by evaluation of the jugular venous pressure (JVP). The internal jugular vein is preferred because there are no valves and it is directly in line with the superior vena cava and right atrium, but the external jugular vein may be easier to visualize when distended. Generally, the venous pulsations are best appreciated with the patient reclined to 30 degrees. To visualize venous pulsations in a patient who is believed to be volume-overloaded, ask the patient to sit with his/her feet dangling over the side of the bed so that venous blood will pool in the lower extremities. If a patient is hypotensive, the supine position may make it easier to visualize the veins. The venous pulsations can be distinguished from the carotid artery by the waveform (a and v waves, and x and y descents) and biphasic pulsation (Table 1.5). The vein also falls with inspiration and obliterates with gentle pressure.

Table 1.5   Jugular venous waveforms associated with cardiovascular diseases.

Diagnosis	Waveform	Description
Normal		Positive deflections are a and v waves; c wave is not always seen; refer to text
Atrial fibrillation		Absent a waves (no regualr atrial contraction)
Complete AV block		Cannon a waves (atria contracting against closed tricuspid valve)
Constrictive pericarditis		Accentuated x descent Sharp deep y descent with rapid ascent
Tricuspid regurgitation (severe)		Prominent v waves (may have single large positive systolic waves with obliteration of the x descent) Rapid deep y descent
Tricuspid stenosis		Large a wave (increased atrial contraction pressure)

Venous pressure is measured by the vertical distance from the top of the column of venous pulsation to the Angle of Louis where the manubrium meets the sternum, normally less than 3 cm. The distance between the sternal angle and the RA is 5 cm which, when added to the vertical column, gives an estimation of the central venous pressure (i.e. 3 cm + 5 cm = 8 cm blood). This method can underestimate the venous pressure, and some recommend that it only be used to distinguish normal from abnormal venous pressure. The most common cause of elevated venous pressure is an elevated right ventricular diastolic pressure.

Normally, the jugular venous pressure falls by at least 3 mm Hg with inspiration. In cases of right-sided volume overload (i.e. constrictive pericarditis or right ventricular infarction), the venous pressure may rise with inspiration known as *Kussmaul's sign*.

Hepatojugular reflux or abdominojugular reflux is indicative of volume overload and is predictive of heart failure and a pulmonary artery wedge pressure greater than 15 mm Hg. This is elicited by applying firm pressure over the right upper quadrant for at least 10 seconds; a positive sign is illustrated if the JVP rises by greater than 3 cm for more than 15 seconds (of normal respirations) followed by a rapid drop in pressure after release of abdominal pressure.

1.2.3 Jugular Venous Waveforms

Although challenging to assess, the jugular venous waveform yields a great deal of information (Table 1.5). The presystolic *a wave* is the dominant wave and is caused by contraction of the right atrium (RA). The RA pressure then falls, causing the *x descent*. The *c wave* occurs when ventricular systole pushes the closed tricuspid valve (TV) into the RA, but is rarely visible. The predominant *x descent* occurs as the RA relaxes and ventricular systole pulls the right atrium and TV downward. The *v wave* occurs in late systole as the right atrium fills (while the TV is closed). When the TV opens and the RA pressure falls rapidly, this is the *y descent*.

1.2.4 Pulses

A weak and delayed carotid pulse, *pulsus parvus et tardus*, suggests severe aortic stenosis. Timing of the carotid pulse is assessed by simultaneous cardiac auscultation.

Table 1.6 Palpation of the Precordium.

Palpation of precordium findings	Clinical associations
Increased amplitude, duration, size	Left ventricular hypertrophy
Lateral and downward displacement	Left ventricular volume overload
	Dilated cardiomyopathy
	Aortic regurgitation
Double systolic impulse	Hypertrophic cardiomyopathy
Lower left parasternal lift during systole	Right ventricular hypertrophy
Left parasternal lift	Severe mitral regurgitation
(after the LV apical impulse)	(large LA causes anterior displacement of RV)
Right parasternal lift	Severe tricuspid regurgitation with large RV
Right sternoclavicular joint pulsation	Aneurysmal dilation of ascending aorta
Pulsation of pulmonary artery	Pulmonary hypertension
in the second left intercostal space	

The carotid upstroke should occur while S1 is heard, though older hypertensive patients with stiff arteries can have a mild delay. A *Corrigan or water-hammer pulse* with an abrupt upstroke and rapid fall-off is characteristic of aortic regurgitation.

The femoral and radial arterial pulses should be palpated simultaneously. A delay in the femoral pulsation and decrease in amplitude indicates aortic coarctation, which can be an unappreciated cause of hypertension. Auscultation of the femoral arteries can reveal a bruit from an arteriovenous fistula, particularly in a patient with prior instrumentation.

1.2.5 Palpation of Precordium

The cardiac impulse gives clues about associated cardiac disease by its timing, duration, and location (Table 1.6). Normally, the left ventricular apical impulse is located at the 4–5th intercostal space in the left midclavicular line, less than 2.5 cm in diameter, and occurs in early systole. The apical impulse can be abnormally displaced, enlarged or delayed depending upon several disease processes.

1.2.6 Heart Sounds

Careful auscultation of cardiac sounds can provide important diagnostic and prognostic information. The exam should take place in a quiet area and should not be rushed. Subtle findings are best appreciated by listening specifically for the sounds that occur in each phase of the cardiac cycle. The carotid pulse should be palpated in order to determine the timing of systole and diastole. Distal pulses (e.g. the radial pulse) should not be used for timing as there is too much time delay to correspond to systole and diastole.

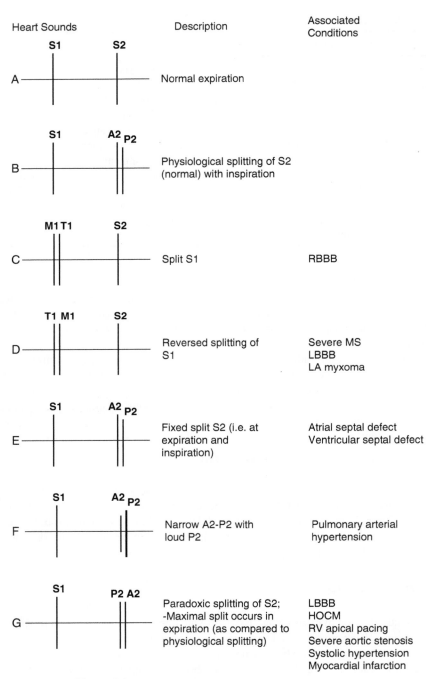

Figure 1.1 Heart sounds: description and associated conditions.

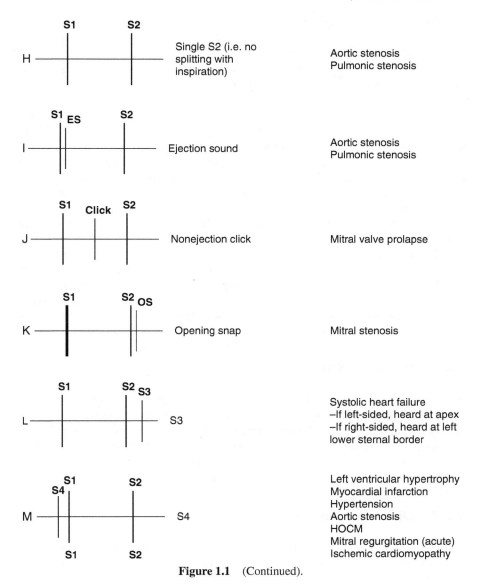

Figure 1.1   (Continued).

The first heart sound (S1) is best heard at the lower left sternal border and reflects closure of the mitral (M1) and tricuspid (T1) valves (Figure 1.1A). A split S1 is heard with a right bundle branch block (Figure 1.1B). Reversed splitting (when the tricuspid component occurs before the mitral component) occurs in severe mitral stenosis, left atrial myxoma, and left bundle branch block (Figure 1.1C). A loud S1 occurs in hyperkinetic states, short PR intervals, and mitral stenosis. S1 can be soft in the setting of late mitral stenosis, contractile dysfunction, beta-blockers, long PR intervals, and mitral regurgitation. The amplitude of all heart sounds may be diminished in the setting of mechanical ventilation, pericardial and pleural effusions, severe COPD, obesity, and pneumothorax.

The second heart sound (S2) is best heard at the second left intercostal space in the supine position, and reflects the closure of the aortic (A2) and pulmonic (P2) valves (Figure 1.1A). *Physiologic splitting of S2* (A2 before P2) occurs with inspiration as venous return to the right ventricle increases, thus prolonging the right ventricular ejection time and delaying the closure of the pulmonic valve (P2) (Figure 1.1D). Simultaneously, the negative intrathoracic pressure of inspiration causes more blood to remain in the lungs, resulting in decreased filling of the LV, faster LV ejection, and earlier closure of the aortic valve (A2). With expiration, the splitting should resolve. Persistent splitting can occur with right bundle branch block or severe mitral regurgitation, but there should still be respiratory variation. A *fixed-split S2* means there is no variation with respiration suggestive of atrial septal defect or ventricular septal defect (Figure 1.1E). In pulmonary arterial hypertension, the A2–P2 interval narrows and P2 is louder (and may be palpable in the second left intercostal space) (Figure 1.1F). Reversed or *paradoxic splitting* (P2 occurs before A2) occurs when aortic valve closure is pathologically delayed as in left bundle branch block, RV apical pacing, HOCM, severe aortic stenosis, systolic hypertension, or myocardial ischemia (Figure 1.1G). The splitting is maximal in expiration and decreases in inspiration. Closure of aortic and pulmonic valves will be quieter in the setting of severe stenosis and this may cause a single S2 to be heard (Figure 1.1H).

1.2.7 Systolic Sounds

An ejection sound is a high-pitched auscultation caused by the initial flow out of the RV or LV (Figure 1.1I). It occurs in early systole and corresponds in timing with the peak of the carotid upstroke. Congenital bicuspid AV or PV disease, aortic or pulmonic stenosis, and aortic root dilation can cause ejection sounds. A nonejection click is caused by mitral valve prolapse (or, more rarely, tricuspid valve prolapse) and is therefore heard in midsystole just after the peak of the carotid upstroke (Figure 1.1J).

1.2.8 Diastolic Sounds

Mitral stenosis causes an opening snap (OS) to occur shortly after S2 but, as the rigidity of the mitral valve increases this sound will decrease or disappear (Figure 1.1K). It is heard best with the bell of the stethoscope with the patient in the left lateral decubitus position.

A third heart sound (S3) is caused by early rapid ventricular filling (Figure 1.1L). This sound may be normal in young people, but is a significant indicator of systolic heart failure in older adults. The left-sided S3 is best heard during expiration with the patient in the left lateral position using the bell of the stethoscope at the apex. The right-sided S3 is best heard during inspiration at the left sternal border or beneath the xiphoid. As heart failure is treated, the S3 disappears, thus this heart sound can be serially assessed during a hospitalization for heart failure.

A fourth heart sound (S4) is caused by late ventricular filling from the "atrial kick" suggesting a high dependency on the atrial contribution to diastolic filling (i.e. maintenance of sinus rhythm may be important in these patients) (Figure 1.1 M). It is best heard with the bell of the stethoscope at the cardiac apex with the patient in the left lateral position. The S4 is frequently present with systemic hypertension, left ventricular hypertrophy, aortic stenosis, hypertrophic cardiomyopathy, acute mitral regurgitation, ischemic heart disease or myocardial ischemia. Left-sided S3 and S4 sounds will increase with isometric exercise.

TAKE HOME POINT #3

S3 and S4 gallops are best heard with the bell of the stethoscope at the cardiac apex with the patient in the left lateral poition.

1.2.9 Cardiac Murmurs

Murmurs may be pathological or benign in origin and accurate identification will guide a clinician to determine the need for echocardiography. Murmur intensity is graded on a scale of 1 to 6 with 4 or higher associated with a palpable thrill (Table 1.7). Location, radiation, and response to maneuvers should always be assessed.

In the absence of symptoms and findings suggestive of cardiovascular disease, echocardiography is not necessary for evaluation of a mid-systolic flow murmur of grade 2 or less intensity. Murmurs of higher intensity, early/late/holosystolic murmurs, continuous murmurs, and all diastolic murmurs should be evaluated by echocardiography with subsequent referral to a cardiologist even in asymptomatic patients.

TAKE HOME POINT #4

Echocardiography should be ordered for all murmurs of higher intensity, early/late/holosystolic murmurs, continuous murmurs, and all diastolic murmurs, even in asymptomatic patients.

Table 1.7 Grading murmur intensity.

Grade 1	Barely audible
Grade 2	Heard with intense listening
Grade 3	Easily heard throughout precordium
Grade 4	Associated with a thrill
Grade 5	Heard with stethoscope partly off chest with thrill
Grade 6	Heard with stethoscope entirely off chest with thrill

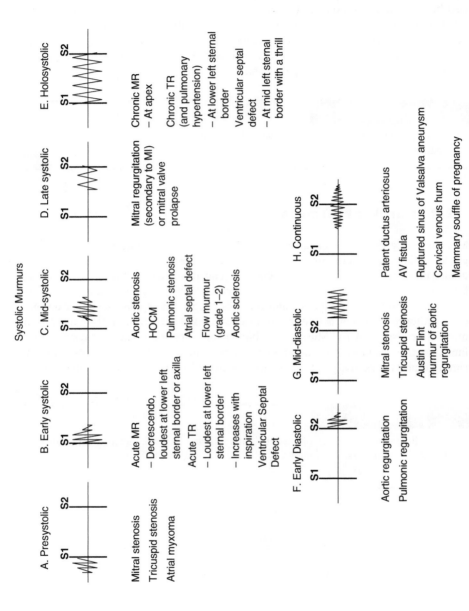

Systolic Murmurs

A. Presystolic

Mitral stenosis
Tricuspid stenosis
Atrial myxoma

B. Early systolic

Acute MR
– Decrescendo,
  loudest at lower left
  sternal border or axilla
Acute TR
– Loudest at lower left
  sternal border
– Increases with
  inspiration
Ventricular Septal
Defect

C. Mid-systolic

Aortic stenosis
HOCM
Pulmonic stenosis
Atrial septal defect
Flow murmur
(grade 1–2)
Aortic sclerosis

D. Late systolic

Mitral regurgitation
(secondary to MI)
or mitral valve
prolapse

E. Holosystolic

Chronic MR
– At apex
Chronic TR
(and pulmonary
hypertension)
– At lower left sternal
  border
Ventricular septal
defect
– At mid left sternal
  border with a thrill

F. Early Diastolic

Aortic regurgitation
Pulmonic regurgitation

G. Mid-diastolic

Mitral stenosis
Tricuspid stenosis
Austin Flint
murmur of aortic
regurgitation

H. Continuous

Patent ductus arteriosus
AV fistula
Ruptured sinus of Valsalva aneurysm
Cervical venous hum
Mammary souffle of pregnancy

Figure 1.2 Assessment of murmurs.

12

1.2.10 Systolic murmurs

Presystolic murmurs can occur with mitral or tricuspid stenosis and occasionally from atrial myxoma (Figure 1.2A). The sound occurs during atrial contraction and is crescendo in nature leading up to a loud S1 (in the case of valve stenosis).

Early systolic murmurs begin with S1 and end in midsystole and are caused by acute tricuspid and mitral regurgitation as well as ventricular septal defects (Figure 1.2B). The murmur of acute tricuspid regurgitation with normal pulmonary pressure is loudest at the left sternal border and increases with inspiration (right-sided murmurs increase with increased venous return). The murmur of acute mitral regurgitation is decrescendo and best heard at the lower left sternal border or axilla.

Mid-systolic murmurs start after S1 and end before S2 (Figure 1.2C). They occur when blood is ejected through the aortic and pulmonic outflow tracts and are crescendo-decrescendo in shape. Aortic and pulmonic stenosis can both cause this pattern as well as hypertrophic cardiomyopathy and atrial septal defects with left to right shunt. A grade 1 or 2 isolated murmur at the left sternal border can be described as a flow murmur resulting from fever, hyperthyroidism, anemia, or pregnancy, and can also be heard in young people.

Aortic sclerosis also causes a mid-systolic murmur with intensity no greater than 2 or 3 and can be differentiated from aortic stenosis by a normal carotid upstroke, preserved A2, and lack of left ventricular hypertrophy; however, a surface echocardiogram is often necessary.

Late systolic murmurs are high-pitched, delayed until after ejection, and are best heard at the apex (Figure 1.2D). These murmurs can occur if myocardial ischemia changes the configuration of the left ventricle or papillary muscles causing late mitral regurgitation. A late systolic murmur can also occur in the setting of late mitral regurgitation secondary to mitral valve prolapse (with or without an audible nonejection click).

Holosystolic murmurs start with S1 and extend up to S2 (Figure 1.2E). They are caused by a large pressure differential between two chambers throughout systole. Typical causes are: (1) chronic MR (loudest at cardiac apex); (2) chronic TR with pulmonary hypertension (loudest at lower left sternal border); and (3) VSD without pulmonary hypertension (loudest at mid-left sternal border, usually with a thrill).

1.2.11 Diastolic Murmurs

Diastolic murmurs should be considered pathological and warrant further evaluation with echocardiography and cardiology consultation.

Early diastolic murmurs start with or are shortly after S2 and are characterized as high-pitched, decrescendo murmurs associated with aortic or pulmonic regurgitation (Figure 1.2F). These murmurs occur in early diastole as this time period corresponds to the greatest amount of regurgitation (due to the largest pressure differential). The best way to hear these soft sounds is by applying firm pressure with the diaphragm over the left midsternal border with the patient sitting forward and holding a breath in full exhalation. The murmur of aortic regurgitation is best heard along the left sternal border if secondary to aortic valve disease or radiating along the right sternal border if secondary to aortic root dilatation. This murmur will enhance with elevation of systolic arterial pressure such as with hand-grip exercise. Pulmonic regurgitation due to chronic pulmonary hypertension is best heard at the left sternal border and is associated with other signs of RV pressure overload.

Mid-diastolic murmurs occur after S2 and end before S1 (Figure 1.2G). They are caused by mitral or tricuspid stenosis, or are heard in the setting of functional stenosis when there is accelerated flow across the valves (i.e. a disproportion between the valve orifice and the flow rate). Mitral stenosis causes a mid-to-late diastolic murmur which may be absent in obese patients or in the setting of low cardiac output. It is best heard as a low-pitched rumbling at the apex in the left lateral decubitus position. In early mitral stenosis, the murmur may be preceded by an opening snap.

The Austin Flint murmur is a mid-to-late diastolic murmur due to severe aortic regurgitation. The murmur occurs when a high velocity aortic regurgitant jet strikes the mitral valve leaflet causing distortion and early closure of the mitral valve during diastole. The murmur is low-pitched and heard best at the apex and should be distinguished from mitral stenosis.

Continuous murmurs raise concern for patent ductus arteriosus (PDA), ruptured sinus of Valsalva aneurysm, and coronary/great vessel/hemodialysis AV fistulas (Figure 1.2H). Benign causes include cervical venous hum and mammary souffle due to pregnancy.

1.3   BEDSIDE MANEUVERS

Simple bedside maneuvers are extremely important for distinguishing different murmurs and should be performed routinely (Table 1.8). Maneuvers that increase left ventricular afterload (i.e. handgrip or the addition of vasopressors) will increase the murmurs of left-sided regurgitant lesions (i.e. MR, AR, or VSD). Squatting causes an increase in ventricular preload and afterload, thus increasing left ventricular volume. In this case, the murmur of HOCM will become softer and shorter because less obstruction is present. The opposite occurs with standing when the ventricular preload drops. During this maneuver, there is less ventricular filling, resulting in increased outflow tract obstruction and a longer and louder murmur. Squatting causes the click and murmur of mitral valve prolapse to move away from S1 because the higher ventricular volume delays the leaflet prolapse (and the opposite occurs with standing). The Valsalva maneuver involves expiration against a closed glottis. The increase in intrathoracic pressure reduces venous return, and decreases cardiac filling. The murmur of HOCM will increase whereas the murmur of aortic stenosis will decrease. Following a premature beat, the next cardiac cycle will have increased LV filling as well as increased contractile function; this causes more forward flow across the aortic valve, a higher gradient and, hence, a louder

Table 1.8   Effect of Maneuvers on Preload, Afterload, Ventricular Filling, and Murmur Intensity.

Maneuver	Effect on preload	Effect on afterload	Ventricular volume	Change in murmurs
Handgrip	–	Increase	Increase	Increase MR, AR, VSD Decrease HOCM
Squat	Increase	Increase	Increase	Decrease HOCM
Stand	Decrease	–	Decrease	Increase HOCM
Valsalva	Decrease	–	Decrease	Increase HOCM, MVP Decrease AS, PS, TR
Beat after a premature contraction	Increase	Decrease	Increase	Increase AS Decrease HOCM No change MR

AR, Aortic regurgitation; AS, Aortic stenosis; HOCM, Hypertrophic obstructive cardiomyopathy; MR, Mitral regurgitation; MS, Mitral stenosis; MVP, Mitral valve prolapse; PS, Pulmonic stenosis; TR, Tricuspid regurgitation; VSD, Ventricular septal defect

murmur of aortic stenosis. The murmur of HOCM will soften, and the murmur of MR will not change (due to less change in volume and gradient across the MV). Inspiration causes decreased intrathoracic pressure, increased venous return, and increased intensity of right-sided murmurs (except for severe tricuspid regurgitation with right ventricular dilation and failure). Left-sided murmurs usually increase with expiration.

TAKE HOME POINT #5

Right-sided murmurs increase with inspiration due to increased venous return. Left-sided regurgitant murmurs (i.e. AR, MR, and VSD) increase with maneuvers that increase left ventricular afterload (e.g. handgrip). The murmur of HOCM decreases with handrip.

KEY REFERENCES

CONSTANT J. Essentials of Bedside Cardiology. 2003. Humana Press Inc: New Jersey.

McGEE SR. Physical examination of venous pressure: A critical review. Am Heart J 1998;136(1):10–18.

ROLDAN CA, SHIVELY BK, and CRAWFORD MH. Value of the cardiovascular physical examination for detecting valvular heart disease in asymptomatic subjects. Am J Cardiol 1996;77:1327–1331.

WEISE J. The abdominojugular reflux sign. Am J Med 2000;109(1):59–61.

Chapter 2

Introduction to Electrocardiography

Zachary D. Goldberger and Timir S. Baman

2.1 INTRODUCTION

The electrocardiogram (ECG) is one of the most important diagnostic (and prognostic) tests in clinical medicine. It is quick, inexpensive, and provides a great deal of clinical information valuable to a hospitalist caring for patients. A quick survey of the 12-lead ECG, or a telemetry strip, can immediately provide valuable insight regarding the diagnosis of an unstable patient or potentially, acute life-threatening conditions (e.g. myocardial infarction); electrolyte imbalance (e.g. hyperkalemia); cardiac structure (e.g. valvular pathology, chamber enlargement); cardiac function (e.g. ventricular aneurysm); underlying comorbities (e.g. hypertension, amyloidosis); endocrine disorders (e.g. hyperthyroidism); and chronic conditions (e.g. chronic obstructive pulmonary disease) among others. The surface ECG also provides clues toward the etiology of an enigmatic arrhythmia without invasive electrophysiology studies and can be helpful in the evaluation of patients with common medical problems such as syncope or weakness. This chapter introduces basic principles of ECG reading and provides examples of important patterns for the inpatient setting.

2.2 INITIAL APPROACH TO THE ECG

Every clinician should have a step-wise, systematic approach to reading a 12-lead ECG. Whatever approach is used should "guarantee" that key findings will not be missed and that there is knowledge of the clinical context in which the ECG was performed.

Inpatient Cardiovascular Medicine, First Edition. Edited by Brahmajee K. Nallamothu and Timir S. Baman.

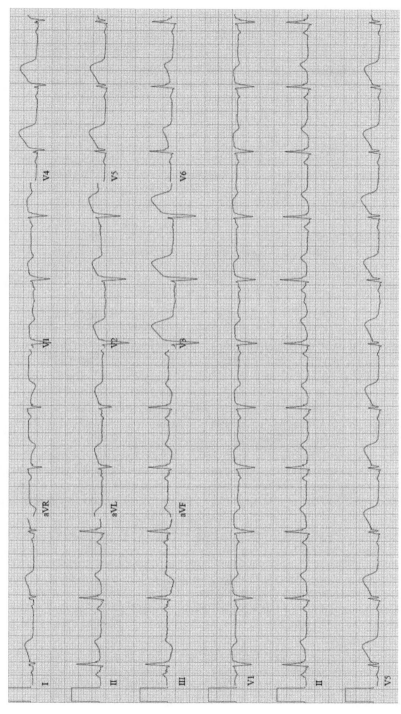

Figure 2.1 Sinus rhythm at ~62 bpm with borderline first degree AV conduction delay (PR 200 ms). An extensive acute anterior MI is present with ST elevations in I, aVL, and across the precordium. The loss of R waves across the affected leads is significant, and will soon evolve into Q waves in these leads. Reciprocal ST depressions in leads II, III, and aVF are present. Cardiac enzymes were markedly elevated. These findings are indicative of a blockage in the proximal left anterior descending coronary artery.

Before a step-wise reading, an overall look at the 12-lead ECG can be helpful to recognize particularly dangerous patterns. Potentially fatal and time-sensitive information can and should be identified immediately. As an example, when taking an all-encompassing look at an ECG such as that shown in Figure 2.1, it is clear that immediate action should be taken.

After quickly recognizing the absence of an emergent clinical situation, a systematic approach can be undertaken. Particular attention should be paid to:

- Rate
- Rhythm
- QRS axis
- Intervals (PR, corrected QT, and QRS width)
- T waves (inversion or peaking)
- ST segments and Q waves
- Chamber enlargement
- Other waves (e.g. the presence of U waves or delta waves).

2.2.1 Rate

Tachycardia is usually defined as a ventricular rate greater than 100 bpm, and brady-cardia as a ventricular rate less than 60 bpm. The presence of tachycardia is important as it can signify the overall clinical condition of the patient. It should not be sur-prising to find tachycardia in a patient who is septic, febrile, post-operative, in pain, or anxious. Resting tachycardia can often signify congestive heart failure, patients with cardiac transplant, or thyrotoxicosis. Resting tachycardia due to arrhythmias, however, should not be overlooked, especially in elderly patients. One study per-formed in an Emergency Department found that more than 80% of subjects ≥51 y/o with a heart rate greater than 141 bpm were not in sinus rhythm. Conversely, subjects ≤50 y/o with a heart rate less than 120 bpm had a 99% probability of having sinus tachycardia. The sinus node's ability to generate rapid rates decreases with increasing age, making rapid sinus rhythms quite unlikely at advanced ages.

Significant bradycardia can also be highly relevant when applied to the appro-priate clinical context. A resting heart rate of less than 40 bpm in a patient who is symp-tomatically light-headed, or who presents with syncope, may be due to an excess of drugs that have atrioventricular (AV) nodal activity (e.g. beta-blockers, calcium-channel blockers, digitalis) or due to intrinsic conduction disease (e.g. sick sinus syndrome, AV block). Conversely, a resting heart rate less than 40 bpm can be considered normal in a conditioned athlete with heightened vagal tone at rest.

AV block, particularly complete heart block, should be considered when significant bradycardia is encountered. The ECG pattern of complete (3rd degree) AV block is characterized by the following traits: (1) a HR usually less than 40 bpm; (2) an atrial rate faster than the ventricular rate; and (3) AV dissociation, where the atrium and ventricle are both electrically independent of each other.

Other forms of AV block should also be considered when bradycardia without complete heart is present. Second degree type I block (also known as Wenckebach

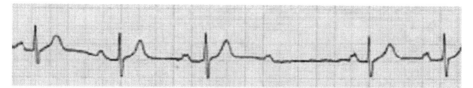

Figure 2.2   Second degree Type I block due to increased vagal tone seen in a 34-year-old athlete.

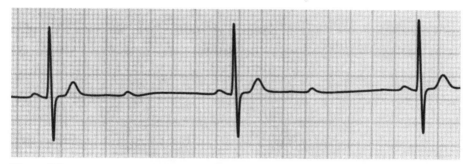

Figure 2.3   2:1 second degree type II block seen in a 78-year-old who presents with symptoms of presyncope.

block) manifests with progressive prolongation of PR intervals followed by a blocked P wave and "dropped" QRS complex (Figure 2.2). AV Wenckebach is sometimes seen in healthy individuals, and can be noted during sleep or periods of heightened vagal tone. Second degree type II block (also known as Mobitz II block) occurs when a single QRS complex is "dropped" without a detriment in PR conduction (Figure 2.3).

Calculation of rate should be performed as precisely as possible. When taking an overall look at the ECG, tachycardia should be readily identifiable. With regular rhythms, a quick estimation of the rate can be calculated by multiplying the total number of QRS complexes present by 6 (the standard ECG paper moves at 25 mm/sec, and takes 10 seconds to print). With irregular rhythms, this is particularly helpful (and necessary) because of the variability in RR intervals. Another quick means of calculating the heart rate is to count the number of large boxes between QRS complexes and divide by 4 (because 300×0.02 seconds $= 60$ and the heart rate is calculated as the number of beats in 60 seconds).

2.2.2   Rhythm

Identifying the inherent rhythm involved is critical, as differentiating between sinus and non-sinus rhythm confers different treatment strategies. An irregular rhythm may signify the presence of atrial fibrillation or atrial flutter with variable block, both of which may necessitate anticoagulation and possibly antiarrhythmics or cardioversion. Conversely, irregular rhythms such as multifocal atrial tachycardia or sinus rhythm with premature beats do not require such treatment strategies. Caution should be taken with rates that are very fast or very slow, as they may appear regular at first glance (Figure 2.4).

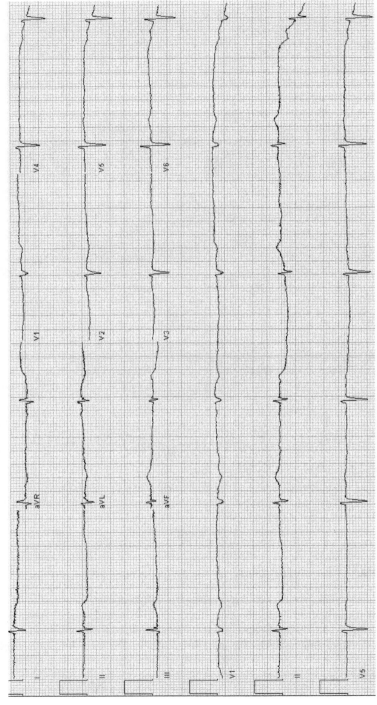

Figure 2.4 Atrial fibrillation with a very slow, relatively regularized ventricular response at approximately 42 bpm. Patient is not on digoxin. Findings are consistent with atrial and AV nodal conduction disease. A pacemaker was implanted. The ECG also shows an unusual rightward axis and slow R wave progression, raising question of COPD.

The term "sinus rhythm" denotes the presence of sinus P waves; however, it does not speak to the presence of a "normal" ECG. For example, the ECG of a patient with complete heart block could be described as "sinus tachycardia at a rate of 60 bpm with a ventricular escape rhythm at 25 bpm and 3rd degree AV block." A sinus P wave should be upright in lead II, as lead II is pointed toward 60 degrees, which is roughly the direction the current takes when originating in the high right atrium toward the AV node. Ectopic P waves originating in the high right atrium may mimic sinus P waves, but will have a subtle morphologic distinction from the true sinoatrial P wave.

2.2.3 Axis

QRS axis configuration can be a difficult aspect of the ECG. As the depolarization current spreads through the ventricles, it changes direction throughout the cardiac cycle—it may be directed toward and away from any given lead at a moment in time. However, the overall electrical axis reflects the summed direction of the mean QRS vectors in the frontal plane (leads I, II, III, aVR, aVL, aVF). A normal axis is often defined as −30 degrees to 100 degrees. An axis less than −30 degrees is termed left axis deviation, and an axis greater than 100 degrees is defined as right axis deviation. Precise calculation of the axis is rarely necessary, and the electrocardiograph can perform this calculation accurately. However, one must be able to quickly determine the overall direction of the mean QRS axis (normal, leftward, or rightward; see Figure 2.5). To determine the axis on an ECG:

- Look at leads I and II.
- Identify the direction of the QRS complexes in those leads.
- If both are upright, the axis is normal; if lead I shows a positive QRS complex and lead II a mostly negative complex (S > R), the axis is leftward; if lead

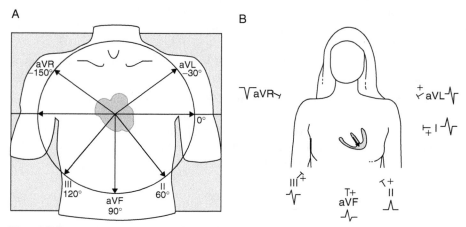

Figure 2.5 **A** Axis determination via frontal plane leads. **B** Normal QRS axis. (Source: Adapted from F. Kusumoto, ECG Interpretation for Everyone, 2012. Reproduced with permission of John Wiley & Sons Ltd.).

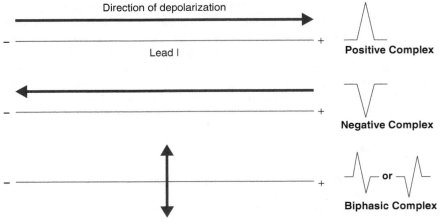

Figure 2.6   What ECG waveforms represent.

I shows a negative QRS complex and lead II a positive complex (R > S), the axis is rightward.

- The presence of biphasic QRS complexes will signify an orthogonal direction in that particular lead (Figure 2.6). For example, lead II is pointed toward 60 degrees. If there is a biphasic complex in lead II, forces are going at 90 degrees toward lead II, meaning at −30 degrees or at 150 degrees. Discerning which one is present involves looking at lead I (if lead I is negative, the axis would be extremely rightward at 150, and if positive, the axis would be −30 degrees). Of note, looking at leads I and aVF to determine axis may be unhelpful, especially if biphasic complexes are present, given leads I and aVF are at 90 degrees to each other. An upright QRS in lead I with a somewhat biphasic complex in aVF would signify an axis close to 0 degrees. However, if a biphasic complex is also present in lead II, the axis is more accurately determined as being less than 0 degrees.
- An undetermined axis may be present if the QRS complex has an unusual morphology, or if biphasic complexes are present in several of the limb leads.

The QRS axis has clinical significance. For example, a shift from normal to rightward axis may reflect acute rightward strain, as is present with an acute pulmonary embolism. Right ventricular hypertrophy may often be seen in cases of pulmonary hypertension and COPD. A leftward axis may represent left ventricular hypertrophy or a left anterior fascicular block.

2.2.4 Intervals

Attention to intervals is another key step in ECG analysis. The upper limit of a normal PR interval is defined as 200 ms (although some texts define it as 210 ms in elderly patients). A short PR interval (less than 90 ms) may indicate the presence of a Wolff-Parkinson-White (WPW) pattern (Figure 2.7). A long PR interval signifies 1st degree AV block, given that the interval itself represents the time it takes for the electrical stimulus to spread through the atria and traverse the AV node. Although a prolonged PR interval suggests AV nodal disease, a mild prolongation is rarely of clinical significance meriting treatment.

A short or long QT interval may be due to an inherited arrhythmogenic condition, and often may herald the risk of sudden death due to a lethal ventricular tachyarrhythmia; or it can be benign, and possibly due to drugs or an electrolyte disturbance. For example, several drugs (e.g. haloperidol, specific antiarrhythmics) may prolong the QT interval. Hypercalcemia, in turn, will shorten the QT interval by virtue of shortening the ST segment.

The QT should be measured in the ECG lead that demonstrates the longest intervals. It is also important to note that, at slow heart rates, a QT interval that appears normal may in fact be prolonged, and at faster heart rates a QT interval that appears prolonged may be normal. As such, it is necessary to correct the QT for heart rate. This formula is defined as the QT interval (ms) divided by the square root of the RR interval (seconds), the latter which can be calculated as 60/HR. If the QT interval is 400 ms at a HR of 60 bpm, the corrected QT interval (QTc) will be 400 ms ($400/\sqrt{60/60}$). If the HR is 80 bpm, the QTc is 461 ($400\sqrt{60/80}$). A prolonged QT interval is defined differently in various sources; however, greater than 450 ms in men and 460 ms in women are generally accepted values. The approach to a patient with an abnormal QT interval is beyond the scope of this chapter and should require cardiology consultation if thought to be clinically relevant.

The QRS width is another important aspect of the ECG, as it represents the time it takes for an electrical stimulus to spread through the ventricles. A narrow complex QRS is defined as less than 120 ms, and a wide complex QRS is ≥120 ms. This becomes especially important when faced with a tachyarrhythmia as a wide complex tachycardia has a significantly different differential diagnosis compared to narrow complex tachycardia. (See Chapters 18 and 19.)

2.2.5 T Waves

The T wave represents ventricular repolarization. It is normally upright in leads I, II, and V3 to V6; inverted in aVr; and variable in the remainder of the leads. T wave inversions (TWI) in leads III, aVL and V1 are often of no clinical consequence. TWIs may signify serious events such as myocardial infarction or ischemia, or central nervous system (CNS) injury but may reflect normal variants as well. As such, T wave changes must be taken in the proper clinical context. For example, healthy individuals may have TWIs in leads V1 through V3, which is termed a persistent juvenile T-wave inversion pattern. Prominent and biphasic TWI can be seen with ST elevations; however, they can also be a benign finding seen in young adult black men and athletes.

Of concern is the presence of TWI as a marker of acute coronary syndromes (ACS). As a general rule, these T-waves are characterized by an isoelectric ST

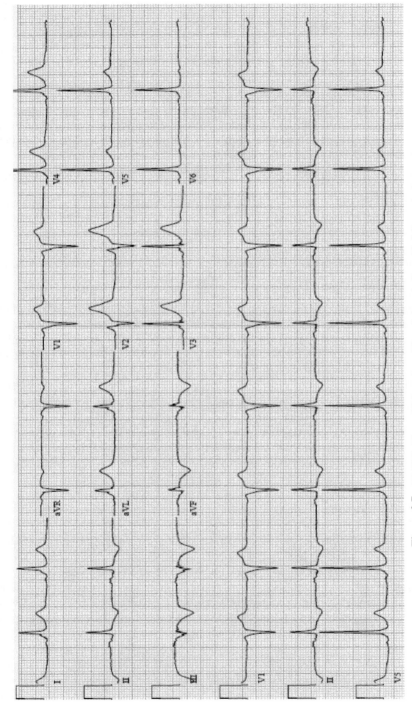

Figure 2.7 Wolff-Parkinson-White pattern. Normal sinus rhythm with delta waves are seen.

24

Table 2.1   Causes of T Wave Inversions.

Normal variants
Bundle branch block
Ventricular paced rhythms
Precordial/limb lead misplacement
Persistent juvenile T-wave pattern
Myocardial ischemia/infarction
CNS events
Ventricular overload
Classic strain patterns
Apical hypertrophic cardiomyopathy (Yamaguchi syndrome)
Digitalis effect
Wolff-Parkinson-White pre-excitation
Idiopathic global TWI
Acute myocarditis
Acute pulmonary embolism

segment that is usually bowed concave followed by a sharp symmetric downstroke. Prominent and deeply inverted T waves are often characteristic of CNS injury or the apical variant of hypertrophic cardiomyopathy. Causes of TWI are seen in Table 2.1. Other abnormalities of T waves include T wave peaking, seen in the early phases of hyperkalemia (Figure 2.8).

2.2.6   ST Segments and Q waves

Careful inspection of the ST segment is paramount in the analysis of the ECG, as myocardial infarction and ischemia may be reflected in deviation of the ST segment from baseline. A normal ST segment is usually isoelectric at the baseline. The J point is defined as the point where the QRS complex meets the ST segment. ST elevations may reflect MI, but can be elevated in a wide variety of settings (e.g. pericarditis, ventricular aneurysm, and other benign clinical conditions) (Figure 2.9 and Figure 2.10).

The presence of Q waves may reflect (1) a recent, evolving, or prior MI, (2) a normal variant in certain leads, or (3) a particular pattern of ventricular depolarization. Normal "septal" Q waves are usually less than 0.04 seconds in width and represent initial septal depolarization as part of a qR depolarization and may be seen in left chest and inferior leads and lateral leads if the heart has a vertical or horizontal electrical axis, respectively.

2.2.7   Ventricular Hypertrophy

The presence of left and right ventricular hypertrophy is suggested by the ECG. Left ventricular hypertrophy needs to be definitively diagnosed by other imaging

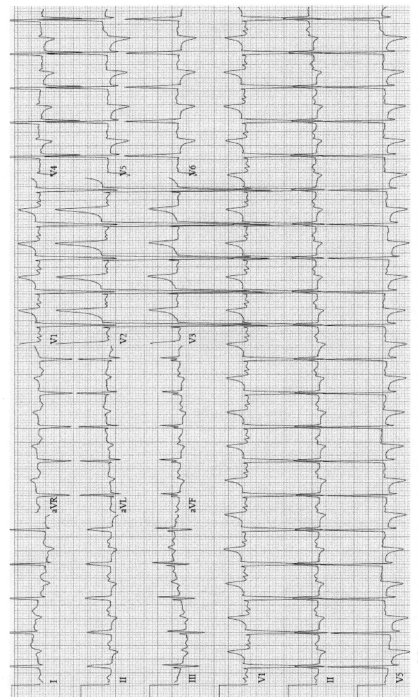

Figure 2.8 Hyperkalemia and LVH. Sinus tachycardia at approximately 120 ms. Note the peaked T waves in V1–V3 consistent with hyperkalemia along with ST depressions and T wave inversions in concert with the prominent voltage due to LVH.

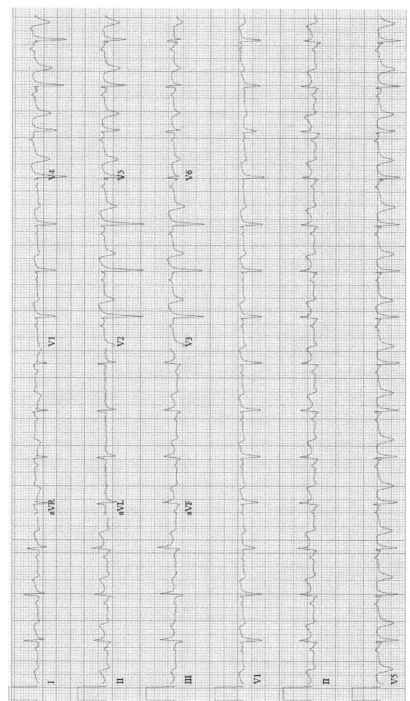

Figure 2.9 This ECG was taken from a 60-year-old man with a history of prior MI, and later found to have a left ventricular aneurysm. The ECG showed persistent inferior ST elevations as well as Q waves and biphasic T waves anteriorly. From the ECG alone one cannot rule out an acute coronary event.

27

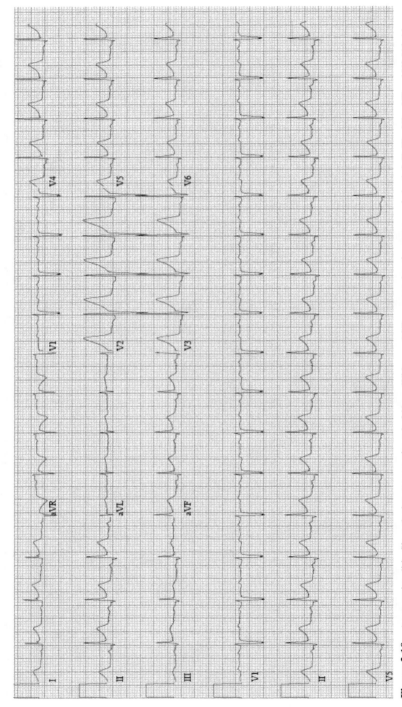

Figure 2.10 Acute pericarditis. Sinus rhythm at approximately 94bpm. Widespread ST segment elevations are seen in leads I, II, III, aVL, aVF and V2–V6. Also present are PR depressions, particularly in lead II, and PR elevation in aVR (reflecting an atrial current of injury).

Table 2.2   Criteria for Left Ventricular Hypertrophy.

Romhilt-Estes Criteria (4 points: LVH likely, 5 points: LVH present)

1. Limb lead R or S amplitude >2.0 mV, or S in V1 or V2 >3.0 mV, or R in V5 or V6 >3.0 mV (3 points)
2. ST segment abnormality: with digitalis, without digitalis (2 points, 1 point)
3. Left atrial abnormality (3 points)
4. Left axis deviation >−30 degrees (2 points)
5. QRS duration >0.09 seconds (1 point)
6. Intrinsicoid deflection in V5 and V6 >0.05 seconds (1 point)

Cornell Criteria

R in aVL + S in V3 ≥2.8 mV (men), ≥2.0 mV (women)

Sokolow-Lyon Criteria

S in V1 + R in V5 or V6 (whichever is larger) ≥35 mm, or R in aVL ≥11 mm

Other

Lead I: R wave >14 mm; Lead aVR: S wave >15 mm; Lead aVL: R wave >12 mm
Lead aVF: R wave >21 mm; Lead V5: R wave >26 mm; Lead V6: R wave >20 mm

---

modalities (e.g. transthoracic echocardiogram), but there are several criteria that suggest LVH: the Romhilt-Estes criteria, the Cornell criteria, and the Sokolow-Lyons criteria (Table 2.2, Figure 2.8).

Right ventricular hypertrophy (RVH) is suggested by (1) a tall R wave in V1, equal to or greater than the S wave, (2) right axis deviation, and (3) T wave in leads V1–V3. The presence of all three of these patterns is strongly suggestive of RVH.

2.2.8 Other Waves

Analyses of the P, QRS, and T waves along with the PR and ST segments are all part of the systematic analysis of the ECG but an inspection for other waves and morphologies is important as well. U waves are small deflections seen after the T wave and represent the final stage of ventricular depolarization. Most commonly, U waves (in concert with ST depression and low amplitude T waves) reflect hypokalemia. Inverted U waves can be seen with myocardial ischemia, often in the setting of left main or left anterior descending coronary artery disease, as well as in coronary spasm. Other causes of U waves include sinus bradycardia (accentuates U waves); T-U fusion complexes exist in some cases of CNS injury, quinidine effect, or long QT syndrome. Finally, U waves may be present in some cases of mitral valve prolapse, hyperthyroidism, or ventricular hypertrophy in leads with prominent R waves.

The electrocardiographic signature of Wolff-Parkinson-White (WPW) pattern is the triad of (1) delta waves, (2) a widened QRS, and (3) a short PR. Secondary ST-T wave abnormalities are also seen (Figure 2.7). The delta wave represents early activation of the ventricles through an accessory pathway, distinct from normal activation via the His-Purkinje system. Patients with WPW may be fully pre-excited or partially pre-excited, depending on the degree of early electrical stimulation of the ventricles. Of note, WPW pattern may become manifest at slow heart rates when the refractory period of the AV node allows for the bypass tract to become a more prominent means of antegrade AV conduction.

2.3 LIMITATIONS

It cannot be overemphasized that, while the ECG can be helpful in both the diagnosis and the management of myriad clinical conditions, the sensitivity and specificity of the ECG in diagnosing several conditions are limited. As such, the presence of a seemingly normal ECG does not rule out life-threatening conditions such as an acute MI or coronary artery disease; similarly, it cannot rule out the presence of chronic conditions such as severe LVH or RVH.

2.4 ECG PATTERNS

A clear, systematic approach is the key to a proper and thorough interpretation of an ECG, and often affords the ability to determine whether a patient has a "normal" ECG. However, much of ECG reading relies on pattern recognition, and the ability to quickly identify unusual or pathologic patterns.

In the supplement that follows this chapter, we have also included the following examples of several patterns that may be encountered in clinical practice, particularly among patients in the inpatient setting.

KEY REFERENCES

BERNE RM, LEVY MN. Cardiovascular Physiology, 8th ed. 2001.

FISCH C. Centennial of the string galvanometer and the electrocardiogram. J Am Coll Cardiol 2000;26:1737–1745.

GOLDBERGER AL, GOLDBERGER ZD, SHVILKIN A. Goldberger's electrocardiography: a simplified approach, 8th ed. 2013. Elsevier (Saunders), Philadelphia.

SURAWICZ B, KNILLANS TK. Chou's Electrocardiography in Clinical Practice, 7th ed. 2001. WB Saunders: Philadelphia.

ALAN E. Lindsay ECG Learning Center: http://library.med.utah.edu/kw/ecg/

ECG Wave Maven: http://ecg.bidmc.harvard.edu//maven

SUPPLEMENTARY ECGS

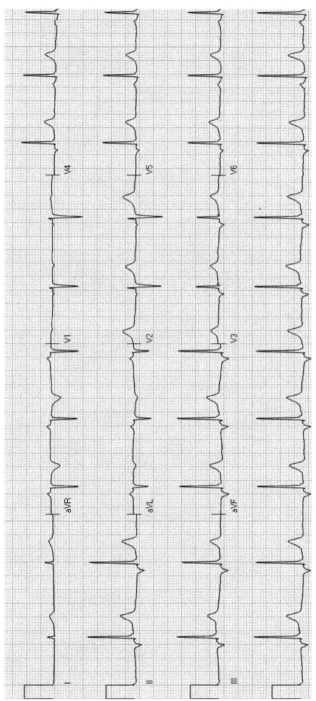

Ectopic atrial rhythm. The rate is approximately 58 bpm Inverted P waves in lead II. Sinus P waves are always upright in lead II reflecting the direction of depolarization from the high right atrium, downward and to the patient's left.

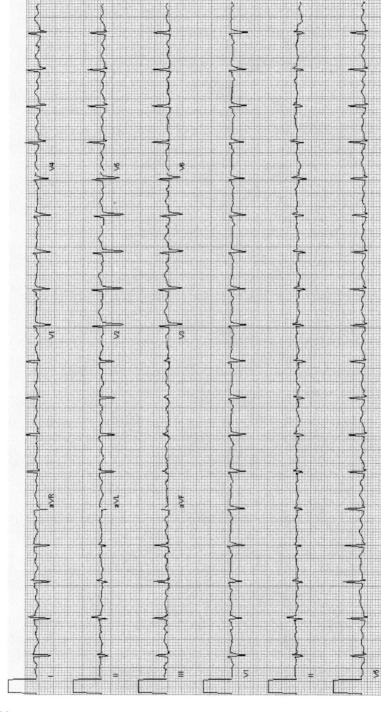

Limb lead reversal: Reversal of the right arm and left arm leads in a normal baseline ECG results in a distinct ECG pattern consisting of (1) an inverted P-QRS-T in lead I; (2) a negative QRS complex in aVL; (3) a positive QRS in aVR; and (4) switching of patterns in leads II and III. This pattern causes spurious right axis deviation and simulates a lateral infarct.

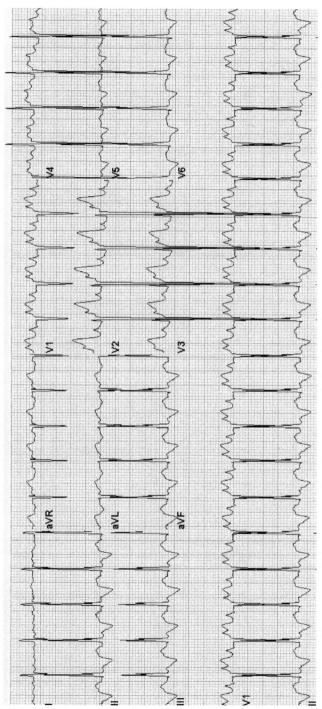

Atrial tachycardia with 2:1 block. This arrhythmia may be due to digitalis toxicity, reflecting increased automaticity of ectopic pacemaker cells with increased AV block. There are ectopic P waves best seen in V1 (arrows) with atrial tachycardia at approximately 187 bpm with a ventricular rate of 113 bpm. However, nowadays most cases of AT with block are not digitalis-related.

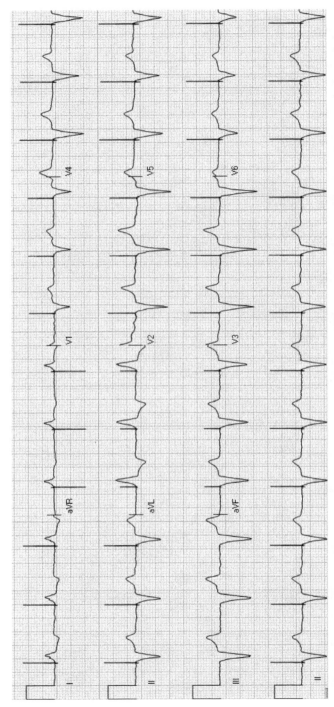

Atrial fibrillation with ventricular pacing with a ventricular rate of 93 bpm. The QRS complexes demonstrate left bundle branch block morphology, reflecting early activation from right ventricular pacing (note the electronic narrow spike). The AF waves simulate "P" waves and may cause a diagnostic misdiagnosis.

Note: reading this as a "ventricular paced rhythm" without atrial fibrillation would be incomplete. The irregularity of atrial fibrillation will be masked by paced rhythms--the inherent risk of stroke and possible need for anticoagulation may still be needed despite the regular rhythm.

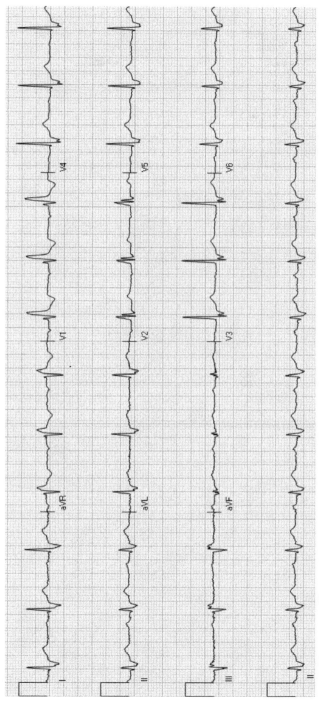

Complete right bundle branch block (RBBB) with probable prior inferior MI. Note the rsR' pattern in V1 with secondary T wave inversions and S waves in leads I, II, aVL, and leads V4–V6 reflecting delayed activation of the right ventricle. Also present are borderline Q waves inferiorly suggesting prior infarct.

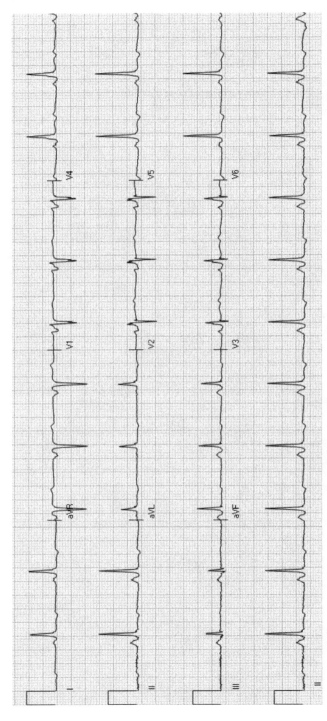

Biatrial enlargement. Normal sinus rhythm at 83 bpm with a biphasic, predominantly negative P wave in V1, with a negative component longer than 40 ms and 1 mm in depth (left atrial enlargement/abnormality), and a tall P wave in lead II (right atrial enlargement/abnormality). There are nonspecific T wave inversions in the infero-lateral leads that could be due to LVH, ischemia, etc.

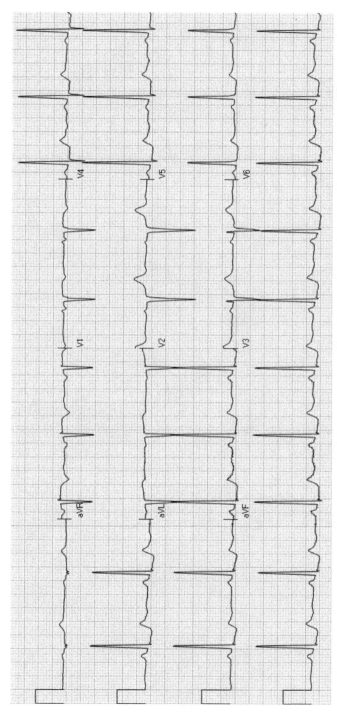

Myocardial infarction/ischemia. Normal sinus rhythm is present with borderline1st degree AV conduction delay (PR=200 ms). There are QS complexes in leads I and aVL, and V1–V2 suggestive of a prior anterior-lateral infarct. Inferolateral ischemia is suggested by ST depressions in leads II, III, aVF, and V4–V6. Right axis deviation is also present due to the loss of lateral forces. In addition, voltage criteria for LVH are present.

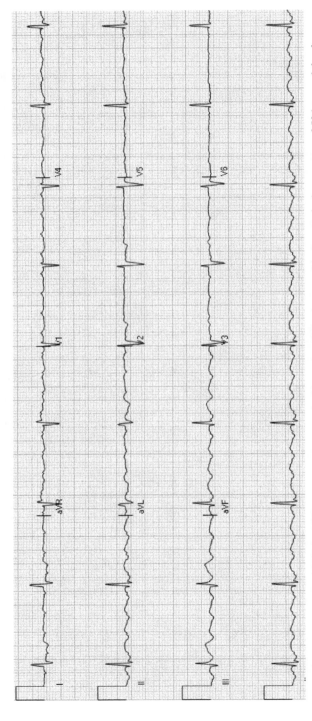

Atrial flutter with 4:1 block. Distinct flutter waves are present in this tracing. What is unusual is the ventricular response of 50 bpm and the slow flutter rate of 200/sec, versus the usual 4:1 flutter rate of 300/sec with a ventricular response of 75 bpm. Slowing of the flutter rate and atrial block could be due to a drug like amiodarone. There are nonspecific ST-T changes and a prior inferior MI cannot be ruled out.

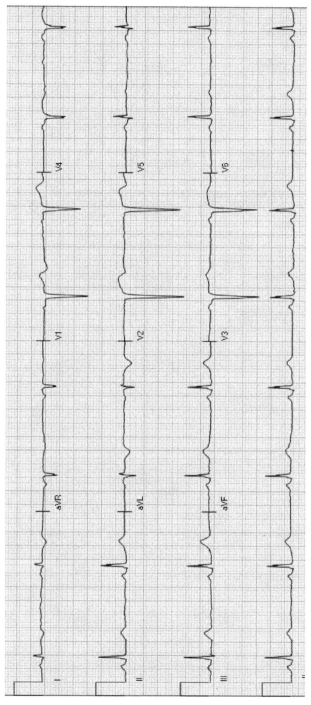

Anterolateral MI of indeterminate age. Sinus bradycardia at a rate of 48 bpm. QS complexes are present in V1–V4, along with Q waves in I, aVL, and V5, and T wave inversions in I and aVL, all suggestive of a prior anterolateral infarction.

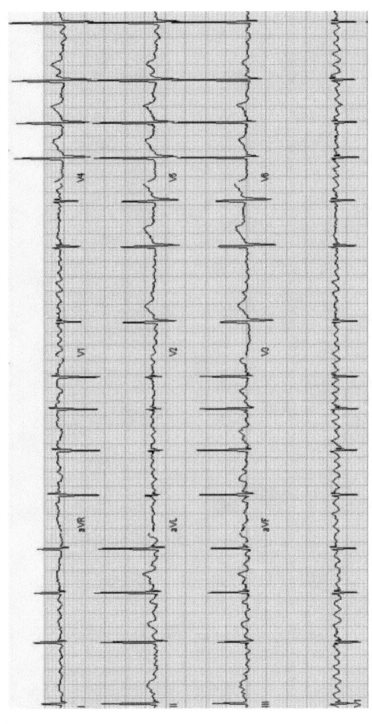

Atrial fibrillation. This ECG shows "coarse" atrial fibrillation with a ventricular response of approximately 90 bpm. Borderline voltage criteria for left ventricular hypertrophy are present, consistent with the hx of hypertension. Features definitively distinguishes atrial fibrillation from atrial flutter here are that (1) the very irregular ventricular response, (2) the morphology of the atrial waves, which are highly variable, and (3) the atrial rate is intermittently very rapid (cycle length less than 180 ms, or 4.5 small boxes on the standard ECG). Atrial activity in atrial flutter is highly patterned and consistent in appearance and the flutter cycle length is usually >180 ms.

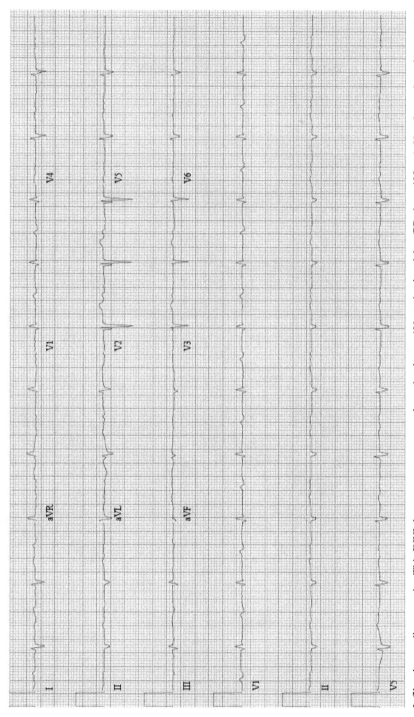

Infiltrative cardiomyopathy. This ECG demonstrates very prominent 1st degree AV conduction delay (PR about 400 ms). Very low voltage is present. The Q waves in the inferior and anterior leads could be due to cardiac infiltration (e.g. with amyloid) vs. actual anterior/inferior MIs. Right axis deviation is present.

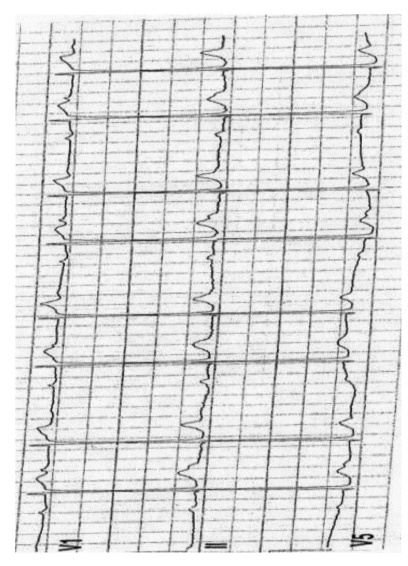

First degree block and AV Wenckebach (Mobitz 1). Grouped beating in this ECG is present, in a pattern of 3:2 AV Wenckebach. Sinus tachycardia at 125 bpm is present, with P waves marching through. This ECG demonstrates the triad of AV Wenckebach: (1) PR prolongation is present prior to a dropped beat; (2) RR intervals shorten slightly; and (3) the interval containing the dropped QRS complex is less than 2 prior PP cycles. Note that the P wave with the dropped beat is buried in the T wave (P waves are marked with arrows).

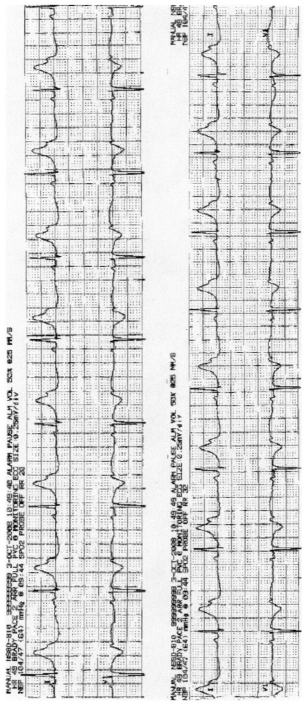

Mobitz II AV block. This continuous telemetry strip demonstrates 2:1 AV block. With 2:1 block, it is difficult to discern between AV Wenckebach and Mobitz II block. However, in this instance there was no evidence of AV Wenckebach pattern emerging over a long period of time, suggesting this is most likely Mobitz II.

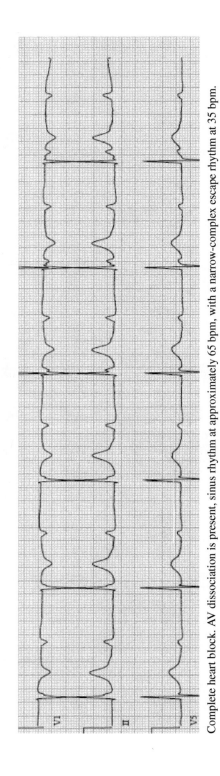

Complete heart block. AV dissociation is present, sinus rhythm at approximately 65 bpm, with a narrow-complex escape rhythm at 35 bpm.

Chapter 3

Non-invasive Cardiac Imaging

Renuka Jain and William F. Armstrong

3.1 INTRODUCTION

Understanding the role of non-invasive cardiac imaging is essential in the inpatient setting. Non-invasive cardiac imaging offers structural information on the heart and adjacent structures, as well as functional information regarding cardiovascular hemodynamics. An appropriately selected imaging modality can be extraordinarily useful in the diagnosis, prognosis, and management of cardiovascular disease but should always be targeted toward a specific clinical question. Recent innovations in cardiac technology have resulted in more detailed representations of the heart and great vessels. This chapter reviews standard non-invasive cardiac imaging with the exception of non-invasive stress testing, which is discussed in the next chapter.

The choice of non-invasive imaging modality is highly dependent upon the clinical question proposed. Table 3.1 lists common clinical questions considered when ordering an imaging study and a set of appropriate imaging tests for that question.

> ### TAKE HOME POINT #1
>
> Always have a clinical question in mind when ordering an imaging study and select the appropriate imaging test for that specific question.

Inpatient Cardiovascular Medicine, First Edition. Edited by Brahmajee K. Nallamothu and Timir S. Baman.

Table 3.1   Common Clinical Questions.

Common clinical questions	Primary modality	Secondary modalities
What is the LVEF?	TTE, MUGA	CT, CMR, PET
Are wall motion abnormalities present?	TTE	PET, CMR
Does my patient have coronary artery disease?	CTA Stress testing	MRA, CTA,
Are congenital abnormalities present?	TTE	CT, CMR
Does my patient have valvular disease?	TTE	TEE (invasive)
Are the pacemaker/defibrillator leads in the right place?	CXR	CT
Does my patient have constrictive or restrictive cardiomyopathy?	TTE	CMR, CT
Is the pericardium normal?	CT, CMR	CXR
Does my patient have aortic dissection?	CT TEE (invasive)	CMR
Does my patient have evidence of myocardial viability?	PET	CMR

Not all tests are appropriate for all patients. In addition to knowing the clinical question, it is useful to review relative and absolute contraindications to imaging modalities prior to choosing a specific study for a particular patient. In this chapter, we focus on non-stress test-related imaging studies as stress tests are discussed elsewhere.

TAKE HOME POINT #2

Ensure that the patient does not have any contraindications to the imaging modality.

3.2 NON-STRESS IMAGING STUDIES

3.2.1 Chest X-Ray (CXR)

The CXR offers valuable but often nonspecific information on cardiovascular disease (Table 3.2). CXR is indicated in any patient with suspicion of structural heart or lung disease. CXR can be performed at the bedside (standard anterior-posterior (AP) projection) or in a radiology lab (standard posterior-anterior (PA) projection and lateral projections). PA CXR is generally more accurate, as the standard 6-foot projection length allows for clearer resolution of borders (Figure 3.1). In addition, most PA CXRs are performed at end-inspiration for maximum delineation of structures; this is difficult to achieve in an AP projection with the patient lying in a hospital bed.

Table 3.2 CXR.

Indications	Heart and lung disease; pericardial evaluation
Contraindications	Pregnancy (relative)
Key structures visualized	Cardiac silhouette, lung parenchyma, ascending aorta silhouette, pericardial calcification
Key structures not visualized	Individual chambers of heart, valves
Limitations	No information on cardiac motion of hemodynamics
	Body habitus or patient positioning can lead to poor image quality

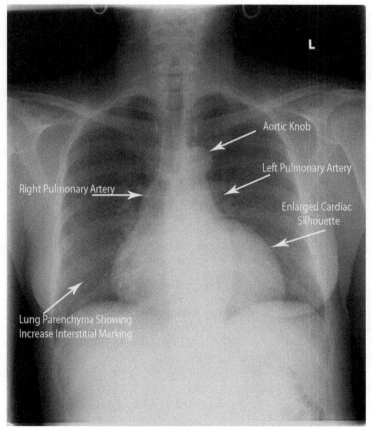

Figure 3.1 CXR PA demonstrating cardiomegaly.

CXR is most useful in the diagnosis of congestive heart failure, primarily by demonstrating evidence of pulmonary congestion (pleural effusions, Kerley B lines, and pulmonary edema), pericardial disease (pericardial calcifications), aortic dissection (enlarged mediastinum), pulmonary hypertension (enlarged pulmonary arteries), and complications of cardiac procedures (pneumothorax, hemothorax). It has a high sensitivity for pneumothorax and hemothorax post-cardiovascular procedures. CXR is also useful for determining location of pacemaker leads and other intravenous catheters. CXR can be helpful in assessing left ventricular dilation, although AP CXR, as compared to PA CXR, tends to overestimate true heart size.

3.2.2 Echocardiography (TTE and TEE)

Transthoracic echocardiography (TTE) is the modality of choice for initial evaluation of cardiovascular structure, function, and hemodynamics (Table 3.3). Transthoracic echocardiography is a real-time 2D ultrasound of the heart and the reflection of ultrasound beams from cardiac structures offers information on their anatomy and motion (Figure 3.2, Figure 3.3, Figure 3.4).

Standard 2D images are acquired from multiple projections and typically consist of parasternal, apical, subcostal, and suprasternal views. In addition to real-time 2D images, Doppler imaging adds information on cardiovascular hemodynamics. Color Doppler imaging is used for assessment of myocardial blood flow and can identify pressure gradients. Pulse wave Doppler and continuous wave Doppler can accurately quantify velocities along a linear path in the ultrasound beam, which can then be used to estimate pressure gradients.

A TTE is very beneficial for the diagnosis of valvular disease, wall motion abnormalities that suggest coronary artery disease, cardiomyopathy, ascending aortic disease, valvular disease, and congenital defects (ventricular septal defect, atrial septal defect, patent foramen ovale). Agitated saline contrast given through a peripheral vein can also delineated intrapulmonary versus intracardiac shunts. Doppler imaging can be used to identify valvular stenosis, valvular regurgitation, and other intracardiac gradients including pulmonary artery pressures and left ventricular outflow tract obstruction. TTE can also be used to estimate or calculate left ventricular

Table 3.3   TTE.

Indications	Structure, function, and hemodynamics
Contraindications	None
Key structures visualized	All heart chambers, all valves, ascending aortic root, aortic arch, pericardium, ventricular septum, inter-atrial septum
Key structures not visualized	Left atrial appendage, distal aorta
Limitations	Body habitus with poor image quality
	Inability to visualize entire aorta to exclude aortic dissection
	Inability to visualize left atrial appendage to exclude thrombus

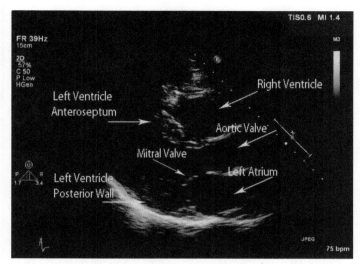

Figure 3.2   Parasternal long-axis view of heart in a normal patient.

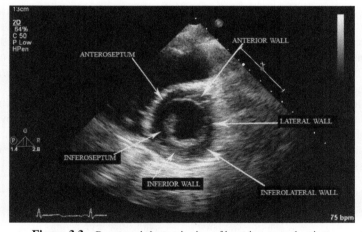

Figure 3.3   Parasternal short-axis view of heart in a normal patient.

ejection fraction (LVEF). Finally, it is valuable for identifying the presence of pericardial fluid and its potential hemodynamic effects on cardiac structures.

There are no contraindications to TTE and no known risks of cardiac ultrasound. However, TTE may be limited by poor image quality often seen in patients with obesity or lung disease. There are also important structures that TTE cannot fully assess, such as the left atrial appendage. It also is limited in examining the entire ascending aorta, aortic arch, and descending aorta with sufficient sensitivity required to exclude aortic dissection. Finally, imaging artifacts can occur during TTE acquisition and hamper interpretation of adjacent cardiac structures.

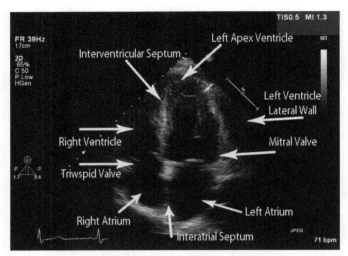

Figure 3.4   Apical 4-chamber view of heart in a normal patient on TTE.

TTE has become routinely applied in clinical care and incidental findings are often reported. In general, referral to a cardiologist is warranted for moderate valve disease with symptoms, severe valve disease even in the absence of symptoms, cardiomyopathy, or congenital abnormality with symptoms or enlargement of the heart.

Transesophageal echocardiography (TEE) offers supplemental information to TTE. TEE is indicated for evaluation of valvular disease if an etiology is not well elucidated by TTE; this is particularly true when examining the mitral valve. It is also one the tests of choice for primary diagnosis of aortic dissection. TEE is the gold standard to assess for thrombus in the left atrial appendage as part of the evaluation of thromboembolic risk prior to cardioversion of atrial flutter or fibrillation. Finally, it is considered the test of choice in patients with concern of endocarditis or intracardiac mass given its superior visualization of valvular structures.

TAKE HOME POINT #3

Because of its safety, portability and rapid image acquisition, TTE is often the test of first choice to identify structural, functional, and hemodynamic abnormalities of the heart.

3.2.3 Cardiac Computed Tomography and Angiography (CTA)

Cardiac CT provides information on the heart as well as surrounding tissue (Table 3.4). CT angiography (CTA) can add additional information on the coronary arteries. A patient is positioned in the CT scanner and medications are usually given (typically beta-blockers) to slow the heart rate while intravenous contrast is injected through the arm. During a

Table 3.4   CT and CTA.

Indications	Structure and function of heart and great vessels
	Delineation of structures adjacent to heart
	Coronary artery opacification
	Coronary calcium
	Left ventricle and right ventricle systolic function
	Ventricular volumes
Contraindications	Uncontrolled heart rhythms
	Renal failure (GFR <30 mL/min)
	Hemodynamic instability
	Inability to hold breath for sustained period of time (>30 seconds)
	Inability to obtain intravenous access
	Claustrophobia
Key structures visualized	Structure of heart and great vessels
	Delineation of structures adjacent to heart
	Opacification of coronary arteries (CTA)
	Evaluation of coronary artery calcium
Key structures not visualized	Valve motion and finer details of valve structure
Limitations	Gating issues
	Artifact from pacemaker leads or other types of prosthetic material
	Motion artifacts common
	Calcium impedes accurate assessment of coronary stenosis

single breath hold, multiple X-ray images pass through the body and are acquired by the scanner. Images are acquired as saggital slices of the thorax and reconstructed for 3D view of the heart. In addition, each coronary artery can be reconstructed from its origin to distal course (Figure 3.5, Figure 3.6). The resolution of cardiac CT is roughly 5 mm; CTA has the ability to characterize coronary artery branches that are greater than 1.5 mm.

All aspects of the heart can be visualized with an optimal cardiac CT except for the valves and myocardium which are not usually well seen. Cardiac CT is rapid and can be used in the emergency room for the evaluation of chest pain and occlusive coronary artery disease. In comparison to conventional coronary angiography, cardiac CTA has a sensitivity of 83% and specificity of 90% in a population with presumed coronary artery disease. Cardiac CTA can also evaluate patency of coronary bypass grafts, although it is often difficult for it to quantify the presence of blockages. In addition, cardiac CT is instrumental in the assessment of anomalous coronary arteries and its courses. Cardiac CT can be used to evaluate for cardiac fistulas (i.e. coronary fistulas, aorto-esophageal fistulas). It is also a reasonable test of choice to diagnose and determine the presence and extent of aortic dissection or aortitis as well as pericardial thickening associated with constrictive pericarditis.

Coronary calcium scoring can also be performed, either on its own or with cardiac CT. When it is used in isolation, it does not require intravenous contrast. Calcification in all three coronary arteries is quantified and an Agatson score is frequently

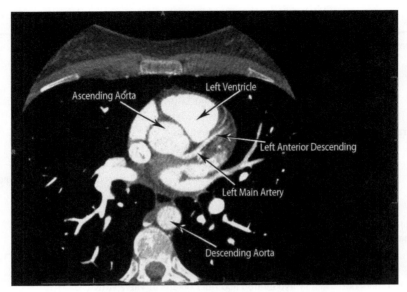

Figure 3.5   Cardiac CT view of heart (normal).

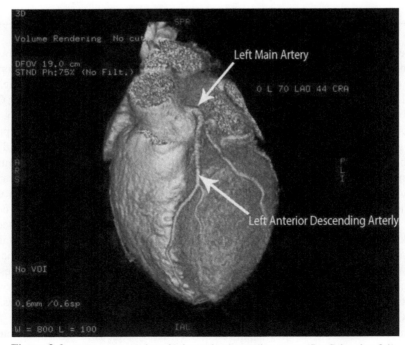

Figure 3.6   CTA reconstruction of left anterior descending artery. (See Color plate 3.1).

Table 3.5   Agatston Score and Cardiac Event Rate in Emergency Room Setting.

Agatston score	Presumed CAD extent	Cardiac event rate %
0	None	0.6
1–99	Mild	6.0
100–399	Moderate	10.0
>400	Severe	13.9

calculated (Table 3.5). The presence of calcification has been shown to correlate with the presence of coronary plaque burden. Although the quantification of coronary calcification does not correlate with the extent of angiographically-significant coronary disease, the overall score does predict cardiac events.

Cardiac CT is contraindicated in patients with kidney failure (GFR < 30 ml) who are not dialysis-dependent and patients who are unable to hold their breath for at least 30 seconds. It is contraindicated in patients with hemodynamic instability and those who cannot travel to the CT scanner. It cannot be performed on patients with atrial fibrillation and uncontrolled heart rates. Cardiac CT is relatively contraindicated in pregnancy, except in cases where benefits outweigh the risks.

Cardiac CT has several limitations. In order to accurately reconstruct the heart, each slice must be obtained in the same phase of the cardiac cycle. Thus, abnormal heart beats are particularly problematic for acquisition of CT – even well-controlled atrial fibrillation will lead to gating issues. Patient motion is also problematic, particularly respiratory motion in patients who cannot hold their breath for image acquisition. Patients with renal insufficiency are at increased risk for renal failure due to the use of contrast. Additionally, cardiac CT has a relatively higher dose of ionizing radiation compared with other imaging modalities, although newer imaging protocols have decreased this concern in recent years. Calcification in coronary arteries also causes significant artifact and impedes assessment of stenosis in coronary arteries in CTA.

Referral to a cardiologist is warranted for structural heart disease, coronary artery abnormalities, or calcium scores that suggest coronary artery disease.

TAKE HOME POINT #4

Cardiac CT offers structural information as well as prognostic information on coronary artery disease using calcium scoring.

3.2.4 Cardiac Magnetic Resonance Image (CMR) and Angiography (MRA)

CMR and MRA are useful to assess cardiovascular structures, cardiac function, and adjacent structures through the use of intravenous gadolinium (Table 3.6). Images are obtained during sequential breath holds, and patient cooperation is necessary to obtain a complete study. Compared with cardiac CT, CMR requires a much longer acquisition

Table 3.6   CMR and MRA.

Indications	Structure of heart and great vessels
	Evaluation of myocardial scar and infiltrative disease
	Delineation of structures adjacent to heart
	Left ventricle and right ventricle systolic function
	Ventricular volumes
Contraindications	Pacemaker/defibrillator leads
	Aneurysm clips
	Uncontrolled heart rhythms
	Renal failure (GFR <30 mL/min)
	Hemodynamic instability
	Inability to hold breath for sustained period of time (>30 seconds)
	Inability to obtain intravenous access
	Claustrophobia
Key structures visualized	Atria, ventricles, pericardium
	Structures adjacent to heart
	Aorta (MRA)
Key structures not visualized	Valve motion and finer details of valve structure
Limitations	Gating issues
	Long acquisition time

time depending on protocols used by individual labs. Images can later be reconstructed along any axis for true 3D views (Figure 3.7). Pressure gradients and intracardiac gradients can also be calculated using CMR. MRA allows for delineation of coronary arteries, aorta, pulmonary arteries, and other vascular structures. CMR and MRA offer the highest resolution images of cardiac structures including pericardium and myocardium. As compared to other imaging modalities, CMR and MRA are least affected by poor body habitus.

Many aspects of cardiac anatomy can be visualized with optimal cardiac CMR and MRA. CMR can measure pericardial thickness and is often used in assessment of pericardial disease. Due to the extremely high resolution and 3D image reconstruction, it is the test of choice in evaluation of complex congenital heart disease. CMR is also frequently used in determination of infiltrative heart diseases including hemochromatosis, sarcoidosis, myocarditis, and amyloidosis, although endomyocardial biopsy is still the gold standard. CMR has been used in acute coronary syndromes to evaluate for wall motion abnormalities and regions of infarction – however, its use is limited in the acute setting due to long acquisition times. In the post-acute coronary syndrome setting, CMR can be useful in determining infarct size, regional wall motion abnormalities, aneurysm/pseudoaneurysm formation, and intracavitary thrombus. CMR is also used in evaluation of hypertrophic cardiomyopathy to evaluate myocardial thickness and scar. Late gadolinium enhancement has been shown to accurately delineate myocardial scar. Thus CMR has potential applications in assessment of myocardial viability post-myocardial infarction.

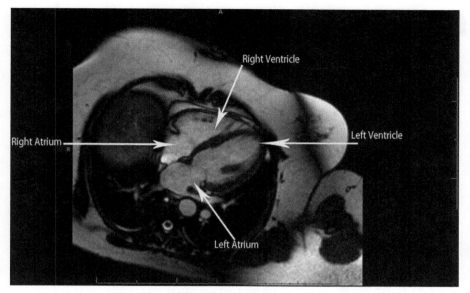

Figure 3.7 CMR view of heart (normal).

MRA is an appropriate method to diagnose and determine extent of aortic dissection and/or aortitis. MRA has been used in the study of coronary artery bypass grafts and native coronary arteries although other imaging modalities are far superior in this regard.

CMR cannot be performed in patients with pacemakers or aneurysm clips, although most CMR (1.5–3.0 Tesla field strengths only) can be safely performed on patients with coronary stents, sternal wires, and prosthetic heart valves. Gadolinium is known to cause nephrogenic systemic fibrosis (thickening and hardening of the skin) in patients with kidney disease; therefore, CMR is not recommended in patients with GFR less than 30 mL/min. Due to long acquisition times (hours), cardiac CMR cannot be used emergently to evaluate for aortic dissection. It also cannot be performed on patients with hemodynamic instability and is difficult to perform on patients that suffer from claustrophobia.

Finally, CMR has several limitations related to its imaging quality. Valve mobility and prosthetic heart valves cannot be optimally assessed by CMR at this time, although the technology is constantly improving in this area. CMR can only assess left ventricular function if images are gated, which can only be obtained with a slow regular heart rate. Beta blockers are often used to slow down the heart rate for image acquisition. Abnormal heart rhythms such as atrial fibrillation or frequent atrial or ventricular ectopy will affect the ability of CMR to accurately assess systolic function, similarly to CT.

Referral to a cardiologist is warranted for infiltrative cardiomyopathies, congenital heart disease, coronary artery abnormalities, or myocardial scar found on CMR or abnormalities in aorta on MRA.

TAKE HOME POINT #5

Cardiac CMR has the highest resolution images of the heart, but has important contraindications and limitations.

3.2.5 Positron Emission Tomography (PET)

Positron emission tomography (PET) allows for assessment of both myocardial perfusion and metabolism using a variety of positron-emitting isotopes (Table 3.7). These radiopharmaceuticals are then injected into a patient placed in a PET camera, which receives the characteristic photons produced by positron emission. Images are reconstructed along standard horizontal long-axis, vertical long-axis, and short-axis views of the left ventricle.

Two radioactive tracers are currently available for assessment of myocardial perfusion (^{82}Rubidium and [^{13}N] ammonia) and are used in stress imaging at limited centers. They can also be used to quantify myocardial blood flow to evaluate for coronary artery disease.

Two additional radiotracers (^{11}Carbon acetate palmitate and ^{18}Flourine deoxyglycose) are used for evaluation of cardiac metabolism. ^{18}Flourine deoxyglycose is most commonly used and requires a hyperinsulinemic state. With serum glucose levels closely monitored prior to injection, patients are given doses of niacin, insulin, and glucose. Patients with diabetes can undergo protocols although serum glucose levels must be acutely controlled. PET metabolism imaging is most useful in evaluating for myocardial viability in patients with evidence of myocardial infarction to determine if revascularization would be of benefit. An area that has abnormal perfusion but normal metabolism is considered viable or "hibernating myocardium." An area with abnormal perfusion and abnormal metabolism is considered scar. Patients with hibernating myocardium are likely to benefit from revascularization while patients with scar are not. PET can also aid in diagnosis of infiltrative

Table 3.7 PET.

Indications	Myocardial metabolism, perfusion, and absolute blood flow
	Left ventricle and right ventricle systolic function
	Ventricular volumes
Contraindications	Claustrophobia
	Uncontrolled diabetes
Key structures visualized	Left ventricle and right ventricle
Key structures not visualized	Cardiac anatomy
Limitations	Long pre-acquisition times to monitor glucose levels
	Gating issues with abnormal heart rhythms or frequent ectopy

Table 3.8 MUGA.

Indications	Left ventricle and right ventricle systolic function
	Ventricular volumes
Contraindications	Claustrophobia
Key structures visualized	Left ventricle and right ventricle
Key structures not visualized	Cardiac anatomy
Limitations	Gating issues with abnormal heart rhythms or frequent ectopy

cardiomyopathies by demonstrating scar in patients with sarcoidosis, amyloidosis, hemochromatosis, and other infiltrative disease processes.

While there are no absolute contraindications to PET, it is difficult to perform in patients with diabetes and uncontrolled glucose levels. In addition, PET provides no information on heart valves, the atria, and structures adjacent to the heart as well as limited information on right ventricle function and perfusion. Assessment of LVEF can be hampered by abnormal heart rhythms, particularly atrial fibrillation, due to abnormal gating.

Referral to a cardiologist is warranted if any abnormalities are identified in myocardial blood flow, perfusion, or metabolism.

3.2.6 Multiple Gated Acquisition Scan (MUGA)

MUGA scans are commonly used for the assessment LVEF, right ventricular ejection fraction (RVEF), ventricular volumes, and regional wall motion (Table 3.8). MUGA can also be used in assessment of diastolic filling pressures and intracardiac shunts although other tests are more commonly used for these clinical questions (TTE, CMR, CT).

MUGA is performed in a nuclear medicine laboratory. A ^{99m}Technetium radioisotope is tagged to red blood cells which then emit gamma rays. When these rays are captured by the gamma camera, images are reconstructed at various frames (defined by time points within the cardiac cycle) and LVEF and RVEF are calculated.

MUGA is considered to be the "gold standard" for assessment of left ventricular ejection fraction, due to its accuracy and precision. As compared to other imaging modalities that calculate LVEF, MUGA is independent of LV geometry. It is often ordered for initial assessment of LVEF in patients who are about to initiate chemotherapy, and can be used to follow LVEF serially in these patients.

There are no absolute contraindications to MUGA. The main limitation is abnormal heart rate. As MUGA calculations are based on acquisitions made through several cardiac cycles, abnormal heart beats or abnormal heart rhythms reduce the accuracy and reproducibility of LVEF.

Table 3.9   Advantages and Disadvantages of Imaging Modalities.

Modality	Advantages	Disadvantages
CXR	Portable Rapid acquisition time	Low specificity
TTE	Portable Rapid acquisition time	Image quality with poor body habitus
CT/CTA	Adjacent structures seen High spatial resolution	Intravenous contrast Motion artifacts common Not portable Ionizing radiation
CMR/MRA	3D images High spatial and temporal resolution No ionizing radiation Least affected by poor body habitus	Lengthy Not portable Unable to use with pacemakers
PET	High resolution Less likely affected by poor body habitus	Long pre-acquisition protocols
MUGA	"Gold standard" LVEF Not affected by body habitus	Not portable

3.2.7   Incorporating Results into Clinical Decision-Making

It is important to remember the limitations of each imaging modality when incorporating results into clinical decisionmaking. If clinical suspicion is high for a certain condition, then a negative imaging study may not rule out the disease process and a secondary imaging study may be warranted. All studies have advantages and disadvantages which must always be taken into consideration (Table 3.9).

TAKE HOME POINT #6

Remember the limitations of each imaging modality when incorporating results into your clinical decision-making.

KEY REFERENCES

GEORGIOU D. et al. Screening patients with chest pain in the emergency department using electron beam tomography: a follow-up study. J Am Coll Cardiol 2001;38:105–110.

LANGERAK SE et al. Value of magnetic resonance imaging for the noninvasive detection of stenosis in coronary artery bypass grafts and recipient coronary arteries. Circulation 2003; 107:1502.

MILLER JM, ROCHITTE CE, DEWEY M, et al. Diagnostic performance of coronary angiography by 64-row CT. N Engl J Med 2008;359:2324–2336.

Chapter 4

Cardiac Stress Testing and the Evaluation of Chest Pain

Njeri Thande and Peter G. Hagan

4.1 INTRODUCTION

Cardiac stress tests are among the most common procedures ordered in the inpatient setting. Indications for ordering a cardiac stress test include: diagnosis of coronary artery disease (CAD) in patients with chest pain or other related symptoms; assessment of functional capacity in patients with established heart disease; and estimation of prognosis. In the hospital setting, the vast majority of stress tests are performed for the first of these indications, and thus will be the largest focus of this chapter.

4.1.1 Rationale for Ordering Cardiac Stress Tests

Prior to referring a hospitalized patient for a cardiac stress test, the referring physician should always consider the following four questions:

1. Do the acute symptoms being evaluated in this patient suggest a noncardiac etiology, possible acute coronary syndrome (ACS), or definite ACS?
2. Is the patient medically stable?
3. Can the cardiac stress test be appropriately performed and, if so, what specific diagnostic or prognostic information will the stress test provide?
4. Which type of stress test would be most appropriate for the clinical situation?

Inpatient Cardiovascular Medicine, First Edition. Edited by Brahmajee K. Nallamothu and Timir S. Baman.

To help clinicians address the questions above, this chapter reviews the indications for cardiac stress testing, the relative advantages and disadvantages of the available stress test modalities, and important contraindications to each.

4.2 CHEST PAIN EVALUATION

The medical evaluation of patients with chest pain always starts with a careful medical history including: characterization of the pain; assessment of vital signs; a focused physical examination; and an electrocardiogram (ECG) and cardiac biomarkers, such as troponin. First and foremost, this medical evaluation should establish the clinical stability of the patient. Patients who have persistent chest pain, recurrent chest pain at rest, hemodynamic instability, heart failure, or ventricular arrhythmias are medically unstable and should never be referred for cardiac stress testing.

TAKE HOME POINT #1

Cardiac stress tests should always be performed in medically stable patients.

ACS includes unstable angina, non-ST segment elevation MI (NSTEMI) and ST segment elevation MI (STEMI), which are each discussed in greater detail elsewhere. These subtypes of ACS represent a spectrum of the same disease process and are differentiated based on the presence of irreversible myocardial injury, as evidenced by abnormal cardiac biomarkers, and the ECG. These conditions are discussed in detail in other chapters. Briefly, most patients who present with MI are not candidates for stress testing but are typically referred directly for cardiac catheterization. STEMIs are an indication for immediate reperfusion with primary percutaneous coronary intervention or thrombolysis and NSTEMIs usually require cardiac catheterization and possibly revascularization, if appropriate.

For patients who present with chest pain and no evidence of ACS, one should determine the likelihood or pre-test probability that the symptoms are due to CAD. Stress testing is most appropriate in those with an intermediate suspicion (10 to 90%) based on their pre-test probability. The assessment of pre-test probability can be based on age, gender and type of chest pain. Table 4.1 summarizes one method of determining pre-test probability of CAD; however, there are many risk stratification scores that use an array of clinical information. Bayes' Theorem then states that the probability of a patient actually having disease is determined by multiplying their pre-test probability with the probability that the test provides a true result. This calculation is often done intuitively and influences the clinical determination of whether a test will be useful or not. For example, a 30-year-old woman with no risk factors for CAD who presents with brief, sharp non-exertional chest pain clearly has a low pretest probability for CAD, in which case a cardiac stress test would not be diagnostically valuable. Even if a stress test were positive in this patient, a false positive result is likely given the very low pretest probability of CAD.

Table 4.1 Pretest Probability of CAD by Age, Gender, and Symptoms*.

Age	Gender	Typical angina	Atypical angina	Nonanginal chest pain	Asymptomatic
30–39	Men	Intermediate	Intermediate	Low	Very low
	Women	Intermediate	Very Low	Very low	Very low
40–49	Men	High	Intermediate	Intermediate	Low
	Women	Intermediate	Low	Very low	Very low
50–59	Men	High	Intermediate	Intermediate	Low
	Women	Intermediate	Intermediate	Low	Very low
60–69	Men	High	Intermediate	Intermediate	Low
	Women	High	Intermediate	Intermediate	Low

*No data exist for patients <30 years old or >69 years old.

Typical angina: substernal, brought on with emotion or exertion, relieved with rest or nitroglycerin.

Atypical angina: only two of the above features.

Nonanginal pain: absence of all of the above features.

High risk = >90%, Intermediate risk = 10–90%, Low risk = <10%.

(Source: Gibbons RJ, Balady GJ, Bricker JT, et al. 2002. Reproduced with permission of Elsevier).

TAKE HOME POINT #2

Diagnostic cardiac stress tests are most useful in patients with an intermediate pre-test probability of CAD as the accuracy of the stress test is highly dependent on the pre-test probability of CAD (Bayes' Theorem).

Cardiac stress tests are most useful as a diagnostic test in patients with an intermediate pre-test probability of CAD because the results of the test have the largest potential effect on diagnosis and future therapies. Cardiac stress tests have very limited diagnostic and prognostic value in asymptomatic, low-risk individuals. False-positive stress tests in these individuals may cause unnecessary follow-up, additional procedures, anxiety, and unwarranted exercise restriction.

4.3 POST-MYOCARDIAL INFARCTION

In contrast to its use as a diagnostic test, cardiac exercise stress testing can be useful after MI or unstable angina to determine risk and prognosis. However, the decision for exercise testing early after MI relies heavily on previous therapies and the clinical status of the patient. Cardiac exercise stress testing after MI helps with: (1) risk stratification and assessment of prognosis; (2) determining functional capacity for activity prescription after hospital discharge; and (3) assessing adequacy of medical therapy and the need to use other diagnostic or treatment options.

Sub-maximal exercise tests are preferred in patients who have not been revascularized and/or did not receive a cardiac catheterization. Sub-maximal exercise stress tests involve a predetermined endpoint such as peak heart rate of 120 bpm, 70% predicted maximum heart rate, or peak metabolic equivalent of task (MET) level of 5. Functional capacity in METs derived from the exercise test can be used to estimate tolerance for specific activities. Most domestic chores and activities require fewer than 5 METs; hence, a sub-maximal test at the time of hospital discharge can be useful in prescribing activity levels for the first several weeks after myocardial infarction.

Symptom-limited exercise tests are generally not recommended soon after myocardial infarction. If necessary, they can be ordered early after discharge (about 14–21 days) if the pre-discharge exercise test was not done or late after discharge (about 3–6 weeks) if the early exercise test was sub-maximal.

4.4   CARDIOVASCULAR STRESS TEST MODALITIES

Stress testing can be performed using electrocardiography with or without adjunctive imaging. The two major imaging modalities are echocardiography and nuclear perfusion imaging; other modalities, such as cardiovascular magnetic resonance (CMR) are much less commonly used.

Determination of which test to obtain depends on the clinical question, patient characteristics (e.g. ability to exercise, body habitus, co-morbidities), baseline electrocardiographic features, the presence of contraindications to pharmacologic agents commonly used for stress testing, and local expertise and technology (Figure 4.1).

4.5   EXERCISE STRESS TEST

Exercise stress testing is a cardiovascular stress test that uses treadmill or bicycle exercise in order to achieve an adequate heart rate. The sensitivity and specificity of exercise stress tests to detect CAD is about 50% and 90% respectively (sensitivity is higher with multivessel CAD compared to 1 vessel CAD). Exercise stress testing is cheap, safe, and provides useful information about ischemia, functional capacity and prognosis. However, when compared to stress imaging, the sensitivity for detecting CAD is not as high nor does it accurately localize the site and extent of ischemia. Absolute and relative contraindications to exercise stress testing are summarized in Table 4.2.

The exercise stress test is the standard initial mode of stress testing used in patients with a normal ECG who are not taking digoxin. However, patients with ST depression at baseline (greater than or equal to 1 mm), complete left bundle-branch block, ventricular paced rhythm, or pre-excitation should usually be tested with an imaging modality (e.g. exercise echocardiography or exercise nuclear imaging). Exercise testing may still provide useful prognostic information in these patients but ECG changes cannot be used to identify ischemia. Patients unable to exercise because of physical limitations (e.g. arthritis, amputations, severe peripheral vascular disease) should undergo pharmacological stress testing in combination with imaging.

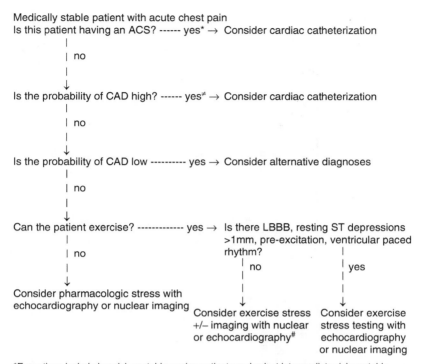

Medically stable patient with acute chest pain
Is this patient having an ACS? ------ yes* → Consider cardiac catheterization

| no

Is the probability of CAD high? ------ yes≠ → Consider cardiac catheterization

| no

Is the probability of CAD low ---------- yes → Consider alternative diagnoses

| no

Can the patient exercise? ------------- yes → Is there LBBB, resting ST depressions
                                              >1mm, pre-excitation, ventricular paced
| no   rhythm?
                                                     | no | yes

Consider pharmacologic stress with
echocardiography or nuclear imaging   Consider exercise stress   Consider exercise
                                      +/– imaging with nuclear   stress testing with
                                      or echocardiography#   echocardiography
                                                                 or nuclear imaging

*Exceptions include low-risk unstable angina patients and select intermediate-risk unstable
angina patients (consult with a cardiologist about these patients).
≠Cardiac stress testing may still be useful in patients with definite CAD for prognosis and risk
assessment.
#Imaging will improve the sensitivity of exercise stress to detect CAD.

Figure 4.1   Algorithm for determining the appropriate cardiac stress test to order.

Beta-blockers and nitrates should be held prior to stress testing for diagnostic purposes since these agents can result in false-negative or non-diagnostic results. However, in stress tests for prognostic purposes, medications need not be held.

A positive exercise stress test is primarily based on ECG findings and the occurrence of ischemic chest pain consistent with angina. Positive ECG findings are defined as greater than 1 mm of horizontal or downsloping ST-segment depression or elevation for at least 60 to 80 milliseconds after the end of the QRS complex. Additional important factors to consider in the interpretation of an exercise stress test are time of onset of symptoms, relationship of symptoms to ECG changes, timing of ECG changes, blood pressure fluctuations, and functional capacity. High-risk features seen on stress testing include: early onset of ST abnormalities (<5 METs); ST changes with classical anginal symptoms; ST changes that persist into recovery; a decrease in systolic blood pressure with increasing workload; and an exercise capacity <5 METs. Men with >10 METs exercise capacity and women with >8 METs have an excellent prognosis regardless of anatomical extent of CAD.

Table 4.2 Cardiovascular Stress Test Modalities.

	Advantages	Disadvantages	Contraindications[4]
Exercise stress with no imaging	Cheap Safe Less time commitment Can assess functional capacity Can assess prognosis	Less sensitive for ischemia compared to imaging No localization or extent of ischemia	*Absolute* Acute myocardial infarction High-risk unstable angina Uncontrolled cardiac arrhythmias Symptomatic severe aortic stenosis Uncontrolled heart failure Acute pulmonary embolu or pulmonary infarction Acute myocarditis or pericarditis Acute aortic dissection *Relative*† Left main coronary stenosis Moderate valvular stenosis Electrolyte abnormalities Severe arterial hypertension‡ Tachy- or brady-arrhythmias Hypertrophic cardiomyopathy and other forms of outflow tract obstruction Mental or physical impairment High-degree atrioventricular block

	Advantages	Disadvantages	Contraindications
Nuclear stress	High sensitivity for ischemia Can assess ventricular size, function and wall motion Can assess myocardial viability	Relative high cost Time commitment Radiation exposure	Same as for exercise stress plus Contraindications to stress agents (Table 4.3) Pregnancy
Stress Echocardiography	Relative low cost Portability Less time commitment Can assess ventricular size, function, wall thickness and motion Can assess valvular disease	Subjective interpretation Difficult interpretation with existing wall motion abnormalities or poor echo images	Same as for exercise stress plus Contraindications to stress agents (Table 4.3)

†If the benefits outweigh the risks, exercise testing can be performed in these situations.

‡In the absence of definitive evidence, ACC/AHA suggests systolic blood pressure of >200 mmHg and/or diastolic blood pressure of >110 mmHg.

TAKE HOME POINT #3

The exercise stress test is the standard initial mode of stress testing used in patients with a normal ECG who are not taking digoxin. Patients with ST depression (greater than or equal to 1 mm), complete left bundle-branch block, ventricular paced rhythm, or pre-excitation on ECG should be tested with an imaging modality

4.6 RADIONUCLIDE IMAGING

Radionuclide imaging uses nuclear imaging to assess the differential uptake of radio-active isotopes combined with pharmaceuticals (radiotracers) in normal, ischemic and infarcted tissue. External detectors (gamma cameras) capture and form images from the radiation emitted by the intravenously injected radiotracers such as thallium-201 and technetium-99 (Figure 4.2).

The most commonly-performed imaging procedure in nuclear cardiology is single-photon emission computed tomography (SPECT) imaging of myocardial perfusion. Following injection of the chosen radiotracer, the isotope is extracted from the blood by viable cardiac myocytes and retained within the tissue. Photons are emitted from the myocardium in proportion to the magnitude of tracer uptake and, in turn, act as a surrogate maker for perfusion. This process can be performed when patients are at rest or after stress. Exercise should be the preferred stressor; however, in patients who cannot exercise, vasodilator stress with adenosine, regadenoson or dipyridamole is the procedure of choice, with dobutamine reserved for patients with a contraindication to vasodilators. However, it is important to recognize that pharmacologic stress can cause serious side-effects. For example, adenosine can cause high grade block and pronounced bronchospastic airway disease. Regadenoson, a newer vasodilator drug, is better tolerated than adenosine, but can also cause high grade block and bronchospastic airway disease. Dipyridamole can induce ischemia due to coronary steal phenomenon. Dobutamine can cause hemodynamic instability, arrhythmias, and induce ischemia. Contraindications to pharmacologic stress agents are summarized in Table 4.3.

The sensitivity and specificity of exercise nuclear stress imaging to detect single-, double-, or triple-vessel CAD is 61, 86, and 94%, respectively. The advantages of nuclear imaging are high sensitivity to detect CAD and an ability to assess left ventricular size, function, wall motion, and myocardial viability. Disadvantages include relatively high cost, high time commitment, radiation exposure, soft-tissue artifact (false-positive anterior defects common in women and false-positive inferior defects common in men), and potential side-effects from pharmacologic agents.

The key elements of interpretation of cardiac nuclear imaging include the usual exercise stress features, the presence, severity, and location of perfusion defects, reversibility on the rest images (implying stress-induced ischemia) or the presence of "fixed defects" corresponding to previous MI. The extent of perfusion abnormality refers to the amount of myocardium or vascular territory that is abnormal, and the severity refers to the magnitude of reduction in tracer uptake in abnormal zone

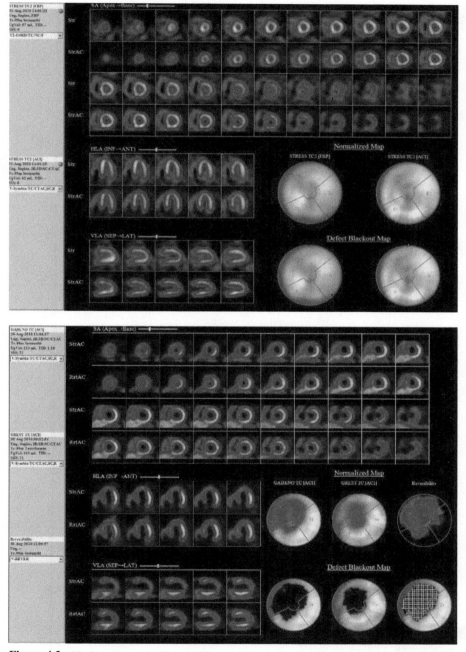

Figure 4.2   Nuclear stress tests. Top panel demonstrates a normal nuclear stress test (only stress images were acquired). Bottom panel demonstrates an abnormal nuclear stress test with a large anterior, anteroseptal and apical partially reversible defect. (See Color plate 4.1).

Table 4.3   Contraindications to Pharmacologic Stress Agents.

Dobutamine	Acute coronary syndrome
	Severe aortic stenosis
	Hypertrophic obstructive cardiomyopathy
	Uncontrolled hypertension
	Uncontrolled atrial fibrillation
	Uncontrolled heart failure
	Known severe ventricular arrhythmias
Adenosine or dipyridamole	Acute coronary syndrome
	Second- or third-degree AV block (without a pacemaker)
	Sick sinus syndrome (without a pacemaker)
	Severe pulmonary hypertension
	Systolic blood pressure less than 90
	Use of dipyridamole or dipyridamole-containing medications (e.g. aggrenox) in the last 48 hours, aminophylline in the last 24 hours, or caffeine in the last 12 hours.
	Known hypersensitivity to adenosine or dipyridamole
	Asthmatic patients with ongoing wheezing*
Regadenoson	Acute coronary syndrome
	Second- or third-degree AV block (without a pacemaker)
	Sick sinus syndrome (without a pacemaker)
	Systolic blood pressure less than 90
	Use of dipyridamole or dipyridamole-containing medications (e.g. aggrenox) in the last 48 hours, aminophylline in the last 24 hours, or caffeine in the last 12 hours.
	Known hypersensitivity to regadenoson
	The safety profile of regadenoson has not been definitively established in patients with reactive airway disease.

*Asthma is a relative contraindication. Patients with adequately controlled asthma can undergo an adenosine stress test and can have pre-treatment with 2 puffs of albuterol or a comparable inhaler.

relative to normal. The extent and severity of perfusion abnormalities have been shown to be independent risk factors for cardiovascular events and mortality. Additional high-risk features of radionuclide imaging are lung uptake and transient ischemic dilation (TID). Both lung uptake and TID provide clues to more extensive CAD than may have been suspected from the perfusion pattern alone. Both signs have been associated with angiographically extensive and severe CAD and with unfavorable long-term outcomes. Contemporary nuclear imaging can also provide information on wall motion and ejection fraction.

TAKE HOME POINT #4

Nuclear stress imaging allows assessment of left ventricular function, assessment of severity and extent of ischemia, and myocardial viability.

4.7 STRESS ECHOCARDIOGRAPHY

Ultrasound beams reflected from cardiovascular structures result in echocardio-graphic images of the heart. Stress echocardiography compares echocardiographic images obtained at the time of stress to baseline images obtained at rest (Figure 4.3). Impairment in regional contractility of the myocardium may reflect a coronary ste-nosis and impaired flow. Stress echocardiography is performed with exercise (tread-mill or bicycle) or pharmacologic agents (dobutamine, adenosine or dipyridamole) if the patient cannot exercise.

The sensitivity and specificity of stress echocardiography is comparable to nuclear imaging. The sensitivity of exercise echocardiography for coronary artery disease in patients with single-, double-, or triple-vessel involvement is 58, 86, and 94%. The advantages of stress echocardiography are: low cost; portability; less time commitment compared to nuclear imaging; and ability to assess multiple parameters including global and regional ventricular function, chamber size, wall thickness, and valvular function. The disadvantages of stress echocardiography are: subjectivity of interpretation; difficulty with interpretation when resting wall motion abnormalities exist; poor image quality in large patients; and possible side-effects from pharmaco-logic agents.

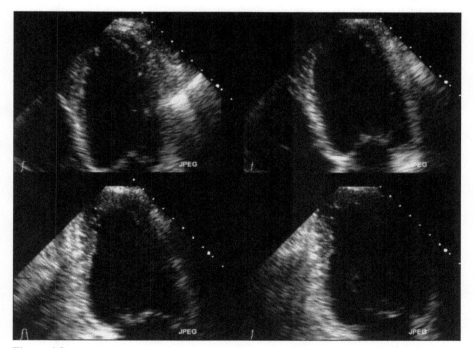

Figure 4.3   Abnormal exercise echocardiogram demonstrating left ventricular dilation at peak stress (lower right image).

The key elements to interpretation of stress echocardiography are the usual exercise stress features on ECG and new or worsening wall motion with stress, which reflects stress-induced myocardial ischemia. However, when the stress level is inadequate or the patient is taking a beta-blocker, stress-induced changes in wall motion may not be detected. Adjunctive diagnostic criteria for a positive stress echocardiography test include left ventricular cavity dilatation and a decrease in global systolic function. These adjunctive diagnostic criteria are more specific for detecting severe coronary artery disease.

TAKE HOME POINT #5

The sensitivity and specificity of exercise echocardiography and exercise nuclear imaging are comparable in studies but may vary between individual operators based on an individual center's experiences.

KEY REFERENCES

CHAITMAN B. Exercise stress testing. In BRAUNWALD E, LIBBY P, BONOW R, MANN D (Eds), Braunwald's Heart Disease: A Textbook of Cardiovascular Medicine, 8th ed. 2008. Saunders Elsevier: Philadelphia, PA.

GIBBONS RJ, BALADY GJ, BRICKER JT, et al. ACC/AHA 2002 guideline update for exercise testing: a report of the American College of Cardiology/American Heart Association Task Force on Practice Guidelines (committee to update the 1997 exercise testing guidelines). JACC 2002;48(8):1531–1540.

KLOCKE FJ, BAIRD MG, LORELL BH, et al. ACC/AHA/ASNC Guidelines for the clinical use of cardiac radionuclide imaging—executive summary: a report of the American College of Cardiology/American Heart Association Task Force on Practice Guidelines (ACC/AHA/ASNC Committee to Revise the 1995 Guidelines for the Clinical Use of Cardiac Radionuclide Imaging). Circulation 2003;108: 1404–1418.

Chapter 5

Perioperative Cardiac Evaluation

Adam M. Rogers and Kim A. Eagle

5.1 OVERVIEW

Hospitalists are regularly asked by surgical colleagues to assess perioperative cardiac risk and treatment options for patients undergoing noncardiac surgery. Patients with known and/or suspected cardiovascular disease are at risk for adverse events during the intraoperative or early postoperative periods. This risk varies significantly based on several factors, and may be reduced by selective use of medical therapy and coronary revascularization.

5.2 RATIONALE FOR PERIOPERATIVE CARDIAC EVALUATION

Perioperative cardiac events include non-fatal acute coronary syndromes, cardiac arrhythmias, non-fatal cardiac arrest, and cardiovascular death. A large recent study estimates the incidence of these events to be approximately 5–7%. The most concerning of these result from ischemic etiologies that may be due to either acute plaque rupture and blood clot formation in a coronary artery or supply-demand mismatch in the setting of fixed coronary stenoses and increased myocardial oxygen demand after surgery. This chapter is focused primarily on ischemic evaluation, but arrhythmias such as atrial fibrillation are also important. These are discussed in detail elsewhere under those specific disease processes.

Inpatient Cardiovascular Medicine, First Edition. Edited by Brahmajee K. Nallamothu and Timir S. Baman.

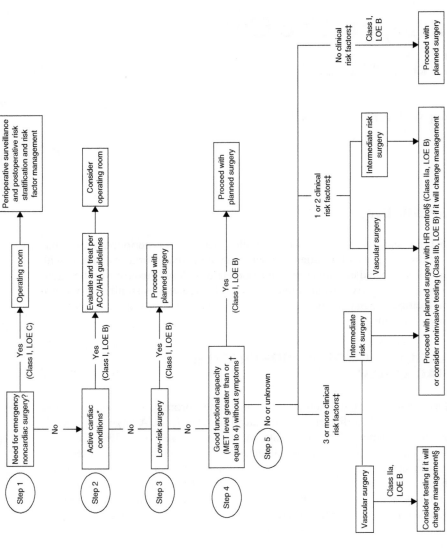

Figure 5.1 Cardiac evaluation and care algorithm for noncardiac surgery based on active clinical conditions, known cardiovascular disease, or cardiac risk factors for patients 50 years of age or greater. *See Table 5.1 for active clinical conditions. †See Table 5.3 for estimated MET level equivalent. ‡Clinical risk markers include ischemic heart disease, compensated or prior heart failure, diabetes mellitus, renal insufficiency, and cerebrovascular disease. §Noninvasive testing may be considered before surgery in specific patients with risk factors if it will change management. §Consider perioperative beta blockade (see discussion) for populations in which this has been shown to reduce cardiac morbidity/mortality. ACC/AHA indicates American College of Cardiology/American Heart Association; HR, heart rate; LOE, level of evidence; MET, metabolic equivalent.

Perioperative cardiac evaluation to minimize ischemic events has evolved greatly in recent years. Contemporary trials suggest a more limited role for perioperative beta-blockade and coronary revascularization – the two most common treatments utilized in these patients. The challenge is for the consultative physician to identify patients with the greatest likelihood of benefit from further diagnostic testing and treatment. Whilst published guidelines have inherent limitations and cannot be applied to all clinical scenarios, the ACC/AHA 2007 guidelines for preoperative evaluation and their 2009 focused update offer a relatively simple algorithm for evaluation and management. The discussion that follows will begin by reviewing this algorithm, which is depicted in Figure 5.1.

5.3 EVALUATION OF RISK

As shown in Figure 5.1, a thorough perioperative cardiac evaluation includes an assessment of both the patient's clinical risk and the degree of risk associated with the surgical procedure. The steps described below should help minimize unnecessary diagnostic testing, which has the potential to delay surgery without improving outcomes.

Step 1:   The first step is to determine whether the noncardiac surgery being performed is emergent. If this is the case, the risk of delaying an emergent noncardiac surgery for the purpose of perioperative cardiac assessment and subsequent treatment outweighs the potential benefit. The emergent noncardiac surgery should proceed with the understanding that the patient may be at risk for adverse cardiovascular events, and postoperative management should include close surveillance for ischemic events as well as long-term risk factor modification.

Step 2:   The second step involves a focused assessment of risk and should proceed after the surgery is determined to be non-emergent. The key goal is to identify active cardiac conditions, such as acute coronary syndromes and acute decompensated heart failure, which pose substantial risk to the patient and require further diagnostic testing or treatment prior to surgery. Table 5.1 includes a list of these active cardiac conditions as described in the 2007 ACC/AHA guidelines.

Step 3:   The next step is to address the risk of surgery. If the planned surgery is categorized as low risk, then the likelihood of an adverse cardiac event is considered sufficiently low to proceed without additional preoperative cardiac testing in most circumstances. Standard postoperative surveillance and medical therapy aligned with pre-existing risk factors should be continued as in all patients (see "Postoperative surveillance" section below). Table 5.2 lists the recommended approach for stratifying surgical procedures into high, intermediate, and low-risk categories.

Step 4:   If the planned surgery is determined to be intermediate or high risk, an assessment of functional status can be used to separate those patients at lower and higher risk for cardiac complications. Patients who are able to achieve greater than or equal to 4 metabolic equivalents (METs) without

Table 5.1 Active Cardiac Conditions for Which the Patient Should Undergo Evaluation and Treatment Before Noncardiac Surgery (Class I, Level of Evidence: B).

Condition	Examples
Unstable coronary syndromes	Unstable or severe angina (CCS class III or IV)* Recent MI[†]
Decompensated HF (NYHA functional class IV; worsening or new-onset HF)	
Significant arrhythmias	High-grade atrioventricular block Mobitz II atrioventricular block Third-degree atrioventricular heart block Symptomatic ventricular arrhythmias Supraventricular arrhythmias (including atrial fibrillation) with uncontrolled ventricular rate (HR greater than 100 bpm at rest) Symptomatic bradycardia Newly recognized ventricular tachycardia
Severe valvular disease	Severe aortic stenosis (mean pressure gradient greater than 40 mm Hg, aortic valve area less than 1.0 cm^2, or symptomatic) Symptomatic mitral stenosis (progressive dyspnea on exertion, exertional presyncope, or HF)

*May include "stable" angina in patients who are unusually sedentary.

[†]The American College of Cardiology National Database Library defines recent MI as more than 7 days but less than or equal to 1 month (within 30 days).

CCS indicates Canadian Cardiovascular Society; HF, heart failure; HR, heart rate; MI, myocardial infarction; NYHA, New York Heart Association.

Table 5.2 Cardiac Risk* Stratification for Noncardiac Surgical Procedures.

Risk stratification	Procedure examples
Vascular (reported cardiac risk often more than 5%)	Aortic and other major vascular surgery Peripheral vascular surgery
Intermediate (reported cardiac risk generally 1–5%)	Intraperitoneal and intrathoracic surgery Carotid endarterectomy Head and neck surgery Orthopedic surgery Prostate surgery
Low[†] (reported cardiac risk generally <1%)	Endoscopic procedures Superficial procedure Cataract surgery Breast surgery Ambulatory surgery

*Combined incidence of cardiac death and nonfatal myocardial infarction.

[†]These procedures do not generally require further preoperative cardiac testing.

Table 5.3   Estimated Energy Requirements for Various Activities.

1 MET	Can you … Take care of yourself?
	Eat, dress, or use the toilet?
	Walk indoors around the house?
	Walk 1 or 2 blocks on level ground at 2–3 mph (3.2–4.8 kph)?
<4 METs	Do light work around the house like dusting or washing dishes?
≥4METs	Climb a flight of stairs or walk up a hill?
	Walk on level ground at 4 mph (6.4 kph)?
	Run a short distance?
	Do heavy work around the house like scrubbing floors or lifting or moving heavy furniture?
	Participate in moderate recreational activities like golf, bowling, dancing, doubles tennis, or throwing a baseball or football?
>10 METs	Participate in strenuous sports like swimming, singles tennis, football, basketball, or skiing?

kph indicates kilometers per hour; MET, metabolic equivalent; mph, miles per hour.

associated cardiac symptoms are considered at lower perioperative risk, and further preoperative risk stratification is unlikely to be high yield. No further preoperative diagnostic testing is usually recommended in this population. Table 5.3 provides a framework for converting several patient activities to their metabolic equivalent levels.

Step 5:   If steps 1–4 are inconclusive, then reviewing key risk factors can help to guide management. These include: (1) history of ischemic heart disease; (2) history of prior congestive heart failure; (3) history of cerebrovascular disease; (4) diabetes mellitus, whether or not the patient is on insulin therapy; and (5) renal insufficiency with creatinine >2 mg/dL. If the patient has none of these risk factors, further preoperative testing or treatment is not recommended. If the patient has one or two, the decision of whether or not to pursue noninvasive diagnostic testing (e.g. stress testing) is determined by overall clinical suspicion, and whether or not the results of such testing are likely to alter management. The same is true for patients with three or more risk factors, although the threshold for noninvasive testing is lower in patients scheduled to undergo vascular surgery. If questions remain at this stage, cardiology consultation may be beneficial.

TAKE HOME POINT #1

Decisions about cardiac testing prior to noncardiac surgery are complex and depend upon the urgency and nature of the surgery as well as the presence of active cardiac symptoms. A previous history of coronary artery disease does not necessarily mean that further testing is required.

5.4 PERIOPERATIVE MEDICAL MANAGEMENT

Beta-blockers have been the primary agents used for cardiac risk reduction in the perioperative setting. However, it is important to recognize that beta-blockers must be carefully administered to the correct subset of patients in order to achieve reduction of adverse cardiac events without inadvertently causing harm. A retrospective study of 783,000 patients 18 years or older undergoing major noncardiac surgery found that perioperative beta-blockade (administered to 16% of the cohort) was beneficial in intermediate or high-risk patients but potentially harmful in low-risk patients. The recent POISE trial also found that intermediate- or high-risk patients treated with high-dose perioperative metoprolol succinate had improved cardiovascular outcomes; however, this apparent benefit was offset by increases in mortality, ischemic stroke, and sepsis compared with those receiving a placebo. An important criticism of the POISE trial relates to the use of high-dose metoprolol succinate (100 mg initial dose within 2–4 hours of surgery, uptitrated to 200 mg/day during the first 18 hours postoperatively), which may have contributed to the number of adverse events observed in this study.

In light of these data, a guideline update was released in 2009 on the role of perioperative beta blockade. Patients already receiving beta-blockers for appropriate indications should have these drugs continued in the perioperative setting. Beta-blockers are recommended for patients undergoing vascular surgery with known or highly suspected coronary artery disease. Their use also is reasonable in vascular surgery patients with multiple cardiac risk markers. The addition of beta-blocker therapy prior to low- or intermediate-risk surgery is of uncertain benefit, and should not be used routinely. In all cases, careful titration of beta-blockers to heart rate and blood pressure targets is paramount to avoid hemodynamic compromise in the perioperative period. For instance, an initial dose of metoprolol tartrate 25 mg by mouth twice daily, uptitrated for a goal heart rate of 55–70 beats per minute and goal systolic blood pressure of 100–120 mmHg.

TAKE HOME POINT #2

Perioperative beta-blocker use is recommended in patients already on outpatient beta-blocker therapy and patients undergoing vascular surgery with known or highly suspected coronary artery disease, but not in all patients. Cautious titration of beta-blocker dose is required.

There is considerable interest in statin use as a potential means of reducing perioperative risk. Most studies addressing this question to date are nonrandomized, though they do demonstrate a tendency toward improved outcomes, particularly in vascular surgery patients. Current guidelines recommend that patients on a statin should continue taking them in the perioperative period; the addition of a statin medication is reasonable in patients undergoing vascular surgery. Additional studies are needed to better elucidate the role of statin therapy in perioperative management.

5.5 PERIOPERATIVE STRESS TESTING AND CORONARY REVASCULARIZATION

Recent data from randomized controlled trials have called into question the benefits of coronary revascularization during the perioperative setting. These studies failed to demonstrate improved outcomes for patients who underwent revascularization prior to surgery compared to those managed medically. Furthermore, coronary stent placement obligates patients to dual antiplatelet therapy for at least one month for bare metal stents and potentially one year for drug-eluting stents. As a result, many elective surgeries are delayed without a proven associated improvement in cardiovascular outcomes.

The utility of preoperative stress testing also becomes less clear since the ultimate intervention that results from an abnormal stress test is coronary revascularization. In addition, acute coronary syndromes during the perioperative setting often arise from non-obstructive vulnerable plaques (i.e. occluding <50% of the coronary artery lumen), which are frequently missed by current imaging modalities. Best practice at this time appears to be to restrict the use of perioperative stress testing to those select circumstances where a positive test would necessitate a change in management, as described in the algorithm above. Consultation with a cardiologist is recommended in unclear situations.

5.6 OTHER STUDIES: PREOPERATIVE ECG AND LEFT VENTRICULAR FUNCTION ASSESSMENT

Preoperative resting 12-lead ECG is reasonable in moderate- to high-risk patients prior to noncardiac surgery, although patients with no known cardiac risk factors undergoing low-risk surgery do not require an ECG. Left ventricular (LV) function assessment before noncardiac surgery is reasonable in patients with dyspnea of unknown origin and in patients with known heart failure with changing clinical status (e.g. worsening dyspnea). Routine use of LV function assessment in perioperative patients is not recommended.

5.7 POSTOPERATIVE SURVEILLANCE

Postoperative surveillance should include regular clinical assessments as part of routine post-procedural care. Patients who develop signs or symptoms of cardiac ischemia should undergo further assessment with electrocardiography and measurement of cardiac enzymes. Routine troponin measurement is not recommended as most positive values are due to physiologic conditions other than acute myocardial infarction. Intraoperative and postoperative ST-segment monitoring (typically with computerized ST-segment analysis via telemetry) can be considered in high-risk patients or patients undergoing vascular surgery where heightened surveillance for postoperative ischemia is deemed appropriate. Prior to discharge, patients with ischemic events should have their risk factors assessed and treated, as outlined in Chapter 9 – Chronic Coronary Artery Disease.

> ### TAKE HOME POINT #3
>
> Routine perioperative troponin measurement is not recommended as most positive values are due to physiologic conditions other than acute myocardial infarction.

KEY REFERENCES

CHOPRA V, FLANDERS SA, FROEHLICH JB, et al. Perioperative practice: time to throttle back. Ann Intern Med 2010;152(1):47–51.

FLEISCHMANN KE, BECKMAN JA, BULLER CE, et al. ACCF/AHA focused update on perioperative beta-blockade. J Am Coll Card 2009;54:2102–2108.

FLEISHER LA, BECKMAN JA, BROWN KA, et al. ACC/AHA 2007 guidelines on perioperative cardio-vascular evaluation and care for noncardiac surgery: a report of the American College of Cardiology/American Heart Association Task Force on Practice Guidelines (Writing Committee to Revise the 2002 Guidelines on Perioperative Cardiovascular Evaluation for Noncardiac Surgery): developed in collaboration with the American Society of Echocardiography, American Society of Nuclear Cardiol-ogy, Heart Rhythm Society, Society of Cardiovascular Anesthesiologists, Society for Cardiovascular Angiography and Interventions, Society for Vascular Medicine and Biology, and Society for Vascular Surgery. Circulation 2007;116(17):e418–e499.

Chapter 6

Cardiac Resuscitation

Dana P. Edelson

6.1 EPIDEMIOLOGY

There are an estimated 200,000 cardiac resuscitation attempts in US hospitals each year, of which one-third occur on general inpatient wards. Unlike the out-of-hospital setting, cardiac arrest in the hospital is often the progression of the patient's underlying acute disease process. As such, hypotension and/or acute respiratory insufficiency are frequent immediate causes and the presenting pulseless rhythm is shockable (e.g. ventricular fibrillation or tachycardia (VF/VT)) in fewer than one quarter of cases. The distinction between shockable and non-shockable rhythms is important not only for treatment but also for prognosis since ~33% of those patients with an initial cardiac rhythm of VF/VT survive to hospital discharge, compared with ~10% for pulseless electrical activity (PEA) or asystole. Interestingly, of the patients who survive to discharge, over 70% have good neurologic outcomes. This chapter reviews cardiac resuscitation from the perspective of the hospitalist who is often a critical member of the resuscitation team.

6.2 PHASES OF IN-HOSPITAL RESUSCITATION

Resuscitations in the hospital can be divided into three phases, with different goals and priorities (Table 6.1).

Inpatient Cardiovascular Medicine, First Edition. Edited by Brahmajee K. Nallamothu and Timir S. Baman.
© 2014 John Wiley & Sons, Inc. Published 2014 by John Wiley & Sons, Inc.

Table 6.1   In-hospital Resuscitation Phases.

Phase	Goal	Priorities
Basic Life Support (BLS) First 3 minutes	Start CPR immediately Defibrillate within 3 minutes	Identify of cardiac arrest Call for help/defibrillator Begin CPR/bag mask ventilation Analyze rhythm (distinguish shockable from non-shockable) Shock if VF/VT Resume compressions
Advanced Cardiac Life Support (ACLS) Ongoing resuscitation	Maintain adequate perfusion until spontaneous circulation is restored	Secure access Secure airway Monitor CPR quality Administer drugs Identify and treat reversible causes
Post-Resuscitation Care – Return of Spontaneous Circulation (ROSC)	Prevent recurring cardiac arrest Maximize neurologic outcome	Optimize oxygenation and ventilation Treat hypotension Consider therapeutic hypothermia Consider coronary reperfusion Treat hyperglycemia Assess prognosis

6.2.1 Basic Life Support (BLS) Phase

The first few minutes of a resuscitation are arguably the most important and yet the most chaotic, as providers arrive and the resuscitation team composes itself. Survival from cardiac arrest is correlated with time to CPR and in the case of VF/VT with time to first shock (Figure 6.1). During the BLS phase, the goal is to initiate chest compressions within 10 seconds and deliver a shock, if indicated, within 3 minutes. Thus, interventions that can delay defibrillation should be deferred until after this first attempt and remaining steps run in tandem, if multiple rescuers are present. (Figure 6.2)

> **TAKE HOME POINT #1**
>
> Cardiac arrests with shockable rhythms of ventricular fibrillation and pulseless ventricular tachycardia require defibrillation within 3 minutes.

Recognition and activation of emergency response. Cardiac arrest should be suspected in any unresponsive patient who is not breathing normally (e.g. gasping or apneic). This should prompt an immediate activation of the hospital's emergency plan and summon a defibrillator to the bedside, with additional rescuers. Cardiac arrest should be confirmed by carotid palpation for 5–10 seconds.

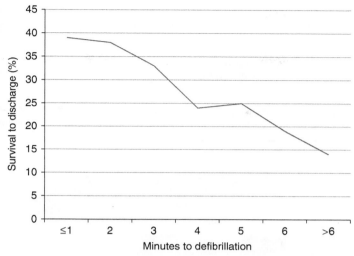

Figure 6.1   Time to defibrillation affects overall mortality.

Initiation of CPR. If no pulse is appreciated within 10 seconds, one rescuer should begin CPR by compressing the lower half of the patient's sternum at a rate of at least 100/min and a depth of at least 2 inches, allowing full chest recoil between compressions. A second rescuer should prepare for ventilation. If the patient does not have an advanced airway in place at the time of cardiac arrest, chest compressions should be paused briefly after every 30 compressions to deliver 2 breaths with a bag-valve-mask, allowing 1 second per breath. In patients with advanced airways, asynchronous ventilation should be provided at a rate of 8–10/min without pausing chest compressions.

Defibrillation. Meanwhile, the arriving defibrillator should be attached and turned on, continuing chest compressions until the monitor is able to pick up a rhythm. The rhythm should be analyzed quickly for the presence of a shockable rhythm. If VF or VT is present, a shock should be administered within 10 seconds of pausing chest compressions, using the manufacturer's recommended energy level (or 200 Joules if unknown). If using a monophasic defibrillator, 360 Joules is administered. If a rescuer able to operate a manual defibrillator, is not readily available, an automated external defibrillator (AED) or AED-mode on a manual defibrillator should be used. However, AEDs can result in prolonged pauses in chest compression and may be associated with worse outcomes for those patients with PEA or asystole when compared to manual defibrillators. Chest compressions should be resumed immediately after defibrillation without rechecking the rhythm or pulse.

6.2.2 Advanced Cardiac Life Support (ACLS) Phase

Following the first rhythm check, the resuscitation moves into the ACLS phase (Figure 6.3) with a goal of maintaining adequate perfusion and restoring a pulse. In this phase, the quality of CPR is paramount as is identifying and treating reversible causes.

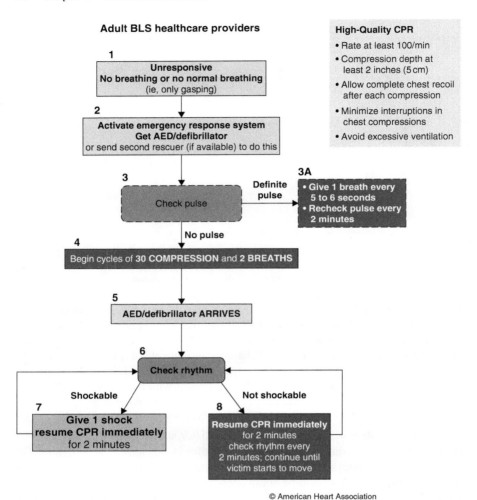

© American Heart Association

Figure 6.2 BLS healthcare provider algorithm. (Source: Berg RA et al. 2010. Reproduced with permission of Wolters Kluwer Health).

Ensuring high CPR quality. The key aspects of CPR quality are listed in Table 6.2. These include ensuring a depth of >2 inches, rate of at least 100/min, allowing full recoil, minimizing pauses in chest compression and avoiding hyperventilation. Interventions previously deferred in the BLS phase, such as advanced airway placement and intravenous or intraosseous (IV/IO) line placement, should be attempted during ongoing chest compressions. If a pause in compressions is required it should be timed with the next scheduled pause for rhythm check, compressor rotation, and possible defibrillation.

CPR Quality
- Push hard (≥2 inches [5 cm]) and fast (≥100/min) and allow complete chest recoil
- Minimize interruptions in compressions
- Avoid excessive ventilation
- Rotate compressor every 2 minutes
- If no advanced airway, 30:2 compression-ventilation ratio
- Quantitative waveform capnography
  - If $PETCO_2 < 10$ mm Hg, attempt to improve CPR quality
- Intra-arterial pressure
  - If relaxation phase (diastolic) pressure <20 mm Hg, attempt to improve CPR quality

Return of Spontaneous Circulation (ROSC)
- Pulse and blood pressure
- Abrupt sustained increase in $PETCO_2$ (typically ≥40 mm Hg)
- Spontaneous arterial pressure waves with intra-arterial monitoring

Shock Energy
- **Biphasic:** Manufacturer recommendation (eg, initial dose of 120–200 J); if unknown, use maximum available. Second and subsequent doses should be equivalent, and higher doses may be considered.
- **Monophasic:** 360 J

Drug Therapy
- **Epinephrine IV/IO Dose:** 1 mg every 3–5 minutes
- **Vasopressin IV/IO Dose:** 40 units can replace first or second dose of epinephrine
- **Amiodarone IV/IO Dose:** First dose: 300 mg bolus. Second dose: 150 mg.

Advanced Airway
- Supraglottic advanced airway or endotracheal intubation
- Waveform capnography to confirm and monitor ET tube placement
- 8–10 breaths per minute with continuous chest compressions

Reversible Causes
- Hypovolemia
- Hypoxia
- Hydrogen ion (acidosis)
- Hypo-/hyperkalemia
- Hypothermia
- Tension pneumothorax
- Tamponade, cardiac
- Toxins
- Thrombosis, pulmonary
- Thrombosis, coronary

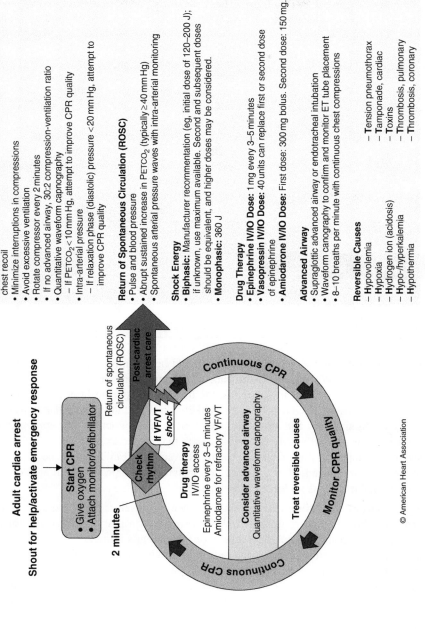

Adult cardiac arrest

Shout for help/activate emergency response

Start CPR
- Give oxygen
- Attach monitor/defibrillator

Return of spontaneous circulation (ROSC)

2 minutes

Check rhythm

If VF/VT shock

Post-cardiac arrest care

Continuous CPR

Drug therapy
IV/IO access
Epinephrine every 3–5 minutes
Amiodarone for refractory VF/VT

Consider advanced airway
Quantitative waveform capnography

Treat reversible causes

Monitor CPR quality

Continuous CPR

© American Heart Association

Figure 6.3 ACLS Cardiac Arrest Circular Algorithm. (Source: Neumar RW et al. 2010. Reproduced with permission of Wolters Kluwer Health).

83

Table 6.2 CPR Quality Components and Strategies for Improvement.

Components	Strategies for achievement
Compression depth >2	Rotate compressors every 2 minutes to avoid fatigue
Full recoil between compressions	Adjust the height of the bed and/or position of the rescuer to balance the upper body strength required with the need to lean on the patient
	Consider incorporation of real-time CPR feedback such as a CPR sensing and feedback device, continuous capnography or arterial waveform tracing
Compression rate >100/min	Consider use of a metronome or song with a beat of 100/min
Minimize interruptions	Secure IV/IO access and airway during ongoing compressions, when possible
	Coordinate pauses for interventions with rhythm/pulse checks and compressor rotation
Avoid excessive ventilation	Count 5–6 seconds between breaths
	Consider using a pediatric bag-valve

TAKE HOME POINT #2

High-quality CPR is critical to cardiac resuscitation and requires adequate rate and depth of chest compressions without leaning, minimization of pauses, and avoidance of hyperventilation.

Drug therapy. Pharmacologic adjuncts should be administered during this phase as well (Table 6.3). While there are no data to show an improvement in survival with the use of any cardiac arrest medications, the use of epinephrine 1 mg IV/IO every 3–5 minutes has been shown to increase the likelihood of achieving a pulse. Vasopressin likely works similarly and may even have benefit in conjunction with epinephrine for prolonged resuscitations. Therefore, rescuers may opt to exchange either the first or second epinephrine dose for vasopressin. Refractory VF/VT should be treated with an antiarrythmic agent after the third defibrillation attempt, of which amiodarone is preferred. Atropine is no longer recommended for cardiac arrest.

Treatment of reversible causes. The presence of pulseless electrical activity as the arrest rhythm should prompt a search for reversible primary etiologies (Table 6.4). This evaluation should include a review of the patient's immediate history for clues, auscultation of breath sounds bilaterally, examination of neck veins, a point of care glucose level and possibly an arterial blood gas, with point of care chemistries and hemoglobin, if available. Routine laboratory studies, even if run on a STAT basis, are unlikely to change management acutely due to delays and will need to be redrawn if the patient is successfully resuscitated. Portable chest X-rays and 12-lead ECGs should not be obtained on a pulseless patient as they require prolonged pauses in

Table 6.3   Adjuvant Drug Therapy During CPR.

Drug	Indication	Dosage
Epinephrine	Vasopressor used to increase likelihood of successful resuscitation	IV/IO dose: 1 mg (10 mL of 1:10,000 solution), followed by 20 mL flush Q 3–5 minutes during resuscitation Endotracheal route: 2–2.5 mg diluted in 10 mL NS
Vasopressin	Alternative/adjunct to epinephrine	One dose of 40 units IV/IO push may replace either first or second dose of epinephrine
Amiodarone	Antiarrythmic used for refractory VF/VT	First dose: 300 mg IV/IO push Second dose (if needed): 150 mg IV/IO push
Lidocaine	Alternative to amiodarone	Initial dose: 1 to 1.5 mg/kg IV/IO For refractory VF may give additional 0.5 to 0.75 mg/kg IV push, repeat in 5–10 minutes; maximum 3 doses or total of 3 mg/kg
Magnesium sulfate	Reversal of cardiac arrest due to hypomagnesemia or Torsade de Pointes	1–2 g (2 to 4 mL of a 50% solution) diluted in 10 mL of D_5W IV/IO

Table 6.4   Common Causes of PEA (Hs and Ts).

Condition	Possible interventions
Hypovolemia	IV fluid
Hypoxia	Advanced airway
	Supplemental oxygen
Hydrogen ions (acidosis)	NaHCO3
Hyper-/Hypokalemia	CaCl
	NaHCO3
	Insulin with glucose
	Albuterol
	Magnesium
Hypothermia	Rewarming
Tension pneumothorax	Needle thoracotomy or chest tube
Tamponade (cardiac)	Pericardiocentesis
Toxins	Specific antidotes
	Hemodialysis
Thrombosis (pulmonary embolus)	Surgical embolectomy
	Fibrinolytics
Thrombosis (acute MI)	Percutaneous intervention (PCI)

compressions. Persistent VF/VT should prompt consideration of acute myocardial ischemia or infarction.

Termination of resuscitation efforts. Sustained spontaneous circulation is achieved in an average of ~50% of in-hospital cardiac arrest patients. Recognition of futility and termination of efforts are therefore an important aspect of resuscitation. While there have been attempts to develop and test resuscitation termination rules in the out-of-hospital setting, there are few data to guide rescuers performing resuscitation in the hospital. However, for hospitals using continuous capnography, one fairly sensitive and specific predictor of death is an end-tidal carbon dioxide ETCO2 <10 mmHg at 20 minutes into the resuscitation.

6.2.3 Post-Resuscitation Care Phase

For those that survive the initial resuscitation attempt, defined as the presence of a spontaneous pulse for >20 minutes, the focus should turn to maintaining hemodynamic stability and increasing the likelihood of survival to discharge with good neurologic function. This generally requires transfer to an intensive care unit and following of the post-resuscitation protocol (Figure 6.4).

Optimize oxygenation, ventilation and hemodynamics. Inspired oxygen should be weaned to the lowest percent that will maintain an oxyhemoglobin concentration of >=94% and hyperventilation should be avoided. Respiratory rates should be titrated to achieve an ETCO2 of 35–40 mmHg or PaCO2 of 40–45 mmHg. An IV fluid bolus of 1–2 L is often helpful in the early post-resuscitation phase to treat hypotension. This should be chilled saline (4 °C) if initiating hypothermia. In addition, a vasopressor infusion is often required and should be prepared immediately upon ROSC in anticipation of a drop in blood pressure. Epinephrine (0.1–0.5 mcg/kg), dopamine (5–10 mcg/kg), or norepinephrine (0.1–0.5 mcg/kg) titrated to maintain a mean arterial pressure >65 are good initial choices.

Therapeutic hypothermia. Patients who are comatosed following cardiac arrest should be considered for induction of hypothermia. While the majority of the benefit has been shown in the out-of-hospital setting for patients with VF arrests, there are some data to support its use following cardiac arrest in the hospital regardless of presenting rhythm. The optimal method to achieve hypothermia is not known but cold saline, surface cooling techniques and endovascular devices have all been described. The goal is to achieve a temperature of 32–34 °C for 12–24 hours. Maintenance within that range may require thermostatic feedback to prevent under- and overshoots of target temperature.

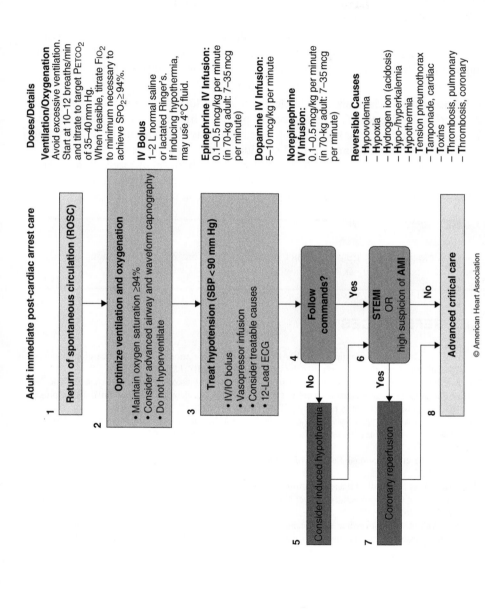

Figure 6.4 Post-cardiac arrest care algorithm. (Source: Peberdy MA, Neumar RW et al. 2010. Reproduced with permission of Wolters Kluwer Health).

87

TAKE HOME POINT #4

If available, therapeutic hypothermia should be considered for comatosed survivors of cardiac arrest, although data in the inpatient setting are limited.

Coronary reperfusion. A 12-lead ECG should be obtained in the early ROSC period and reviewed for signs of acute myocardial ischemia. If suspected, early coronary angiography followed by appropriate revascularization of culprit lesions should be considered.

Prognostication. There are no reliable predictors of long-term outcomes in the first 24 hours following ROSC. The absence of pupillary light and corneal reflexes after 72 hours is fairly specific for poor outcome in patients who have not received hypothermia. In addition, unprocessed EEG findings and somatosensory evoked potentials may also be useful after 24 hours. As a result, withdrawal of care within 24, and possibly even 72, hours following ROSC is likely premature. Engaging families and other decision-makers early on in these discussions is important.

TAKE HOME POINT #5

Neurologic prognostication should not be attempted before 24 hours following ROSC and may require waiting at least 72 hours.

KEY REFERENCES

BERG RA et al. Adult basic life support: 2010 American Heart Association guidelines for cardiopulmonary resuscitation and emergency cardiovascular care. Circulation 2010;122:S685–S705.

MEANEY PA et al. CPR Quality: Improving Cardiac Resuscitation Outcomes Both Inside and Outside the Hospital: A Consensus Statement From the American Heart Association. Circulation 2013; in press. (available online but not yet in print)

MORRISON LJ et al. Strategies for improving survival after in-hospital cardiac arrest in the United States: 2013 consensus recommendations: a consensus statement from the American Heart Association. Circulation 2013;127(14):1538–63.

NADKARNI VM et al. National Registry of Cardiopulmonary Resuscitation Investigators. JAMA 2006; 295(1):50–57.

NEUMAR RW et al. Adult advanced cardiovascular life support: 2010 American Heart Association Guidelines for Cardiopulmonary resuscitation and emergency cardiovascular care. Circulation 2010; 122:S-729–S767.

PEBERDY MA et al. Post-cardiac arrest care: 2010 American Heart Association guidelines for cardiopulmonary resuscitation and emergency cardiovascular care. Circulation 2010;122:S768–S786.

Chapter 7

Acute Coronary Syndromes: Unstable Angina and Non-ST Elevation Myocardial Infarction

Gerald C. Koenig and Stanley J. Chetcuti

7.1 INTRODUCTION

Acute coronary syndromes (ACS) cover the spectrum of clinical conditions ranging from unstable angina (UA) to non-ST-segment elevation myocardial infarction (NSTEMI) to ST-segment elevation myocardial infarction (STEMI). UA and NSTEMI are pathophysiologically- and clinically-related conditions differing in severity. Both conditions may be characterized by electrocardiographic (ECG) ST-segment depression or prominent T-wave inversion; however, NSTEMI is also characterized by positive biomarkers indicative of necrosis (e.g. cardiac troponin – TnI or TnT, and CK-MB) in the absence of ST-segment elevation and in an appropriate clinical setting (chest discomfort or anginal equivalent).

Acute coronary syndromes, with emphasis on unstable angina and NSTEMI, are a major cause of emergency medical care and hospitalization in the United States with approximately 1.5 million admissions with a primary or secondary diagnosis of ACS each year. The estimated direct and indirect cost for ACS in the U.S. was $450 billion in 2008.

7.2 ETIOLOGY AND PATHOPHYSIOLOGY

Etiologies of ACS are characterized by an imbalance between myocardial oxygen supply and demand. The most common cause of UA/NSTEMI is reduced myocardial perfusion caused by plaque rupture and thrombus formation. Less common

Inpatient Cardiovascular Medicine, First Edition. Edited by Brahmajee K. Nallamothu and Timir S. Baman.

mechanisms include dynamic obstruction, progressive atherosclerosis or restenosis of previously-treated coronary lesions, and inflammation. Hypercontractility of vascular smooth muscle or endothelial dysfunction may lead to intense focal spasms within segments of the epicardial coronary arteries (Prinzmetal's angina). Other dynamic obstructions may be caused by diffuse microvascular dysfunction or induced by specific vasoconstrictor substances (e.g. cocaine-induced coronary spasm). Progressive atherosclerotic obstruction may occur in stable calcified lesions or following percutaneous coronary intervention (PCI), resulting in severe narrowing without spasm or thrombus. Secondary mechanisms to UA/NSTEMI may be caused by: (a) increased myocardial oxygen requirements due to systemic diseases (fever, thyrotoxicosis, tachycardia); (b) reduced coronary blood flow from non-obstructive causes (hypotension, arrhythmia); or (c) reduced myocardial oxygen delivery (anemia, hypoxemia).

TAKE HOME POINT #1

Most patients with ACS have plaque rupture leading to thrombus formation.

7.3 CLINICAL PRESENTATION

Presentations of unstable angina are based on the duration and intensity of angina as graded by the Canadian Cardiovascular Society classification scheme (class 0 – asymptomatic; class 1 – angina with strenuous exercise; class 2 – angina with moderate exertion; class 3 – angina with mild exertion; and class 4 – angina at any level of exertion). NSTEMI generally presents as more intense prolonged angina or angina equivalent.

The ACS spectrum requires early recognition of symptoms, as well as the appropriate classification of the likelihood of acute ischemia (Table 7.1), as it has substantial clinical and economic consequences. The *five most important factors* derived from the initial history, ranked in order of importance, are: (1) the nature of the anginal symptoms; (2) prior history of CAD; (3) gender; (4) age; and (5) the number of traditional risk factors present. Classically, the chest discomfort is described as a pressure sensation arising in the substernum that often radiates to the left upper extremity and neck or jaw, exacerbated by activity or emotional stress, and relieved by rest and/or nitroglycerin. Associated symptoms include diaphoresis, dyspnea, nausea, vomiting and unexplained fatigue. Atypical presentations are more common among women and the elderly.

ACS, as associated with coronary heart disease, has well established *major risk factors*, including smoking, family history, adverse lipid profile, diabetes mellitus, and elevated blood pressure. However, the presence or absence of these risk factors is far less important than symptoms, ECG findings, and cardiac biomarkers.

The *physical examination* is focused on identifying possible precipitating causes of myocardial ischemia and to assess hemodynamic consequences. Findings indicating large areas of ischemia and high risk that demand a more aggressive management pathway include: diaphoresis; cool extremities; tachycardia; third or

Table 7.1 Likelihood Signs and Symptoms Represent ACS Secondary to CAD (Source: Adapted from Anderson et al. 2007. With permission of Wolters Kluwer Health).

Feature	High Likelihood *Any of the following*:	Intermediate Likelihood *Absence of high-likelihood features and presence of any of the following*:	Low Likelihood *Absence of high- or intermediate-likelihood features but may have*:
History	Chest or left arm pain or discomfort as chief symptom reproducing prior documented angina Known history of CAD, including MI	Chest or left arm pain or discomfort as chief symptom Age >70 years Male sex Diabetes Mellitus	Probable ischemic symptoms in absence of any of the intermediate likelihood characteristics Recent cocaine use
Examination	Transient MR, hypotension, diaphoresis, pulmonary edema, or rales	Extracardiac vascular disease	Chest discomfort reproduced by palpation
ECG	New, or presumably new, transient ST-segment deviation (≥0.05 mV) or T-wave inversion (≥0.2 mV) with symptoms	Fixed Q waves Abnormal ST segments or T waves note documented to be new	T-wave flattening or inversion in leads with dominant R waves Normal ECG
Cardiac markers	Elevated cardiac TnI, TnT, or CK-MB	Normal	Normal

fourth heart sounds; murmurs; basilar rales; and hypotension. Other conditions that may be considered in the differential diagnoses of ACS should also be evaluated for, including unequal pulses ± aortic regurgitation (aortic dissection), pericardial friction rub (acute pericarditis), and diminished breath sounds (pneumothorax).

TAKE HOME POINT #2

Risk factors are far less important than symptoms, ECG findings and cardiac biomarkers in evaluating patients with suspected ACS.

7.4   EVALUATION AND DIAGNOSTIC STUDIES

Several *risk assessment schemes* have been developed in evaluating patients with UA/NSTEMI and are an integral prerequisite to decision-making. The Global Registry of Acute Coronary Events (GRACE) risk tool uses eight variables to predict in-hospital mortality (and death or MI) in patients with STEMI, NSTEMI or UA, and is used to guide treatment type and intensity (Figure 7.1). As a part of this assessment,

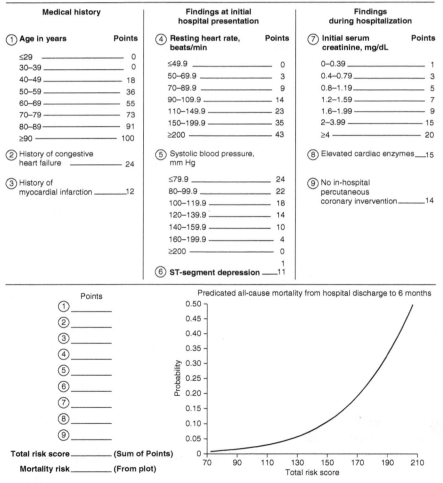

Figure 7.1   GRACE prediction score sheet and nomogram for all-cause mortality (Source: Anderson et al. 2007. Reproduced with permission of Wolters Kluwer Health).

several diagnostic studies also are instrumental in its evaluation. An online tool is available for calculating the GRACE risk tool: http://www.outcomes-umassmed.org/GRACE/acs_risk/acs_risk_content.html

7.4.1 Electrocardiography

Specific pattern characteristics and magnitude of pattern abnormalities increase the likelihood of ACS. Findings associated with UA/NSTEMI include: (a) new or dynamic ST-segment depression (>0.5 mm); (b) T-wave inversion (≥3 mm); and (c) nonspecific ST-segment changes (≤0.5 mm) and T-wave changes (≤2 mm). The latter is much less specific and may also be related to drugs (e.g. phenothiazines, tricyclic antidepressants, digitalis, etc.), hyperventilation, repolarization abnormalities associated with left ventricular hypertrophy or conduction disturbances. Serial ECG tracings or continuous ST-segment monitoring early on during hospitalization are encouraged as myocardial ischemia may be dynamic.

7.4.2 Cardiac Biomarkers

Cardiac biomarkers detect myocardial necrosis and are recommended to be measured for all patients presenting with signs and symptoms suggestive of ACS. *Cardiac troponins* (cTnI or cTnT) allow for high accuracy, sensitivity and specificity in diagnosing myocardial injury. Recent expert groups have defined myocardial necrosis as an elevation of troponin above the 99th percentile of normal. Myocardial infarction, which is necrosis related to ischemia, is further defined by the elevation of troponin and one of the following criteria: ischemic ST and T-wave changes, new left bundle-branch block, new Q-waves, PCI-related marker elevation, or positive imaging for loss of viable myocardium. Cardiac troponins are detectable about 6 hrs after myocardial injury and measurable for up to 2 weeks. Mortality risk is directly proportional to the level of troponin elevation and its prognostic information is independent of other clinical and ECG risk factors. *Creatine kinase-MB*, the prior standard marker for the diagnosis of MI, is less sensitive and less specific than the cardiac troponins. However, because of its shorter half-life, CK-MB is useful to detect eventual infarct extension and recurrent MI. *Myoglobin* is a nonspecific, very early marker that can be used to provide high-negative predictive value for MI.

Besides markers of myocardial necrosis, markers of inflammation are also under investigation. *C-reactive protein* (CRP) levels appear to be related to long-term mortality after ACS in an independent and additive fashion to troponin levels. The role of other markers, such as amyloid A, interleukin-6, fibrinogen, plasminogen activator inhibitor-1 (PAI-1), and B-type natriuretic peptide (BNP), are yet undefined.

7.4.3 Non-Invasive Testing

A *chest radiograph* should be used to evaluate for other causes of chest pain and screen for pulmonary congestion, implicating a worse prognosis in ACS. *Echocardiography* allows for the rapid determination of left ventricular function, regional wall motion, and valvular function. Stress testing to risk stratify should be performed in low-risk and intermediate-risk patients free of complications and not referred for coronary angiography. Choice of stress test is based on the resting ECG, ability to exercise, and local expertise. Treadmill stress testing is suitable for patients with the following criteria: (a) good exercise tolerance; and (b) ECG free of ST-segment abnormalities, bundle branch block, left ventricular hypertrophy, intraventricular conduction delay, paced rhythm, pre-excitation, and digitalis effect. Stress testing with adjunctive imaging using either echocardiography or nuclear stress imaging should be used in patients with ECG abnormalities that prevent accurate interpretation. Pharmacological stress testing can be performed in patients who cannot achieve an adequate treadmill exercise threshold. Recent data suggest that cardiac computed tomography (CT) may also be used to rule out ACS in patients and allow for earlier discharge from the hospital.

7.4.4   Cardiac Catheterization

Cardiac catheterization is an invasive procedure that defines regional and global left ventricular function, valvular function, and coronary artery anatomy. The procedure is routinely performed 1–2 days after hospital admission in patients treated with an "initial invasive strategy", which is directed toward immediate coronary revascularization. Patients considered for this approach should be at higher risk. Alternatively, the "initial conservative strategy" involves reserving cardiac catheterization for patients with recurrent angina on aggressive medical therapy or for those with ischemic stress testing results. Both initial invasive and initial conservative strategies have been shown to be equivalent under various scenarios. Specific recommendations for the choice of initial strategy in managing UA/NSTEMI are listed in Table 7.2. Clinical pathways for each endorsed by recent guidelines are summarized in Figure 7.2 (Initial Invasive Strategy) and Figure 7.3 (Initial Conservative Strategy).

TAKE HOME POINT #3

Patients can undergo an initial invasive or initial conservative strategy based on the presence of key clinical characteristics and preference.

7.5   TREATMENT

Optimal management of ACS involves immediate relief of ischemia and prevention of serious adverse outcomes. These goals may be achieved by an approach that includes *anti-ischemic therapy*, *anti-thrombotic therapy*, *ongoing risk stratification*, and use of a *definitive treatment strategy* (i.e. initial invasive strategy or initial conservative strategy).

Table 7.2   Factors Associated with Invasive versus Conservative Strategy in UA/NSTEMI.

	Patient characteristics
Invasive strategy is preferred when any of these high-risk features are present:	Recurrent angina or ischemia occurs at rest or with low-level activities while on medical therapy
	Elevated cardiac biomarkers are present, including troponin
	New EKG changes such as ST-segment depression
	Signs or symptoms of heart failure
	High-risk findings on noninvasive stress testing
	Hemodynamic instability
	High-risk ventricular arrhythmias like sustained ventricular tachycardia
	Recent PCI (within 6 months)
	Prior CABG
	High-risk GRACE or TIMI risk scores
	Reduced left ventricular systolic function of less than 40%
Conservative strategy is preferred when:	Low TIMI or GRACE risk scores
	Patient preference in the absence of high-risk features

7.5.1   General Measures

Bed rest is recommended in the presence of ongoing ischemia. When symptom free, mobility to a chair or bedside commode may be allowed. Use of *supplemental oxygen* is recommended with an arterial saturation <90%, respiratory distress, and other high-risk features for hypoxemia. *Continuous ECG monitoring* for arrhythmias allows for prompt detection and treatment of potentially fatal rhythm disorders and ongoing ischemia.

7.5.2   Anti-Ischemic Agents

Nitrates

In patients with signs and symptoms of ongoing ischemia after three sublingual nitroglycerin tablets in 10 min, intravenous nitroglycerin should be started at 10 mcg/min and increased every 3–5 min until ischemia is relieved or hemodynamically tolerated. In the absence of refractory symptoms, intravenous nitroglycerin should be converted to an oral or topical form within 24 hrs. Use of sildenafil, or other PDE-5 inhibitors, in the preceding 24–48-hr period represents a strong contraindication to the use of nitrates in any form.

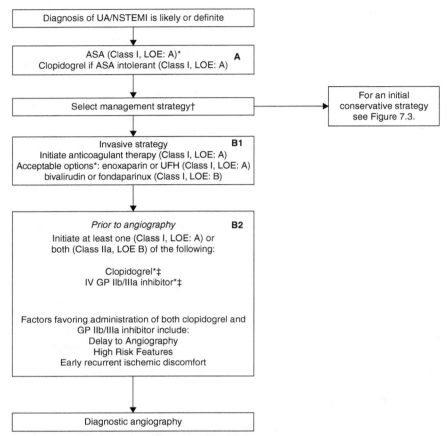

Figure 7.2 Algorithm for patients with UA/NSTEMI managed by an early invasive strategy (Source: Anderson et al. 2007. Reproduced with permission of Wolters Kluwer Health).

Morphine and other analgesics

Morphine sulfate has potent analgesic and anxiolytic effects, as well as hemodynamic effects, that are potentially beneficial in UA/NSTEMI. Morphine sulfate (1–5 mg IV) is reasonable to administer in patients whose symptoms are not relieved with nitroglycerin therapy or whose symptoms recur despite adequate anti-ischemic therapy. Use of nonsteroidal anti-inflammatory drugs, both nonselective agents and cyclooxygenase-2-selective agents (except for aspirin), should be discontinued when possible.

Beta-blockers

In the absence of contraindications, oral β-blocker therapy should be initiated within the first 24 hrs after onset of ACS with a goal heart rate of 50 to 60 beats/min. In high-risk patients, β-blockers may be initially given intravenously followed by oral

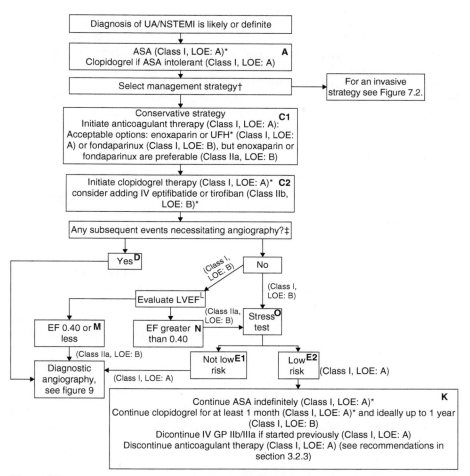

Figure 7.3   Algorithm for patients with UA/NSTEMI managed by early conservative strategy (Source: Anderson et al. 2007. Reproduced with permission of Wolters Kluwer Health).

delivery. Contraindications to β-blockade include severe bradycardia (heart rate <50 beats/min), marked first degree or any second- or third-degree atrioventricular conduction block, persistent hypotension, pulmonary edema, history of broncho-spasm, evidence of a low-output state, and cardiogenic shock.

Other agents

Calcium channel blockers are recommended for patients with persistent or recurrent symptoms after treatment with full-dose nitrates and β-blockers, contraindications or intolerances to β-blockade, or Prinzmetal's variant angina. Angiotensin-converting enzyme (ACE) inhibitors or angiotensin II receptor blockers (ARBs) are recommended to patients with pulmonary congestion or reduced LV systolic function

(EF $\leq$40%) within the first 24 hrs in the absence of hypotension or other known contraindications. Selective aldosterone receptor blockers, i.e. eplerenone, are indicated in patients with MI complicated by LV dysfunction and either CHF or diabetes mellitus in the absence of severe renal dysfunction or hyperkalemia. A recently-approved anti-ischemic agent, ranolazine, exerts its effects without reducing heart rate or blood pressure and may be used for refractory angina. Finally, the intra-aortic blood pump (IABP) has been used in MI patients with refractory angina and hemodynamic instability during ACS.

Anti-thrombotic agents

Anti-thrombotic therapy is essential during ACS to modify the disease process and prevent subsequent cardiac events. A combination of antiplatelet therapy (aspirin plus an additional agent) and anticoagulant therapy is considered most efficacious, but should be balanced against bleeding risks.

Antiplatelet therapy. Aspirin is recommended in doses ranging from 75 to 325 mg daily in the management of all patients with ACS and should be continued indefinitely, unless side-effects are present. Thienopyridines, such as ticlopidine and clopidogrel, and now prasugrel, inhibit adenosine diphosphate (ADP)-induced platelet activation and aggregation. Use of ticlopidine has been superseded by clopidogrel because of the faster onset of action and fewer side effects (gastrointestinal problems, neutropenia, and thrombotic thrombocytopenia purpura). An oral loading dose (300–600 mg) of clopidogrel is typically used to achieve rapid platelet inhibition, followed by a maintenance dose of 75 mg daily for at least 9 months after an ACS, in addition to aspirin therapy. Prasugrel, an irreversible P_2Y_{12} ADP receptor antagonist, can achieve higher levels of platelet inhibition than clopidogrel, and is correspondingly shown to reduce rates of major cardiovascular events. An oral loading dose of 60 mg is used with a maintenance dose of 10 mg daily. However, the efficacy of prasugrel is offset by a higher risk of bleeding than clopidogrel, with patients aged $\geq$75 yrs, those weighing <60 kg and those with a history of stroke or transient ischemic attack at the greatest risk. Glycoprotein IIb/IIIa inhibitors offer an intravenous alternative to oral agents like the thienopyridines and can be discontinued more quickly. Abciximab is approved for patients with UA/NSTEMI in whom an initial invasive strategy with PCI is planned within 12 hrs. When abciximab is used, platelet counts should be monitored due to its association with thrombocytopenia. Otherwise, eptifibatide or tirofiban are the preferred choice and should be administered, along with aspirin and heparin, to patients with continuing ischemia or high-risk features (i.e. positive troponin, diabetes, ST-segment changes, recurrent angina, previous aspirin use, or TIMI risk of $\geq$4).

Anticoagulant agents

Current guidelines recommend one of four anticoagulant agents to be administered to ACS patients as soon as possible after presentation: unfractionated heparin (UFH); low-molecular-weight heparin (LMWH); direct thrombin inhibitors; and factor Xa inhibitors.

Unfractionated heparin. UFH is a glycosaminoglycan with multiple different polysaccharide chain lengths that acts to inhibit thrombin and factor Xa. Weight-adjusted dosing of UFH should be used (60 U/kg bolus (maximum 4,000 U), and 12 U/kg/hr infusion (maximum 1,000 U/hr)) with frequent monitoring of activated partial thromboplastin time (aPTT) every 6 hrs initially until titration achieves a goal of 1.5–2.5x control. UFH is typically continued at least 48 hrs after presentation.

Low-molecular-weight heparin. LMWH (enoxaparin, dalteparin, nadroparin) is obtained through the depolymerization of the polysaccharide chains of heparin. These agents are able to inactivate both thrombin and factor Xa, therefore inhibiting both the action and generation of thrombin. Key advantages over UFH include less thrombocytopenia, greater bioavailability, less binding to plasma proteins, ease of subcutaneous administration, and stability of anticoagulant effects making laboratory monitoring unnecessary. Weight-adjusted dosing of LMWH is recommended with enoxaparin (1 mg/kg SQ every 12 hrs) or dalteparin (120 IU/kg SC every 12 hrs).

Direct thrombin inhibitors. DTIs bind reversibly to thrombin, inhibit clot-bound thrombin, and do not cause thrombocytopenia. Bivalirudin is the most commonly-used agent and may be used for treatment of ACS patients selected for an initial invasive strategy. Other direct thrombin inhibitors, e.g. lepirudin (recombinant hirudin) and argatroban, are typically recommended for patients with heparin-induced thrombocytopenia who are not candidates for bivalirudin. Oral direct thrombin inhibitors, such as rivaroxaban, have been studied as secondary prevention therapies after ACS but are not yet FDA approved for this indication.

Factor Xa inhibitors. These agents act more upstream in the coagulation cascade to prevent multiplier effects and thereby reduce thrombin generation. *Fondaparinux* is a synthetic pentasaccharide (2.5 mg SQ daily) that is the most commonly-used indirect factor Xa inhibitor, and is recommended as treatment for ACS patients who will be managed by either a conservative strategy or an initial invasive strategy, unless CABG is planned within 24 hrs.

Other agents. Lipid-lowering therapy with statins is recommended to be initiated in all patients with UA/NSTEMI, regardless of baseline LDL levels. Expert groups have suggested titration to a dose necessary to obtain LDL-C levels of <70 mg/dL.

TAKE HOME POINT #4

High-risk ACS patients should receive both antiplatelet and anticoagulant therapy acutely unless their bleeding risks are excessive.

7.6 HOSPITAL DISCHARGE AND POST-HOSPITAL CARE

Following the initial care of ACS patients with no complications, most can be discharged safely either the day after using an initial invasive strategy, or soon after noninvasive stress testing suggests a low-risk state when an initial conservative strategy is utilized.

The ultimate goals of hospitalization include evaluating for risk factor modification and instituting long-term therapies that will reduce the risk of recurrent coronary events. Patients should also be prepared for how to resume usual activities and medical follow-up care should be established.

Most patients are discharged on an anti-ischemic regimen similar to the inpatient regimen, with the following being strong recommendations: aspirin (75–325 mg daily); clopidogrel (75 mg daily for 9 months); beta-blocker; ACE-inhibitor (for those with CHF, LVEF <40%, hypertension, or diabetes); lipid lowering agent (statin) and diet therapy; and sublingual nitroglycerin. Secondary prevention with the control of known cardiac risk factors should also be implored, including tight glycemic control (HbA1c <7%) in diabetic patients, hypertensive control (goal blood pressure <130/85 mmHg), smoking cessation, initiation of physical activity, and maintenance of optimal weight.

After discharge, patients should be seen in the outpatient setting within one to two weeks (higher-risk patients) or within two to six weeks (lower-risk and revascularized patients) to assess recovery and reinforce secondary preventative measures. Referral to cardiac rehabilitation services should be strongly considered in eligible patients.

TAKE HOME POINT #5

Most patients should be discharged on a regimen that includes aspirin, beta-blocker, thienopyridine, and statin with additional agents added based on the clinical scenario.

KEY REFERENCES

American Heart Association. Heart disease and stroke statistics – 2008 update. American Heart Association.

ANDERSON JL, ADAMS CD, ANTMAN EM, et al. ACC/AHA 2007 guidelines for the management of patients with unstable angina/non ST-elevation myocardial infarction: a report of the American College of Cardiology/American Heart Association Task Force on Practice Guidelines. Circulation 2007;116: e148–304.

FUSTER V, BADIMON JJ, CHESEBRO JH. The pathogenesis of coronary artery disease and the acute coronary syndromes. N Engl J Med 1992;326:242–250,310–318.

LIBBY P, THEROUX P. Pathophysiology of coronary artery disease. Circulation 2005;111:3481–3488.

Chapter 8

Acute ST Elevation Myocardial Infarction

Michael C. Reed and Brahmajee K. Nallamothu

8.1 INTRODUCTION

Acute coronary syndrome is due to an insufficient supply of myocardial oxygen for the demand placed on the heart. There are three types of acute coronary syndrome (ACS): unstable angina; myocardial infarction without ST elevation (NSTEMI); and myocardial infarction with ST elevation (STEMI). The latter two are associated with a typical rise and fall of cardiac biomarkers such as troponin. Patients with STEMI are differentiated from the other forms by a typical pattern evident on their presenting electrocardiogram (ECG) and have a high likelihood of thrombus completely occluding a major epicardial coronary vessel. Patients with STEMI are ideally managed with emergent reperfusion therapy with either fibrinolysis or "primary" percutaneous coronary intervention to re-establish blood flow to infarcted myocardium. Substantial delays in initiating reperfusion therapy lead to worse outcomes, making the management of STEMI a medical emergency.

8.2 EPIDEMIOLOGY

Approximately 500,000 patients suffer STEMI each year in the United States. Mortality varies with the presence or absence of adverse risk factors but overall in-hospital mortality is between 8 and 10%. Mortality is affected by a number of factors including the use of timely reperfusion therapy and subsequent left ventricular systolic function (i.e., ejection fraction).

Inpatient Cardiovascular Medicine, First Edition. Edited by Brahmajee K. Nallamothu and Timir S. Baman.
© 2014 John Wiley & Sons, Inc. Published 2014 by John Wiley & Sons, Inc.

8.3 PATHOPHYSIOLOGY

Most cases of STEMI result from sudden intra-coronary plaque disruption leading to thrombosis with complete occlusion of a coronary artery. The involved plaque may not be obstructive or even symptomatic prior to rupture. Plaques vulnerable to rupture typically contain lipid-rich cells, macrophages and other inflammatory cells beneath a thin fibrous cap. Upon disruption of the fibrous cap, the plaque contents are released into the blood stream and trigger platelet activation and aggregation, and thrombus formation. This process may result in occlusion of the involved coronary artery.

TAKE HOME POINT #1

Vulnerable plaques may not be obstructive or even symptomatic prior to rupture and coronary occlusion resulting in STEMI.

8.4 EVALUATION

8.4.1 History and Physical Examination

The history and physical examination should be detailed enough to establish the diagnosis of STEMI, but should also be concise in order to prevent unnecessary delay in reperfusion therapy (Table 8.1).

The chest discomfort associated with STEMI typically lasts more than 30 minutes, but may wax and wane if intermittent, spontaneous reperfusion occurs from endogenous fibrinolysis. It is typically substernal, but may originate in or radiate to the jaw, arm, neck, or epigastrum. A crushing pain, such as "an elephant sitting on my chest" is classic, but the discomfort may be more diffuse or milder, and confused with indigestion or heartburn. Associated symptoms may include nausea, vomiting, diaphoresis, fatigue, and dyspnea. Onset of symptoms is important: patients with pain which began >12–24 hours prior to hospital arrival that has subsequently subsided may no longer be candidates for emergent reperfusion therapy since the likelihood of substantial myocardial salvage is much less at that point.

Prior history of angina, myocardial infarction, percutaneous coronary intervention, coronary artery bypass surgery, or stress testing should be obtained. The patient should be questioned about risk factors such as hypertension, diabetes mellitus, hypercholesterolemia, family history of coronary disease, smoking, and cocaine use.

Severe tearing pain radiating to the back, especially in elderly or hypertensive patients, should raise the suspicion for aortic dissection. Other potential mimics of STEMI that should be considered include: acute pericarditis; coronary vasospasm; stress-induced cardiomyopathy (Takotsubo Syndrome); old infarction with left ventricular aneurysm formation; and early repolarization.

Because therapy for STEMI includes antiplatelet, anticoagulant, and fibrinolytic agents, risk of bleeding should be evaluated. History of gastrointestinal bleeding, peptic ulcer disease, prior stroke, transient ischemic accident, intracranial hemorrhage, head trauma, or recent surgery should be obtained.

Table 8.1   Brief Initial Evaluation for Acute STEMI.

History
    Chest pain: time of onset, type, associated symptoms
    History of MI, CVA, PCI, CABG
    Risk factors for CAD
    Bleeding risk
    Contraindications to fibrinolysis

Physical exam
    Airway, breathing, circulation
    Vital signs
    Evidence of CHF (JVD, rales, peripheral edema, cool extremities)
    Focal neurologic deficits

Electrocardiogram
    ST elevation ≥0.1 mV in 2 contiguous leads
    Anterior (V1–V4)
    Lateral (V5–V6, I, aVL)
    Inferior (II, III, aVL)
    Right ventricular (V1, right-sided V4)
    True posterior (V7–V8, ST depression V1–V3)
    New or presumed new LBBB (obtain old ECG)
    Arrythmia

Laboratory analysis
    Troponin, CK, CKMB
    CBC with platelets
    PT, PTT
    Electrolytes
    Creatinine
    Glucose
    Lipid panel
    B-hcg if women of child-bearing age
    Urine tox if suspect cocaine

Decide on strategy for reperfusion

Physical examination should focus on patient stability (ABC: Airway, Breathing, Circulation), vital signs, jugular venous pressure elevation, murmers, rubs, gallops, rales, peripheral pulses, cool or edematous extremities, and focal neurologic defects.

8.4.2 Electrocardiogram

A 12-lead electrocardiogram (ECG) should be performed immediately in patients suspected of having an ACS because it helps determine the presence of STEMI and candidacy for reperfusion therapy. Patients with ST segment elevation of greater than

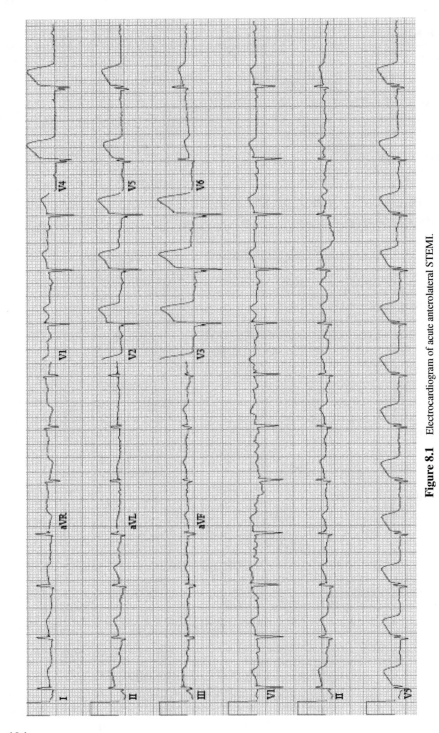

Figure 8.1   Electrocardiogram of acute anterolateral STEMI.

0.1 mV in at least two consecutive leads or a new or presumed new left bundle branch block (LBBB) are candidates for reperfusion therapy (Figure 8.1). It is important to note that within the first few minutes after symptom onset, the first ECG may not show ST segment elevation, but will show hyperacute (peaked) T waves. A repeat ECG is an invaluable tool in this setting. In patients with an inferior STEMI (Figure 8.2), a right sided ECG should be obtained to screen for right ventricular involvement, indicated by ST elevation in lead V4 on the right sided ECG. An ECG with deep ST depressions in V1–V4 accompanied by upright T waves and tall R waves in V1 and V2 may represent a true posterior infarction. In this situation, an echocardiogram or an ECG using posterior leads V7 and V8 may be helpful.

TAKE HOME POINT #2

Patients with a myocardial infarction and 0.1 mV of ST elevation in contiguous leads or new LBBB are candidates for reperfusion therapy.

There are several other conditions which can cause ST elevation which must be distinguished from acute STEMI prior to implementation of reperfusion therapy (Table 8.2). Comparison to an old ECG is essential in this setting.

8.4.3 Laboratory Evaluation

Initial laboratory evaluation should include cardiac biomarkers (troponin, CK-MB, CK), CBC, PT, PTT, creatinine, electrolytes, glucose, and lipid panel. However, reperfusion therapy should not be delayed while awaiting the results of lab studies since it may take several hours for cardiac biomarkers to be elevated in the blood.

TAKE HOME POINT #3

Cardiac biomarkers may not be elevated initially in patients who present early in the course of a STEMI.

8.4.4 Other Diagnostic Studies

Chest radiography is indicated in all patients with STEMI, but should not delay reperfusion therapy. If, based on the clinical evaluation, aortic dissection becomes suspected a trans-esophageal echocardiogram or computed tomography (CT) scan should be obtained urgently prior to anticoagulation or reperfusion therapy. A surface echocardiogram may be useful in some settings if the diagnosis of STEMI is uncertain or to exclude mechanical complications (see Section 8.6 below).

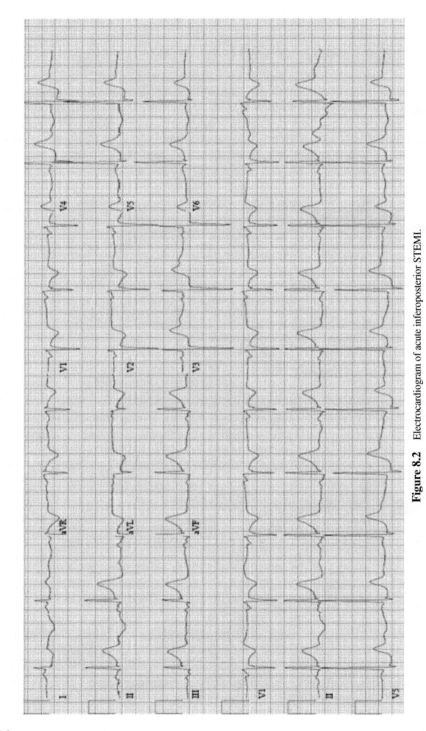

Figure 8.2 Electrocardiogram of acute inferoposterior STEMI.

Table 8.2   Differential Diagnosis of ST-Elevation on Clinical History and Electrocardiogram.

Cause	Clues
Acute STEMI	Reciprocal changes, clinical history
Stress-induced cardiomyopathy (Takotsubo Syndrome)	Emotional stress, apical ballooning on echocardiogram or ventriculogram
Aortic dissection	Hypertension, tearing pain radiating to the back
Ventricular aneurism	Q-waves, absence of acute chest discomfort
Early repolarization	Most marked in V4, often with notched J point
Left ventricular hypertrophy	Concave
Left bundle branch block or ventricular paced rhythm	Discordant ST segment changes <5 mm from QRS direction
Acute pericarditis	Diffuse ST elevation and PR depression
Hyperkalemia	Tall, peaked T waves, loss of P wave amplitude, widened QRS
Pulmonary embolus	Sinus tachycardia, S1Q3T3, right bundle branch block
Brugada syndrome	rSR' in V1 and V2 with down-sloping ST elevation

8.5 TREATMENT

Treatment for STEMI can be divided into initial therapy, reperfusion therapy, antiplatelet and anticoagulant therapy, and post-reperfusion therapy (Table 8.3).

Table 8.3   Inpatient Management of STEIM.

Initial management
O2, IV access, cardiac monitor
Aspirin 325 mg chewable PO or 300 mg PR
Morphine IV PRN
NTG SL PRN

Reperfusion therapy
PCI vs. lytics (see Figure 8.3)

Antiplatelet therapy
Aspirin
   325 mg chewable PO or 300 mg PR initially, then 81 mg PO daily indefinitely
Theinopyridine
   Clopidogrel 300 mg PO initially, then 75 mg PO daily for 12 months
   Prasugrel 60 mg PO initially, then 10 mg PO daily for 12 months
     Caution if prior TIA or stroke, age >75 years, or weight <60 kg

(continued)

Table 8.3   Continued.

Initial management

Glycoprotein IIb/IIIa Inhibitor in the setting of PCI
   Abciximab
   Eptifibitide
   Tirofiban

Anticoagulant therapy
If primary PCI, discontinue therapy after PCI
If fibrinolysis performed or no reperfusion therapy given, continue therapy until hospital
  discharge
Agents
   Unfractionated heparin
   Bivalirudin
   Low molecular weight heparin (if age is <75 years and renal function is not impaired)
   Fondaparinux (if renal function is not impaired)

Post-reperfusion inpatient management
General
   Admit to ICU and monitor for complications
   Ambulate in 12–24 hours
   Check echocardiogram to evaluate systolic function
Beta-blocker
   Within 24 hours and indefinitely in the absence of heart failure, low cardiac output,
     atrioventricular block, active wheezing, or increased risk for cardiogenic shock (age >70,
     SBP <120 mmHg, HR >110 bpm or <60 bpm, time since symptom onset >12–hours)
   Patients initially not candidates should be re-evaluated prior to discharge
ACE-inhibitor (or angiotensin receptor blocker if intolerant)
   Within 24 hours and indefinitely if not hypotensive. Most benefit is in patients with
     impaired left ventricular systolic function or an anterior STEMI.
HMG-CoA reductase inhibitor (i.e. statins)
   High dose therapy initially and later titrated based on lipid panel and drug tolerance.
Aldosterone-blocker (i.e., spironolactone)
   If EF <0.40 and either symptomatic CHF or diabetes and without renal failure of
     hyperkalemia.
Pain control
   Morphine, nitroglycerine if ongoing ischemia
   Avoid nonsteroidal anti-inflammatory agents

Post-discharge follow-up management
Cardiac rehabilitation
   Ultimate goal of 30 minutes exercise 7 days per week
Risk factor modification
   Smoking cessation
   Goal BP <140/90, <130/80 if diabetes or chronic kidney disease
   Goal LDL substantially <100, consider <70 mg/dL
   Goal HbA1c <7%

8.5.1   Initial Therapy

Initial therapy should include applying oxygen, obtaining IV access, connecting the patient to continuous cardiac monitor, and stabilizing of the airway, breathing, and circulation. Antiplatelet therapy with a chewable aspirin 162–325 mg should be given promptly. In the absence of hypotension, a right ventricular infarction, or the use of a PDE5 inhibitor (e.g., sildenafil) in the last 24 hours, sublingual or intravenous nitroglycerine may be given to help relieve chest discomfort. Morphine sulfate IV is the analgesic of choice for relief of chest pain in STEMI.

8.5.2   Reperfusion Therapy

All acute STEMI patients who present within 12 hours after the onset of symptoms should undergo a rapid evaluation for reperfusion therapy with either primary PCI or fibrinolysis (Figure 8.3). Patients who present more than 12 hours after the onset of symptoms are less likely to benefit from reperfusion therapy, but may still be candidates for revascularization based on clinical factors such as the presence of ongoing chest discomfort (particularly for PCI). Each medical community should have a system in place for pre-hospital identification and activation and for inter-hospital transfer protocols to route patients to the hospitals best able to care for them.

Two types of hospital systems exist: PCI-capable hospitals and non-PCI-capable hospitals. Primary PCI is preferred if the medical-contact-to-balloon time at a skilled

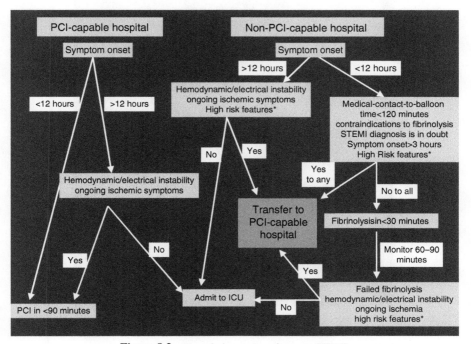

Figure 8.3   Reperfusion strategy for acute STEMI.

A

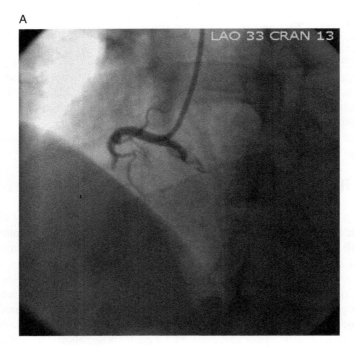

B

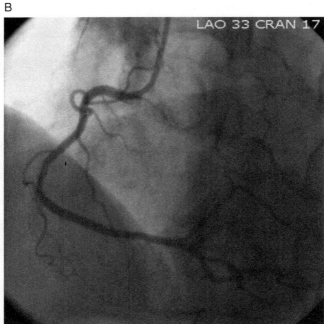

Figure 8.4   Coronary angiography of a right coronary artery in a patient with an acute inferior STEMI **A** before and **B** after PCI.

lab is <90 minutes (Figure 8.4). Patients who arrive at a hospital without PCI capability should be transferred to a PCI-capable facility if the initial medical-contact-to-balloon-time will still be less than 120 minutes. Additional reasons to consider transfer for a patient to a PCI-cabable center include: contra-indications to fibrinolysis, an uncertain diagnosis of STEMI, late presentation (e.g. >3 to 6 hours after the onset of symptoms), and high-risk features (e.g. hemodynamic instability or ≥2 mm ST-elevation in 2 anterior leads).

Fibrinolysis within 30 minutes of arrival is a reasonable alternative if there are no contra-indications to fibrinolytic agents and if there is an expected delay in the time to PCI (defined as medical-contact-to-balloon time at a skilled lab is >120 minutes) – particularly in patients presenting early (<3 hours after symptom onset) and without high-risk features. Fibrin-specific agents, such as tissue plasminogen activator (t-PA) and reteplase, have shown superiority in randomized clinical trials.

Failure to restore myocardial perfusion after fibrinolytic therapy is defined as ST-elevation less than 50% resolved 90 minutes after drug initiation in the lead showing the worst initial ST-elevation. Failed myocardial perfusion should prompt transfer to a PCI-capable facility for rescue PCI (Table 8.4). Other scenarios which should also prompt transfer to a PCI-capable facility include: (1) hemodynamic or electrical instability; (2) ongoing ischemic symptoms; or (3) high-risk features.

Coronary artery bypass grafting (CABG) is rarely used in the setting of failed fibrinolysis or PCI, although it might be considered in patients with left main or 3 vessel coronary artery disease.

Table 8.4   Reasons to Transfer a Patient Post-Fibrinolysis to a PCI-Capable Facility.

Failed fibrinolysis
  ST-elevation less than 50% resolved 90 minutes after the initiation of a thrombolytic agent in the lead showing the worst initial ST-elevation
Hemodynamic or electrical instability
Ongoing ischemic symptoms
High-risk features
  ≥2 mm ST elevation in 2 anterior leads
  ≥1 mm ST elevation in the inferior leads with one of the following:
    SBP <100 mmHg
    HR >100 bpm
    Killip class II to IV CHF
    2 mm ST depression in anterior leads
    1 mm ST elevation in right-sided V4R

TAKE HOME POINT #4

In acute STEMI less than 12 hours after the onset of symptoms, reperfusion therapy with PCI should be administered with a door-to-balloon-time of less than 90 minutes. When PCI is not possible, reperfusion therapy with fibrinolysis should occur with a door-to-needle time of less than 30 minutes.

8.5.3 AntiPlatelet Therapy

An initial dose of 162–325 mg chewable aspirin should be administered on arrival. In the event of severe vomiting, a 300 mg suppository can be administered. A dose of 81 mg aspirin should be continued indefinitely in all patients with STEMI.

P2Y12 inhibitors (i.e. clopidogrel, prasugrel, or ticagrelor) should be given to all patients with STEMI regardless of the type of reperfusion therapy they receive. Clopidogrel is the most widely-used of these agents and strong evidence supports its use in patients treated with both fibrinolytic therapy and primary PCI. Prasugrel has been more recently introduced and its advantages include greater platelet inhibition and less variability across patients. However, prasugrel is associated with a higher risk of bleeding and is contraindicated in the following patients: history of TIA or stroke, weight <60 kg, or age >75 years. A new agent, ticagrelor, has now been approved for use in the United States. As opposed to clopidogrel and prasugrel, ticagrelor is given twice a day. If patients receive a bare metal or drug-eluting stent, dual antiplatelet therapy with both aspirin and a P2Y12 inhibitor should be continued for 12 months. Continuation of dual antiplatelet therapy is crucial to help prevent stent thrombosis, a devastating complication with a high mortality. If patients do not receive a stent, clopidogrel should be used and continued for at least 14 days and ideally for 12 months. P2Y12 inhibitors should be held for 5–7 days for patients who require bypass surgery, although platelet function testing may be used to individualize this decision.

> **TAKE HOME POINT #5**
>
> Continuation of dual antiplatelet therapy with aspirin and a P2Y12 inhibitor is crucial to help prevent stent thrombosis, a devastating complication with a high mortality. It should even be used in patients who receive fibrinolytic therapy or no reperfusion therapy.

Glycoprotein (GP) IIb/IIIa inhibitors (abciximab, eptifibitide, tirofiban) may be used in STEMI patients who receive PCI. It is important to be conscious of bleeding in patients who have received a GP IIb/IIIa inhibitor since these drugs have no reversal agent and rarely cause severe thrombocytopenia.

8.5.4 AntiCoagulant Therapy

In patients who receive PCI, unfractionated heparin is the most commonly used anticoagulant, but bivalirudin may be used as an alternative – particularly in patients with heparin-induced thrombocytopenia or with increased risk of bleeding. Less commonly, low-molecular weight heparin or fondaparinux may be used to support a PCI. Anticoagulants are typically stopped after PCI to minimize the risk of bleeding.

In patients who receive fibrinolysis or who do not receive reperfusion therapy, anticoagulants should be continued for a minimum of 48 hours and preferably for the duration of the hospitalization. Due to the risk of heparin-induced thrombocytopenia with prolonged infusion of unfractionated heparin, the preferred anticoagulants after fibrinolysis are low-molecular weight heparin (if the patient age is <75 years and renal function is not impaired) or fodaparinux (if renal function is not impaired).

Long-term anticoagulation with warfarin may be considered in patients who have a documented left ventricular thrombus or atrial fibrillation, provided that the benefit outweighs the risk of bleeding.

8.5.5 Post-Reperfusion Inpatient Care

Patients should be admitted to an intensive care unit and monitored for re-infarction or mechanical complications. Left ventricular systolic function should be assessed. Patients should be encouraged to ambulate after 24 hours if tolerated. Pain should be managed with morphine and nitroglycerin, but NSAIDs should be avoided.

Oral beta-blockade should be administered within 24 hours and continued indefinitely in the absence of heart failure, low cardiac output, atrioventricular block, active wheezing, or increased risk for cardiogenic shock (age >70, SBP <120 mmHg, HR >110 bpm or <60 bpm, time since symptom onset >12 hrs).

In the absence of hypotension, an ACE-inhibitor (or an angiotensin receptor blocker if intolerant to an ACE-inhibitor) should be administered within the first 24 hours – particularly in patients with impaired left ventricular systolic function or an anterior STEMI.

The routine use of intravenous beta-blockers or ACE-inhibitors does not improve outcomes and may be potentially harmful.

Intensive statin therapy, e.g. atorvastatin 80 mg per day, should be administered regardless of the cholesterol panel.

An aldosterone blocker, such as aldactone, should be considered in patients who have a left ventricular ejection fraction <0.40, who have either symptomatic heart failure or diabetes, and who are without renal failure or hyperkalemia. Careful measurements of renal function and potassium are required in these patients.

8.5.6 Outpatient Management/Secondary Prevention

Close follow-up with either the patient's cardiologist or their primary care provider should occur. Patients should be referred to cardiac rehabilitation with the ultimate goal of achieving 30 minutes of physical activity per day, 7 days per week. Patient willingness to quit smoking should be assessed, and they should be advised to quit and provided with medical and social resources to succeed in smoking-cessation. Goal LDL is <100 mg/dL and <70 mg/dL, although the addition of other cholesterol-reducing agents beyond statins has not been shown to improve mortality. Goal blood pressure is <140/90 mmHg and <130/80 mmHg in patients with diabetes or chronic kidney disease.

8.6 COMPLICATIONS

Complications can occur after STEMI (Table 8.5) and are most often responsible for early mortality. Complications can be divided into the following categories: hemodynamic, mechanical, arrhythmias, recurrent chest pain, and other.

Common hemodynamic complications include cardiogenic shock from left ventricular systolic dysfunction or right ventricular infarction. In the setting of hypotension or pulmonary congestion, all patients should have an urgent echocardiogram to evaluate left and right ventricular function and to rule out a mechanical complication. Maintaining a high suspicion for mechanical complications when something goes wrong with a patient is critical to ensuring prompt diagnosis and treatment, since many require urgent surgical intervention.

The time course for mechanical complications is bimodal: within the first 24 hours and again between 3–5 days. Immediately life-threatening mechanical complications include papillary muscle rupture leading to acute mitral regurgitation (1% incidence), ventricular septal rupture (1–3% incidence), and left ventricular free wall rupture 0.8–6.2% incidence) (Figure 8.5, Figure 8.6, and Figure 8.7). These complications require immediate surgical management. Another mechanical complication is left ventricular aneurism – particularly following an anteroapical myocardial infarction. Left ventricular mural thrombus may form within an aneurism and require a short period of anticoagulation with warfarin.

Table 8.5   Complications after Acute STEMI.

Hemodynamic
   Low output state
   Pulmonary edema
   RV infarction
Mechanical
   Papillary muscle rupture
   Ventricular septal rupture
   LV free wall rupture
   LV aneurism
Arrythmia
   Ventricular fibrillation, ventricular tachycardia
   Supraventricular
   Atrio-ventricular block
Chest pain
   Post-infarct pericarditis
   Recurrent ischemia or infarction
Other
   Stroke
   Bleeding
   DVT/PE

A

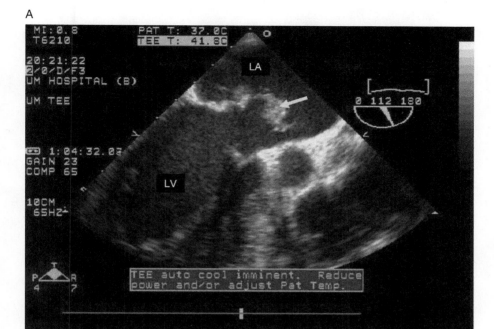

B

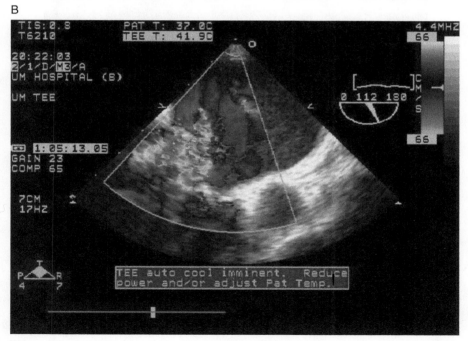

Figure 8.5   **A** Echocardiogram of papillary muscle rupture (arrow) with **B** severe mitral regurgitation. (See Color plate 8.1).

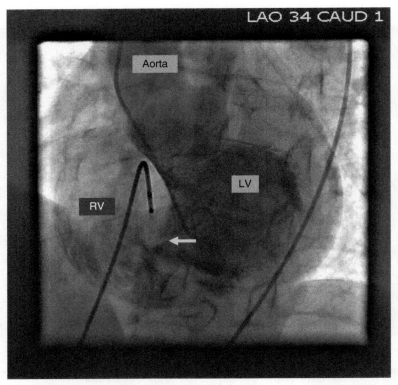

Figure 8.6   Left ventriculogram showing a ventricular septal rupture (arrow) 3 days after an anterior STEMI. Note the contrast flow from the left to the right ventricle.

Atrial and ventricular arrhythmias can occur following STEMI. Advanced atrioventricular block may occur following an inferior STEMI or an anterior STEMI and may require a temporary and occasionally permanent pacemaker. Ventricular fibrillation and unstable ventricular tachycardia, and atrial tachyarrhythmias should be managed according to Advanced Cardiac Life Support protocols, including the use of lidocaine or amiodarone as needed. It is critical to distinguish ventricular tachycardia from accelerated idioventricular rhythm – a wide complex ventricular rhythm with a rate typically 90–110 bpm which occurs commonly in the setting of myocardial reperfusion – since the latter is benign. Long-term considerations for implantable cardioverter defibrillators (ICDs) should be made in consultation with a cardiologist, particularly in patients with ventricular tachycardia or severely impaired left ventricular systolic function. Early implantation of ICDs for primary prevention after STEMI has not been shown to improve mortality in high-risk subgroups.

Chest pain after a myocardial infarction may be due to recurrent ischemia or infarction and referral for cardiac catheterization should be considered – particularly in the setting of pain refractory to medical therapy or dynamic ECG changes. Acute pericarditis can occur early or late after infarcts – particularly after a large anterior

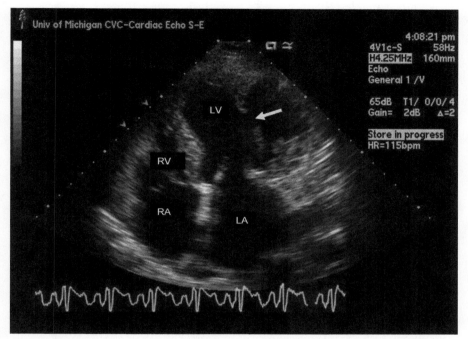

Figure 8.7   Echocardiogram of free left ventricular rupture (arrow) following a posterolateral STEMI.

STEMI – and may be associated with a pericardial friction rub. Anticoagulation should be used with caution in the setting of acute infarct pericarditis as it may lead to development of a hemorrhagic pericardial effusion and pericardial tamponade. Symptomatic patients may benefit from treatment with high-dose aspirin or colchicine, with NSAIDs and corticosteroids used cautiously. A late presentation of pericarditis weeks after STEMI may be due to postcardiac injury (Dressler's) syndrome, an immune-mediated reaction that is not isolated to STEMI but can occur after any substantial cardiac injury.

Other complications include post-fibrinolytic or post-cardiac catheterization bleeding, venous thromboembolism and stroke. Abrupt changes in metal status or focal neurologic changes should prompt emergent evaluation for stroke or intracranial hemorrhage, particularly after administration of fibrinolytic agents.

KEY REFERENCES

ANTMAN EM, ANBE DT, ARMSTRONG PW, BATES EB, et al. 2004. ACC/AHA guidelines for the management of patients with ST-elevation myocardial infarction. Available at: www.acc.org/ qualityandscience/clinical/statements.htm.

ANTMAN EM, HAND M, ARMSTRONG PW, BATES EB, et al. Focused update: ACC/AHA 2004 guidelines for the management of patients with ST-elevation myocardial infarction. J Am Coll Cardiol 2008;51:210–217.

KUSHNER FG, HAND M, SMITH SC, KING SB, et al. Focused updates: ACC/AHA guidelines for the management of patients with ST-elevation myocardial infarction (updating the 2004 guideline and 2007 focused update); and ACC/AHA/SCAI guidelines of percutaneous coronary intervention (updating the 2005 guideline and 2007 focused update): A Report of the American College of Cardiology Foundation/ American Heart Association Task Force on Practice Guidelines. J Am Coll Cardiol 2009; 54:2205–2241.

STEG PG, GOLDBERG RJ, GORE JM, FOX KA, et al. Baseline characteristics, management practices, and in-hospital outcomes of patients hospitalized with acute coronary syndromes in the Global Registry of Acute Coronary Events (GRACE). Am J Cardiol 2002;90:358–363.

WANG K, ASINGER RW, MARRIOTT HJ. ST-segment elevation in conditions other than acute myocardial infarction. N Engl J Med 2003;349:2128–2135.

Chapter 9

Chronic Coronary Artery Disease

Amir B. Rabbani and P. Michael Grossman

9.1 INTRODUCTION

Coronary artery disease (CAD) remains the single leading cause of mortality world-wide. The American Heart Association estimates over 10 million Americans suffer from angina, the most common symptom associated with chronic CAD, and there are 500,000 new cases of angina per year. A dramatic reduction in mortality due to CAD in recent years can be attributed to aggressive risk factor modification as well as secondary treatment strategies in chronic CAD.

Chronic CAD may be asymptomatic or associated with angina pectoris (or angina "equivalents"). Angina pectoris from chronic CAD is defined as symptoms that occur predictably with activity due to chronic narrowing of the coronary arteries leading to ischemia. In contrast, acute coronary syndromes (which are addressed elsewhere) arise from unstable plaque rupture and thrombus formation, and may be associated with rest angina, new onset angina, or accelerated angina. While most chronic CAD can be managed in the outpatient setting, the high frequency of this comorbidity in hospitalized patients makes it important for hospitalists to understand and treat.

9.2 PATHOPHYSIOLOGY

The primary mechanism for chronic CAD is atherosclerosis, which begins early in adulthood. Endothelial dysfunction, accumulation of lipid-laden smooth muscle cells, inflammation of the vessel wall, foam cell formation, and connective tissue

Inpatient Cardiovascular Medicine, First Edition. Edited by Brahmajee K. Nallamothu and Timir S. Baman.

deposition all contribute to its development. Endothelial dysfunction is believed to be an important early step accelerated by physical (e.g. branch-points in the coronary vessels, hypertension) and chemical (e.g. diabetes, smoking) factors. Early in the atherosclerosis progresses, plaque deposits do not encroach on the lumen of the artery (Glagov effect) as the vessel grows to accommodate it. In the absence of acute coronary syndromes, it is only during the late phase of atherosclerosis that extensive plaque deposition (usually >70% of vessel lumen diameter) is present and symptoms of angina develop. The extent of angina is not always consistent with the extent of plaque deposition, particularly in patients with single-vessel disease.

TAKE HOME POINT #1

Extent of CAD does not always correlate with extent of angina symptoms.

9.3 RISK FACTOR ASSESSMENT

Risk factors for the development of coronary artery disease can be broken down to modifiable and nonmodifiable risk factors. Modifiable risk factors include dyslipidemias (elevated LDL, low HDL), tobacco exposure, hypertension, and diabetes mellitus. Nonmodifiable risk factors include advanced age, male gender, and family history. Occasionally, patients with severe aortic stenosis or hypertrophic cardiomyopathy may experience angina-like pain in the absence of identifiable epicardial coronary disease. The Framingham risk score incorporates age, gender, LDL-cholesterol, HDL-cholesterol, blood pressure, smoking status, and diabetes to derive an estimated risk of having an event related to CAD.

9.4 CLINICAL MANIFESTATION

The clinical history is an important tool in identifying and managing patients with chronic CAD. Anginal symptoms are frequently classified as typical or atypical. Typical angina is described as a vice-like, crushing, or heavy sensation that is associated with exertion or stress. Patients may describe discomfort rather than "pain." Symptoms may radiate to the jaw, the neck, or the arm (typically the ulnar aspect of the left arm). Typical angina usually begins gradually and usually reaches its maximum intensity over a period of minutes before subsiding. It is unusual for angina to reach maximum intensity over seconds. Chest discomfort while walking in the cold, uphill or after a meal also is suggestive of angina. Preconditioning may allow some patients who develop angina with exertion to continue exertion after a rest period without symptoms. The Canadian Cardiovascular Society (CCS) classification of effort angina provides a grading system (Table 9.1).

TAKE HOME POINT #2

The clinical history is an important tool in identifying patients with chronic CAD.

Table 9.1   Canadian Cardiovascular Society (CCS) Classification of Severity of Angina.

Class I	No angina with regular daily activity
	Angina after strenuous exertion
Class II	Angina limits early physical activity, angina comes on after one flight of stairs
	Meals or cold may make angina worse
Class III	Unable to perform daily activities due to pain
Class IV	All physical activity causes angina or angina at rest

Table 9.2   Newer Biomarkers for Diagnosis and Prognosis for Coronary Artery Disease.

Lipoprotein(a)	Modified form of LDL which apolipoprotein(a) covalently bound to apolipoprotein B
	Several studies have associated Lp(a) and CVD (Reykjavik Study)
Apolipoprotein B	Primary apolipoprotein responsible for carrying LDL to tissue
	Reflects number of LDL particles rather than LDL content
Apolipoprotein A-1	Major protein component of HDL
	Reflects HDL particle number rather than HDL content
High-sensitivity CRP	Adds to the predictive capacity of established risk factors, may even be independent risk factor
	In JUPITER trial, patients with LDL <130 and hsCRP >2 had modest but significant benefit with lipid-lowering therapy

9.5 PHYSICAL EXAMINATION

As mentioned, the clinical history plays a prominent role in identifying patients with chronic CAD, but the physical exam is often normal. Indirect findings raising suspicion for coronary disease include signs of hyperlipidemia such as: corneal arcus and xanthelasma; carotid bruits; decreased peripheral pulses; an S4 or S3; or displaced apical impulse (which would suggest LV dysfunction).

9.6 LABORATORY AND ECG ASSESSMENT

Laboratory investigation focuses on metabolic abnormalities and biomarker assessment. All patients with suspected CAD should have total cholesterol, LDL, HDL, triglycerides, estimated glomerular filtration, and fasting blood glucose checked. Newer biomarkers, such as high-sensitivity CRP, have been associated with overall poorer prognosis but there is no consensus yet for recommended testing (Table 9.2).

Resting ECG may be normal in many patients with stable CAD. The presence of an abnormal ECG raises the risk for future cardiovascular events. Nonspecific ST-T wave inversions, particularly in V1–V3, are associated with increased risk. LVH, AF, LBBB and AV block convey a poorer overall prognosis in the setting of angina.

9.7   NONINVASIVE TOOLS FOR RISK STRATIFICATION

Exercise stress testing provides diagnostic and prognostic information (see Chapter 4). One of the strongest prognostic indicators is determined by maximum exercise capacity. Transient myocardial ischemia seen on the ECG also conveys poorer prognosis (excluding leads with Q waves or aVR). The Duke treadmill score takes into account both of these objective variables and integrates the subjective presence or absence of angina symptoms to indicate the likelihood of CAD. The generated score places patients into categories of low (score >5), intermediate (score −10 to 4), and high risk (score <−11). Patients in the high-risk category often have multivessel or left main disease.

TAKE HOME POINT #3

Exercise capacity and ischemic ECG changes during exercise testing are among the strongest predictors of overall mortality.

Adjunctive imaging with myocardial perfusion imaging or echocardiography improves the sensitivity and specificity of exercise stress testing with ECG alone. Overall, high risk features of noninvasive testing (conferring >3% annual mortality) include severe LV systolic dysfunction (EF <35%) at rest, high risk treadmill score, and severe exercise-induced LV dysfunction. Large stress-induced perfusion defect on imaging (particularly anterior), stress-induced multiple perfusion defects of moderate size, and a large, fixed perfusion defect with LV dilation also predict poor prognosis. Table 9.3 reviews several of these key findings.

Table 9.3   Noninvasive Risk Stratification.

High risk	Intermediate risk	Low risk
Severe LV dysfunction (<35%), or severe dysfunction with stress	Mild-to-moderate LV dysfunction at rest (35–50% EF)	Treadmill score >5
High risk treadmill score (<−11)	Treadmill score −11 to 5.	Normal or small perfusion defect with stress
Stress-induced large perfusion defect or multiple moderate size defects	Stress-induced moderate perfusion defect	Normal stress echo wall motion with stress
Large, fixed perfusion defect with TID	Limited stress echo ischemia with wall motion only at higher dobutamine doses	
>2 segments echo wall motion abnormalities or wall motion at low cardiac workload		

9.8 EMERGING NONINVASIVE TESTS FOR RISK STRATIFICATION

Coronary calcium scoring (with electron beam or multidetector CT) has been studied in several large trials. While the calcium score provides additional prognostic information, particularly in combination with the Framingham risk score, its routine use is not recommended. At present, use of CT coronary angiography in symptomatic patients may be a reasonable alternative to evaluating intermediate risk patients (rather than traditional stress testing) or could be useful when stress test results are equivocal. Contrast-enhanced MR (CMR) stress imaging improves upon the sensitivity and specificity of MPI and stress echo with sensitivity and specificity of 91% and 81% but its use is limited to experienced centers.

9.9 MEDICAL TREATMENT OF CHRONIC STABLE CORONARY DISEASE

For hospitalists, the goals for medical management for chronic stable CAD are to reduce the risk of adverse cardiovascular events, improve mortality, and reduce anginal symptoms if present. Unless contraindicated, all patients with known CAD should be started on aspirin therapy. In aspirin-allergic patients, clopidogrel is a safe and equally effective alternative. The routine use of dual antiplatelet therapy with aspirin and clopidogrel as secondary prevention has not been shown to improve outcomes (Table 9.4), but may be appropriate for select high-risk patients.

Beta blocker therapy should be used as a first-line agent for chronic anginal symptoms, and is the only anti-anginal agent shown to reduce mortality in patients with previous myocardial infarction or LV systolic dysfunction (i.e. ejection fraction <40%). Their benefit is less certain in patients with stable CAD without myocardial infarction or LV systolic dysfunction. ACE inhibitors reduce morbidity and mortality in patients with LV systolic dysfunction or in patients with diabetes and hypertension (class I recommendation). In low-risk patients without diabetes and hypertension, ACE inhibitors have not been shown to reduce mortality (class IIa recommendation).

Table 9.4 Recommended Pharmacotherapy for Chronic Stable Angina.

Class I	Class IIa	Class IIb
Aspirin	Plavix when ASA	Low-intensity
Beta blockers	contraindicated	warfarin in
Ace inhibitors in patients with	Long acting non-	addition to aspirin
diabetes or LV dysfunction	dihydropyridine CCBs when	
SLNTG for immediate anginal	BBs contraindicated	
relief	LDL lower <100 or <70 for	
CCB or long-acting nitrates for	high-risk patients	
anginal relief when BBs are	Ace inhibitors for CAD or other	
contraindicated	vascular disease	
CCBs or LANs in combination		
with BBs		

Calcium channel blockers, long-acting nitrates and ranolazine are agents that should be used in patients with refractory symptoms. Nitrates should not be used in the setting of 5-PDE inhibitors, such as sildenafil, and a daily 12-hour "nitrate-free" period should be maintained to avoid nitrate tolerance. Ranolazine should not be used in patients with a prolonged QT or who are taking QT-prolonging medications.

LDL-lowering therapy with statins is a mainstay of treatment of chronic CAD. The goal LDL for patients with CHD is <100 mg/dl, and for high-risk individuals is <70 mg/dl. Statin therapy has been shown to increase survival, improve myocardial perfusion on nuclear studies and decrease ischemia on ambulatory ECG monitoring in patients with stable angina. Other agents that reduce LDL have not shown similar benefits and should only be considered for those intolerant of statins or unable to reach goal with statins only.

TAKE HOME POINT #4

A daily aspirin and beta blockade is indicated for all patients with stable CAD who are eligible. Statin therapy is strongly encouraged.

9.10 ROLE FOR REVASCULARIZATION FOR CHRONIC ANGINA

In addition to risk factor modification and pharmacologic therapy, coronary revascularization remains an important part of the therapeutic armamentarium available for the treatment of chronic CAD (Table 9.5). Recent evidence has demonstrated that optimal medical therapy should be the first-line treatment for chronic CAD and non-surgical disease (e.g. absence of left main disease or multivessel disease with proximal involvement of the left anterior descending coronary artery). Revascularization, either with PCI or CABG, can be safely reserved for those patients with ongoing symptoms despite a regimen of optimal medical therapy that includes antiplatelet agents, anti-ischemic agents, ACE inhibitors or angiotensin receptor blockers and statins.

TAKE HOME POINT #5

Revascularization can be safely deferred for many patients with stable CAD.

Strong indications for coronary angiography include: Canadian Cardiovascular Class III or IV angina despite optimal medical therapy; left ventricular dysfunction in the setting of angina; a high-risk, strongly positive stress test at a low cardiac workload; or life-threatening arrhythmias in the setting of SCD or VT. Coronary angiography should also be considered in patients with uncertain diagnosis of MI or ischemia after stress testing and in patients for whom it is important to know a definitive diagnosis (could be high-risk clinical features or a high-risk occupation). Selected asymptomatic patients with a positive stress test can also be treated conservatively. Patients most likely to benefit from revascularization are those who present with a positive stress test at a low cardiac workload, if ventricular arrhythmias or hypotension occur during stress, or if a large area at risk is seen on the ECG, nuclear perfusion, or echocardiogram.

Table 9.5 Guidelines for Revascularization with PCI or CABG.[i]

Class	Indication
I	CABG for LM disease
	CABG for 3 v disease, especially with LV dysfunction
	CABG for 2 v disease with proximal LAD involvement with positive stress test or LV dysfunction
	PCI for 2 v or 3 v disease with proximal LAD involvement, normal LV function, and no diabetes
	PCI for 2 v or 3 v disease without proximal LAD involvement, but with high-risk stress or large area of myocardium at risk
	PCI or CABG for patients who have not been treated successfully with medical therapy and who can undergo revascularization with acceptable risk
IIa	Repeat CABG for multiple graft stenosis
	PCI or CABG for 2 v or 3 v disease without proximal LAD but with moderate area of viable myocardium and demonstrable ischemia
	PCI or CABG for single vessel CAD with proximal LAD disease
IIb	Compared with CABG, PCI for patients with 2 v or 3 v disease with significant proximal LAD disease with diabetes or systolic dysfunction
	PCI for patients with LM disease with suitable anatomy, lower SYNTAX score and higher surgical risk[ii]
III	PCI or CABG for patients with single or 2 v disease without proximal LAD, mild symptoms unlikely due to myocardial ischemia, or who have not had an adequate trial of medical therapy
	PCI for stenosis <50–60% except for LM disease

[i] ACC/AHA/SCAI 2011 Guidelines on Percutaneous Croonary Intervention.
[ii] Serruys PW et al. NEJM 2009;360:961–972.

Coronary artery bypass grafting is generally preferred in the setting of >50% left main trunk stenosis, for three vessel disease and abnormal LV function or diabetes, and for two vessel disease with significant proximal left anterior descending artery involvement. The choice of PCI versus CABG is less clear in the setting of two or three vessel disease with significant proximal left anterior descending artery disease with normal LV function and in the absence of diabetes. PCI or CABG are also both class I indications for patients with one or two vessel CAD without significant LAD involvement but with a large area of viable myocardium at risk and high-risk criteria on noninvasive imaging. Increasingly, the choice of PCI versus CABG is being driven by anatomic considerations that can be assessed using scoring algorithms, such as the SYNTAX score.

KEY REFERENCES

SMITH SC et al. AHA/ACCF Secondary Prevention and Risk Reduction Therapy for Patients with Coronary and Other Atherosclerotic Vascular Disease: 2011 Update. Circulation 2011;124:2458–2473.
BODEN WE et al. Optimal Medical Therapy With or Without PCI for Stable Coronary Artery Disease. NEJM 2007;356:1503–1516.
LEVINE GN et al. 2011 ACCF/AHA/SCAI Guidelines for PCI. Circulation 2011;124:e574–651.

Chapter 10

Peripheral Arterial Disease

Yogendra M. Kanthi, Christos Kasapis, and Hitinder S. Gurm

10.1 INTRODUCTION

Peripheral artery disease (PAD) is broadly defined as the array of diseases that involve the medium-to-large caliber branches of the aorta, including the renal arteries and arteries to the extremities. PAD can be separated into aneurysmal and occlusive disease. It is a common manifestation of atherosclerosis and strongly correlates with major cardiovascular events, as 25% of patients with PAD can have concomitant coronary artery disease (CAD) or cerebral atherosclerosis. Additional causes include the spectrum of disorders associated with vasculitides and vasospasm. This chapter focuses on atherosclerotic PAD of the lower extremities while Chapter 11 addresses thoracic aortic diseases.

10.2 EPIDEMIOLOGY, ETIOLOGY, AND NATURAL HISTORY

Atherosclerosis is the most common cause of PAD. PAD affects more than 5 million adults in the United States, and its prevalence increases with age. The risk factors associated with PAD include cigarette smoking, diabetes mellitus (DM), hyperlipidemia, hypertension, hyperhomocysteinemia and chronic renal insufficiency. Smoking increases the prevalence of PAD by 1.5 to 2-fold for every decade increase in age. DM increases the prevalence of PAD by approximately 2 to 4-fold. In addition, diabetics with PAD have 5 to 10-times higher need for major amputation compared to non-diabetics. Hyperlipidemia has an observed 10% increase in the

Inpatient Cardiovascular Medicine, First Edition. Edited by Brahmajee K. Nallamothu and Timir S. Baman.

likelihood of developing PAD for every 10 mg/dL risk in total cholesterol. There is a 2 to 4-fold increase in the prevalence of coronary and cerebrovascular disease in patients with PAD. CAD is the most common cause of death in patients with PAD, accounting for approximately half of all deaths, whereas cerebrovascular disease accounts for 10–20% of deaths. Only 20–30% of patients with PAD die of noncardiovascular causes. Risk factor modification, similar to that used for CAD, is of paramount importance in the management of PAD. Many patients with PAD are asymptomatic and critical limb ischemia is the initial clinical presentation in only a minority of patients. This is important to identify since urgent therapies are often required. Symptomatic claudication, which is defined as activity-induced tightness, cramping or fatigue, occurs in as many as one-third of patients with PAD and atypical leg pain in an additional 40–50%. The location of claudication and atypical leg pain often depends upon the location of the disease within the artery.

TAKE HOME POINT #1

Many patients with PAD are asymptomatic and critical limb ischemia is rare.

10.3 CLINICAL MANIFESTATIONS AND EVALUATION

The diagnostic work-up of patients with suspected PAD can be seen in Figure 10.1.

10.3.1 Signs and Symptoms

A history should include a vascular review of symptoms to assess for claudication, rest pain, walking impairment and impaired wound healing in the lower extremities. Claudication must be differentiated from pseudoclaudication and other nonvascular causes of claudication (see Table 10.1). Sedentary patients may not experience symptoms until exerted by a 6-minute walk test, on a treadmill or with repeated chair raises or leg elevation. Screening for the presence of PAD has been recommended in some high-risk groups (see Table 10.2), but its relevance for hospitalists is less clear. The severity of stenosis is correlated with the amount of exercise required to elicit claudication symptoms. Pain symptoms typically present one segment below the level of obstruction. They are gradual in onset and relieved rapidly with rest. **Distal aortic disease manifests with gluteal claudication, iliac disease with thigh pain and superficial femoral artery (SFA) disease with calf claudication.** When impotence and diminished femoral pulses are combined with gluteal claudication, this is known as Leriche Syndrome. **Critical limb ischemia (CLI) presents with rest pain, non-healing ulcerations, or gangrene.**

Physical examination is focused on the vascular system and requires careful evaluation for signs of acute or chronic peripheral ischemia *with the patient's shoes and socks removed.* Attention should be paid to the quality of carotid and peripheral pulses (femoral, popliteal, posterior tibial and dorsalis pedis) with regard to upstroke,

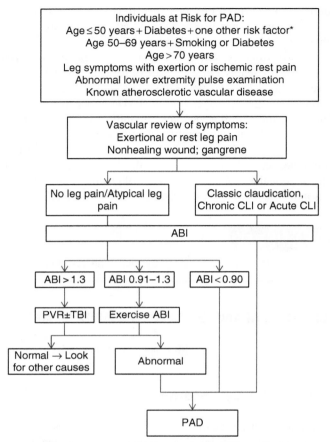

Figure 10.1   Diagnosis of Peripheral Artery Disease (PAD). ABI, Ankle-brachial index; CLI, Critical limb ischemia. *Risk factors include: cigarette smoking, diabetes mellitus, hypertension, hyperlipidemia, hyperhomocysteinemia, chronic renal insufficiency. (Source: Adapted from Hirsch AT, Haskal ZJ, Hertzer NR, et al. 2006. With permission of Elsevier).

amplitude and presence of bruits. Other signs of PAD include hair loss, coolness, skin pallor, scaling, and ulcerations and dystrophic nails. The abdomen should be palpated for evidence of an aortic aneurysm and blood pressure checked in both arms.

10.3.2   Diagnostic Testing

The diagnostic evaluation for PAD starts with ABIs. Table 10.3 lists the advantages and disadvantages of additional imaging modalities that are used in conjunction with ABIs.

Ankle/Brachial Index (ABI)

Measurement of ankle and brachial blood pressures is an accurate and practical non-invasive laboratory test for detecting PAD. The ABI, which is the ratio of these two

Table 10.1 Differentiation of Vascular Claudication from Pseudoclaudication (Nonvascular Causes).

Characteristic	Intermittent claudication	Spinal stenosis	Arthritis	Venous congestion
Character of discomfort	Cramping, fatigue, tiredness	Same symptoms as with claudication or with tingling, weakness or with clumsiness	Aching	Tightness, stretching pain
Location of discomfort	Buttock, hip, thigh, calf, foot	Buttock, hip, thigh	Hip, knee, ankle	Groin or thigh
Exercise-induced discomfort	Yes	Variable	Variable	Variable
Discomfort with standing	No	Yes	Yes, changes with shift in position	Yes, changes with shift in position
Relief of discomfort	Rapid relief with rest	Relief with sitting or otherwise changing position	Slow relief with avoidance of bearing weight	Slow relief with leg elevation
Other	Associated with atherosclerosis and weak pulses	History of lower-back problems	Discomfort at joint spaces	History of deep vein thrombosis, signs of venous congestion

Information is from the American Heart Association and the American College of Cardiology (Hirsch et al.) and from Schmeider and Comerota 2001.

Table 10.2   Populations to screen for peripheral artery disease (PAD).

Populations to screen for PAD
Age ≤50 + diabetes + one other risk factor*
Age 50–69 + diabetes or smoking
Age ≥70 + abnormal pulse exam or known atherosclerosis

*Risk factors include: cigarette smoking, diabetes mellitus, hypertension, hyperlipidemia, hyperhomocysteinemia, chronic renal insufficiency.

Table 10.3   Noninvasive and Invasive Diagnostic Imaging for Peripheral Artery Disease.

	Duplex ultrasound	Invasive artery angiography	Computed tomographic angiography	Magnetic resonance angiography
Advantages	Noninvasive	Gold standard High resolution images	Noninvasive High resolution images Three-dimensional	Noninvasive No radiation, no iodinated contrast exposure Three-dimensional
Disadvantages	Operator-dependent, limited by dense calcification	Invasive Radiation and contrast exposure Two dimensional	Radiation and contrast exposure Limited by dense calcification	Lack of resolution in high grade stenosis or calcification, nephrogenic systemic sclerosis, artifacts with stents/clips, cost

Table 10.4   Ankle Brachial Index Calculation and Interpretation.

Interpretation of calculated index
>1.30 – non-compressible vessels
1.00–1.29 – normal
0.91–0.99 – borderline
0.71–0.90 – mild obstruction
0.41–0.70 – moderate obstruction
0.00–0.40 – severe obstruction

measurements of blood pressure, can be performed at the bedside with ease and correlates well with disease severity (Table 10.4). It should be measured in both the right and left ankle, with the highest systolic pressure compared with the highest systolic pressure obtained in either upper extremity. A resting ABI of less than 0.90 is diagnostic of PAD with 95% sensitivity and 99% specificity for excluding PAD. Its sensitivity and specificity are increased by simultaneous Doppler velocity waveform (VWF) measurements. Based on the principle that blood flow accelerates through stenotic areas, Doppler VWF uses the peak systolic and end-diastolic velocities through an arterial segment to estimate the degree of stenosis. "Exercise" ABI can be useful in unmasking significant PAD in patients with a high index of suspicion but normal resting ABIs (e.g. isolated iliac stenosis). With treadmill exercise testing, a decrease in ABI of 15–20% from baseline is diagnostic of PAD. With noncompressible, calcified vessels (most commonly in patients with diabetes, renal failure or advanced age), the ABI is less useful and measuring a toe-brachial index (TBI) may be warranted, with values less than 0.7 considered diagnostic for PAD. The ABI with Doppler VWF can be effectively used as a serial test to monitor progression of PAD.

TAKE HOME POINT #2

ABIs are the first step in evaluating patients with PAD.

Pulse Volume Recordings (PVR)

Measurement of PVR is based on the concept that blood flow into the lower extremities is pulsatile. The resulting changes in lower limb arterial volume with each cardiac cycle can be measured using a plethysmographic technique. Blood pressure cuffs are placed at the thigh, upper calf, lower calf, midfoot and toe. The magnitude of the pulse upstroke and pulse volume correlates with blood flow and a sequential decrease suggests the presence of a significant stenosis in the more proximal arterial segment. Both PVR and Doppler VWF techniques can provide accurate information even in patients with noncompressible, calcified vessels. They also assess the location and severity of PAD as well as to follow the progression after a revascularization procedure.

Magnetic Resonance Angiography (MRA)

MRA can diagnose lower extremity PAD with high accuracy. The noninvasive nature of MRA, lack of nephrotoxic iodinated contrast dye or radiation exposure, and its ability to generate three-dimensional reconstructed images of peripheral arteries are among the advantages over conventional angiography. The main limitations are the lack of resolution in high-grade stenosis or calcification due to turbulent flow, use of gadolinium contrast which has been reported to rarely cause nephrogenic systemic fibrosis, high cost, limited availability, and contraindications in patients with implanted pacemakers or defibrilators and artifacts in patients with stents or metal clips.

Computed Tomographic Angiography (CTA)

New CTA technology allows rapid imaging of the entire lower extremity and abdomen in one breath and can provide three-dimensional reconstructed images. It provides better visualization of eccentric stenosis and collateral vessels than conventional angiography but with lower resolution. CTA has several advantages over MRA: patients with pacemakers and defibrillators can be imaged safely and there are fewer artifacts with metallic clips or stents. The lower cost, higher resolution and ability to provide images of calcification in the vessel wall are additional advantages.

Conversely, disadvantages of CTA include the use of iodinated contrast with risk of nephrotoxicity as well as exposure to ionizing radiation.

Arterial Angiography

Invasive, arterial angiography is considered the "gold standard" method for evaluation of PAD, especially when noninvasive tests are inconclusive or revascularization is being considered. It is invasive, with the inherent risks associated with any invasive procedure and arterial access, and requires iodinated contrast dye (although carbon dioxide can be used). It is useful when planning surgical or percutaneous revascularization.

10.4 TREATMENT

The mainstays of treatment for symptomatic PAD include exercise, risk factor modification, pharmacotherapy and, if warranted, endovascular or surgical therapies (see Figure 10.2).

10.4.1 Exercise

Exercise has been shown to significantly improve walking time and overall walking ability in patients with PAD and intermittent claudication. It is the least expensive intervention and may be more effective than antiplatelet therapy in improving maximum walking time and may have equivalent efficacy to surgery. The recommended exercise program for patients with intermittent claudication involves walking to near-maximal pain three times a week for a minimum of 30 minute sessions for a period of six months. A meta-analysis of several randomized trials demonstrated a greater symptomatic benefit and improvement in pain-free and maximal walking distance with a supervised, as opposed to non-supervised, exercise program.

TAKE HOME POINT #3

Exercise therapy is a critical therapy in patients with claudication that may exceed antiplatelet treatments and match surgery in terms of efficacy.

10.4.2 Risk Factor Modification

Cardiovascular disease is the major cause of mortality in patients with PAD. It is imperative that aggressive modification of atherosclerotic risk factors be pursued in all patients with PAD (see Table 10.5). Smoking cessation can reduce the risk of amputation and decrease the 5-year mortality rate by 50%. Aggressive treatment of

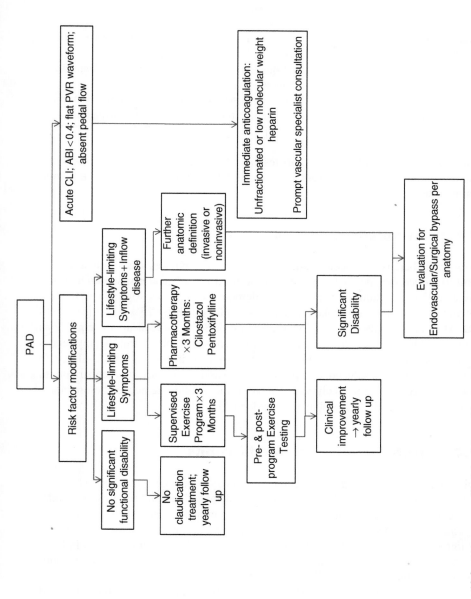

Figure 10.2 Management of Peripheral Artery Disease (PAD). ABI, Ankle-brachial index; CLI, Critical limb ischemia. (Source: Adapted from Hirsch AT, Haskal ZJ, Hertzer NR, et al. 2006. With permission of Elsevier).

133

Table 10.5   Modifiable Risk Factor Management for Peripheral Artery Disease.

Risk factor	Goal
Smoking	Cessation
Exercise	30–45 minutes of sustained aerobic exercise three to five times each week
Blood pressure (BP)	Systolic BP <140 mm Hg; diastolic BP <90 mm Hg Patients with diabetes or renal disease: Systolic BP <130 mmHg; diastolic BP <80 mm Hg
Diabetes mellitus	Hemoglobin A1c <7% Daily foot assessment for complications of ischemia
Low-density lipoprotein (LDL)	<100 mg/dL; if risk very high, LDL <70 mg/dL

hypertension, hyperlipidemia and diabetes mellitus should be implemented. Diabetic patients should conduct daily foot assessment for early identification of ischemic complications.

10.4.3   Antiplatelet Therapy

Antiplatelet therapy has been studied in several large clinical trials and has been found to reduce the risk of limb loss and the need for surgical revascularization in patients with claudication. A meta-analysis demonstrated that aspirin reduces the risk of myocardial infarction, stroke and cardiovascular death by 25% in patients with PAD. This analysis also showed low daily dose of 81 mg of aspirin was equally as effective as higher doses. All patients with PAD should be on aspirin therapy unless contraindicated. Clopidogrel is an effective alternative in the setting of allergy to aspirin. Clopidogrel reduced composite cardiovascular events in comparison to aspirin in a large randomized clinical trial but further studies are needed before clopidogrel replaces aspirin as first-line therapy for PAD.

10.4.4   Anti-Claudication Medications

Table 10.6 reviews different anti-claudication medications. Cilostazol is a phosphodiesterase type III inhibitor that is a direct arterial vasodilator and suppresses platelet aggregation. Treatment with cilostazol for 3–6 months has been shown to improve maximal walking distance by 50–67% and improve quality of life indicators without any impact on cardiovascular morbidity and mortality. It is contraindicated in heart failure because of an increase in mortality seen in this subgroup with other phosphodiesterase inhibitors. Pentoxifylline is a methylxanthine derivative that is an inferior alternative to cilostazol but has been shown to marginally increase pain-free and maximal walking distance. Several other agents have been evaluated and have not been proven effective in the treatment of PAD.

Table 10.6 ACC/AHA Guidelines for Pharmacologic Management of Claudication.

Medication, class of evidence	Level of evidence	Dose	Side effects
Class I			
Cilostazol	A	100 mg twice daily	Contraindicated in heart failure; can cause headache, dizziness, diarrhea, palpitations, pharyngitis
Class IIb			
Pentoxifylline	A	400 mg thrice daily	Contraindicated in recent cerebral or retinal hemorrhage; can cause headache, dizziness, dyspepsia, nausea, vomiting
Arginine	B	2–3 gm thrice daily	Contraindicated in diabetes, hepatic or renal insufficiency; can cause diarrhea, flushing
Propionyl levocarnitine	B	0.5gm twice daily – 1 gm thrice daily	No significant side effects
Ginkgo biloba	B	120–160 mg daily	No significant side effects
Class III			
Prostaglandins	A	Beraprost 40 micrograms thrice daily	Headache, flushing, diarrhea
Vitamin E	C	50 mg daily	No significant side effects
Chelation (EDTA)	A	1.5–3 gm twice weekly (intravenous)	Hypocalcemia, renal failure, gastrointestinal distress

Information is from the American Heart Association and the American College of Cardiology (Hirsch et al.). Class I evidence is defined as evidence for and/or general agreement that the treatment is beneficial, useful, and effective; class IIb as conflicting evidence or divergence of opinion about the usefulness/efficacy (or efficacy that is less well-established by evidence/opinion); and class III evidence as evidence and/or general agreement that the treatment is not useful/effective and in some cases may be harmful. Levels of evidence are classified as follows: (A) data derived from multiple randomized clinical trials or meta-analyses; (B) data derived from a single randomized trial or nonrandomized studies; (C) the consensus opinion of experts, data from case studies, or the standard of care.

10.4.5   Endovascular and Surgical Therapies

These therapies are indicated in patients with "lifestyle limiting" claudication, rest pain or critical limb ischemia resulting in ischemic ulceration or gangrene. Revascularization can be achieved percutaneously or surgically. The choice to use either approach is typically based on the patient's clinical condition as well as the location and severity of their atherosclerotic lesions. While attempts are made to avoid it as much as possible, under certain circumstances amputation is required if blood flow cannot be re-established and there is severe limb ischemia.

TAKE HOME POINT #4

The choice between endovascular and surgical therapies depends upon the clinical condition and anatomic location and severity of the lesions.

Catheter-based, percutaneous endovascular revascularization can be offered to selected patients as a less-invasive and equally effective alternative to surgical therapy. The procedure-related morbidity and peri-procedural risk associated with catheter-based interventions is much lower than that with surgery. Percutaneous intervention is preferred in patients under 50 years of age given the high risk of graft failure with surgical revascularization due to aggressiveness of underlying disease in this subset of patients. Based on the extent and anatomic location of the lesion, decisions to use stents or balloon angioplasty may vary.

Surgical revascularization is primarily offered to bypass long or complex segments of diffuse arterial disease, with critical limb ischemia or after failure of conservative or endovascular therapy. Patients are carefully selected if they have a reasonable likelihood of symptomatic improvement, favorable limb arterial anatomy and low cardiovascular risk for surgical revascularization. Amputation is not desirable but is sometimes necessary in patients who cannot be successfully revascularized.

10.5 OTHER CONDITIONS AND VASCULAR EMERGENCIES

Acute arterial occlusion occurs rarely, but it is important for the hospitalist to recognize. Acute arterial occlusion occurs typically following embolization of thrombotic material from either the heart (approximately 80%) or an "upstream" vessel like the abdominal aorta. Given the importance of the heart as a source of emboli, it is important to perform a careful cardiac history and physical exam with the focus on ruling out atrial fibrillation as a potential source of embolization. The most common location where embolization occurs is the femoral artery bifurcation. At times, there can also be the development of spontaneous thrombosis in atherosclerotic plaque within areas with PAD.

Symptoms and signs of acute arterial occlusion depend upon the type of occlusion (emboli or thrombus), site of occlusion and the extent of collaterals. Emboli often require more urgent attention due to the lack of time for collateral development and more significant ischemia. For the hospitalist, it is important to look for the 5 Ps: pulselessness, paralysis, paresthesia, pain, and pallor. When these are present, consultation with a vascular surgeon should be considered urgently to maximize limb salvage. Vascular surgeons will help to guide further testing and the possible involvement of an endovascular expert. Key findings that should prompt urgent consultation of vascular surgeons include: (1) acute leg pain correlated with a cool distal extremity; (2) diminished or absent distal pulses; and (3) an ankle systolic blood pressure of less than 50 mm Hg. Acute therapy should include anticoagulation with intravenous heparin to minimize extension of thrombus as well as recurrent embolizations. Locally-delivered thrombolytic therapy and surgical embolectomy or revascularization are often required.

TAKE HOME POINT #5

Look for the 5 P's in patients with suspected arterial occlusion: pulselessness, paralysis, paresthesia, pain, and pallor.

Vasculitis syndromes result from inflammatory processes in the vessel wall that can be due to either immune-complex deposition or cell-mediated reactions. Most causes of these syndromes are unknown. The various forms of vasculitis syndromes are distinguished from each other by the pattern of involved vessels as well as histological and laboratory findings. These include: (1) polyarteritis nodosa (small-to-medium blood vessels like the renal, hepatic and skeletal muscle); (2) giant cell or temporal arteritis (medium-to-large blood vessels, especially the cranial vessels); (3) Takayasu's arteritis (aorta and its large branches); and (4) Buerger's disease (small-to-medium blood vessels in the distal upper and lower extremities) that is classically associated with smokers. These conditions often require consultation of rheumatologic specialists for diagnostic testing and discussions about the use of immunosuppressant therapy.

KEY REFERENCES

HIRSCH AT, HASKAL ZJ, HERTZER NR, et al. ACC/AHA 2005 guidelines for the management of patients with peripheral arterial disease (lower extremity, renal, mesenteric, and abdominal aortic). J Am Coll Cardiol 2006;47:1239–1312.

MAHAMEED AA, BARTHOLOMEW JR. Disease of peripheral vessels. In: ERIC TOPOL (Ed.) *The Topol Solution: Textbook of Cardiovascular Medicine*, 3rd edition, 2007. Lippincott, Williams & Wilkins: Philadelphia.

SCHMIEDER FA, COMEROTA AJ. Intermittent claudication: magnitude of the problem, patient evaluation and therapeutic strategies. Am J Cardiol 2001;87(12A):3D–13D.

WHITE C. Intermittent claudication. N Engl J Med 2007;356:1241–1250.

Chapter 11

Thoracic Aortic Diseases

Anna M. Booher and Thomas T. Tsai

11.1 THORACIC AORTIC ANEURYSM

Thoracic aortic aneurysm has an incidence of approximately 5.6–10.2 patients per 100,000 patient years, making it far less common than other cardiovascular conditions. However, due to the increased mortality associated with aneurysmal disease, including aortic rupture or dissection, hospitalists must always consider these in their differential diagnosis, especially during atypical clinical presentation.

The aorta is dilated if it exceeds the normal limits of age and body size and is aneurysmal if it exceeds >50% of this normal limit. Most commonly, thoracic aortic disease is asymptomatic and typically discovered during an imaging study performed for an unrelated indication. Over 60% of thoracic aortic aneurysms involve only the aortic root or ascending aorta, 10–20% involve the descending aorta only, while 10% are isolated to the arch. Others involve one or more of these segments in combination.

11.1.1 Pathophysiology, Etiology, and Natural History

The pathophysiologic basis for thoracic aortic aneurysms is complex and related to underlying conditions that predispose patients to aortic dilation. A specific genetic mutation or predisposition to excess inflammatory mediators lead to decreased contractile function of vascular smooth muscle cells. These inflammatory mediators are then responsible for breakdown of elastic fibers and resultant progressive aortic dilation.

Inpatient Cardiovascular Medicine, First Edition. Edited by Brahmajee K. Nallamothu and Timir S. Baman.

Table 11.1   Etiology of Thoracic Aortic Aneurysm.

Etiology	Details
Degenerative aneurysms	May be accelerated by hypertension, age, smoking
Atherosclerotic	More commonly involves the descending aorta and arch
Bicuspid aortic valve	>50% may have tubular/ascending aneurysm while 20% have sinus of Valsalva involvement
	Faster rate of growth than aneurysms associated with a three leaflet valve
Familial thoracic aortic aneurysm syndromes	
Marfan Syndrome	Most common inherited connective tissue disease
	Mutation in Fibrillin 1 gene leads to decreased tensile strength of the aorta
	An estimated 75% of patients will have a dilated aortic root
Loeys-Dietz Syndrome	Aggressive vasculopathy linked to TGFBR1 or 2 mutation
	Early detection and intervention is important
Aortitis	
Infectious	Syphilis (historical), Salmonella, staphylococcal sp, mycobacterium
Non-infections/inflammatory	
	More common:
	Giant cell and Takaysu's arteritis
	Less common:
	Behcets, Cogans syndrome, replapsing polychondritis
	Rare:
	Rheumatoid arthritis, spondyloarthropathies
Trauma	Typical location is at the aortic isthmus
	Complications include rupture, pseudoaneurysm, chronic dissection with secondary aneurysm formation
Chronic aortic dissection	Aneurysm may form due to growth and pressure differential of false lumen

Examples of the various etiologies of thoracic aortic aneurysm disease are listed in Table 11.1. Although the genetics of this disease are multifactorial and not fully elucidated, it is thought that the predominant inheritance of thoracic aortic disease is autosomal dominant with reduced penetrance. Nearly 20% of patients who develop a thoracic aortic aneurysm will have a family history of aortic disease and a familial pattern should be suspected in patients who present at a young age. Younger patients with thoracic aortic dilation should also be evaluated for a bicuspid aortic valve. The presence of a bicuspid valve is highly associated with aneurysm in this population, and these patients may be at higher risk for aortic complications. In older patients, the most common etiology of thoracic aortic aneurysm is degenerative processes associated with increased age; however, hypertension, tobacco abuse, hyperlipidemia, and other genetic factors can result in acceleration of growth. Thoracic aortic aneurysms grow at an average rate of 1–1.5 mm/yr. However, aneurysms that are larger than 5 cm in the ascending aorta and 6 cm in the descending aorta will grow at a faster rate and require more immediate attention.

11.1.2   Clinical Presentation

The vast majority of patients who present with thoracic aortic aneurysms are asymptomatic and the diagnosis is typically made on an imaging test performed for an unrelated indication. Patients may present with chest pain, symptoms of heart failure due to aortic root involvement and subsequent aortic valve insufficiency, local mass effect including compression of trachea or bronchus (wheezing, cough), compression of the esophagus (dysphagia) or hoarseness due to involvement of the recurrent laryngeal nerve. A physical exam may reveal a murmur of aortic valve regurgitation or stenosis, or an early systolic click in the presence of a bicuspid aortic valve.

11.1.3   Evaluation and Diagnostic Studies

Typical chest X-ray findings include a widened mediastinum, deviation of the trachea or displacement of the aortic knob or displaced calcification of the aortic wall. However, none of these findings on chest X-ray are particularly sensitive or specific for thoracic aortic aneurysm. Invasive angiography is the historical gold standard but has largely been replaced by cross-sectional imaging modalities. Table 11.2 highlights the common modalities used to image the thoracic aorta and their respective advantages and disadvantages. Computed tomography (CT) with contrast is typically the most easily accessible and time-efficient modality and is preferred in acute settings (Figure 11.1). Other available modalities for imaging the thoracic aorta include transesophageal and transthoracic echocardiography (Figure 11.2) and magnetic resonance imaging (MRI). Serial imaging utilizing similar imaging modalities is valuable as changes in size over time can dictate the necessity and timing of intervention.

   If an aneurysm not requiring surgery is found to involve the aortic root or ascending aorta, then a surface echocardiogram should be performed to evaluate for concomitant aortic valve disease or bicuspid aortic valve disease, which can often be associated with thoracic aortic aneurysms. Once an aneurysm is diagnosed, appropriate surveillance imaging should be performed at 6 months to 1 year for the first year to document aneurysm size stability and then every 1–3 years subsequently depending on the etiology of the aneurysm, the rate of growth and the severity of the concomitant valvular disease.

TAKE HOME POINT #1

Most patients with thoracic aortic aneurysms are asymptomatic and diagnosed on an imaging study carried out for unrelated indications.

Table 11.2 Imaging the Thoracic Aorta

Modality	Advantages	Disadvantages
CT angiography	Rapid image acquisition (20–30 s), can use in unstable patients.	Need for iodinated contrast
	3D reconstruction allows multiple views/orientations	Radiation exposure (10–20 mSv) – of concern in young patients requiring serial imaging
	Ability for post image processing	Image artifacts, particularly in aortic root, may be improved by ECG gating
		Aortic size can be overestimated due to oblique cuts through lumen
MRI/MR angiography	No radiation or iodinated contrast exposure	Caution with use of gadolinium in renal failure
	3D, multi-planar and high resolution	Need for breath hold
	Dynamic and functional cardiac information available	Time consuming (10–30 min at minimum) depending on center expertise
	May be appropriate for serial imaging over many years	Not for use in unstable patients (distance of equipment/staff for resuscitation from patient)
Echocardiography Transthoracic	No radiation or iodinated contrast exposure	Cannot visualize entire aorta
	Can be performed at the bedside, immediate information available	May be limited by technical difficulties, patient body habitus, lung disease
	Excellent evaluation of valve function, pericardial effusion and LV function	
Transesophageal	Can visualize aorta from root to GE junction.	Semi-invasive
	Doppler interrogation of true and false lumen	Requires conscious sedation and patent/secure airway
	Evaluation of valvular dysfunction	
	Performed at beside	

11.1.4 Treatment

Since most thoracic aortic aneurysms are asymptomatic, the primary indication for treatment is to prevent the development of life-threatening complications, such as

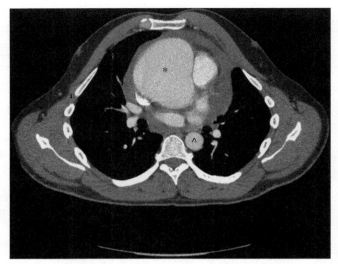

Figure 11.1   CT angiography demonstrating ascending aortic aneurysm. Note size differential between ascending aorta (*) and descending aorta (^).

dissection or rupture. The likelihood of these complications depends on the size of the aneurysm and its location as well as the skill of the surgeon. In asymptomatic patients, the thresholds for elective surgical intervention are listed in Figure 11.3. In general, non-genetically mediated aneurysms should be considered for surgical intervention when the size is >5.5 cm. In experienced centers, these thresholds might be lower: e.g. when the ascending aorta and arch are ≥5.0–5.5 cm or ≥5.5–6.0 cm in the descending aorta. In patients with the Marfan syndrome and other genetically triggered conditions, the cutoff is lower (4–5 cm) due to their typically younger ages and higher likelihood of developing life-threatening complications over time.

Another important consideration is the rate of growth over time. Most centers consider a rate of growth of ≥0.5 cm per year in the ascending and ≥1 cm per year in the descending aorta as a high risk marker and an indication for surgical or endovascular intervention. Symptomatic patients with a thoracic aortic aneurysm should be evaluated promptly for surgical intervention, particularly if the size is >5 cm.

For smaller aneurysms, treatment modalities can include medical therapy. Aggressive blood pressure control with beta blockers is first-line therapy. There are emerging data in the Marfan syndrome population that treatment with angiotensin receptor blockers decreases the rate of growth of ascending aortic aneurysms, largely via tempering the effects of TGF-B. Aggressive use of HMG CoA Reductase inhibitors (statins) have been shown to be of benefit in abdominal aortic aneurysms and should be used in thoracic aortic disease, particularly if the disease is atherosclerotic in origin (Table 11.3; Figure 11.3).

Another important aspect of therapy is lifestyle limitations and modifications. In general, patients with thoracic aortic aneurysms >4–4.5 cm should not lift, pull or

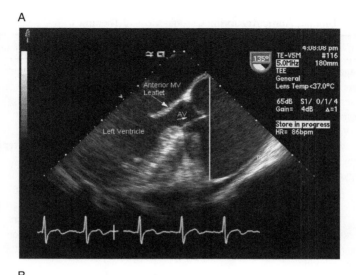

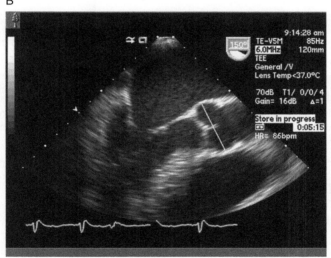

Figure 11.2 **A** TEE of ascending/aortic aneurysm. Long axis, mid esophageal TEE view of large aneurysm at sinus of Valsalva measuring 10.5 cm. **B** TEE of normal size aortic root for comparison. Long axis view of normal appearing aortic root measuring 3.2 cm. AV, aortic valve. MV, mitral valve.

push anything over 30–50 pounds. Digging or shoveling, hammering, chopping wood, and any type of exertion that involves sudden use of force should be discouraged. Mild-to-moderate aerobic activity should be encouraged to promote overall cardiovascular health. Smoking cessation should be encouraged.

Referral to an aortic center of excellence should be considered for all patients with the Marfan syndrome or any genetically triggered aneurysm. Additionally, referral should be considered in patients with an ascending aorta >4.5 or descending

Table 11.3   Thoracic Aortic Aneurysm: Chronic Medical Therapy.

Medication	Dosage	Goal of therapy
First-line agent: B-blockers	Titrate to effect	Heart rate <60 bpm

Second-line agents:
  Angiotensin receptor
  blockers or ACE inhibitors
	Start at a low dose and
	  titrate to BP goals
		Blood pressure
		  <130/80 mmHg

Third-line agent
Calcium channel blocker
  (dihydropyridine)
	Start at a low dose and
	  titrate to above goals
		As needed to lower systolic
		  BP into range of
		  <130 mmHg

Statins	Highest dose that patient
	  can tolerate to reach goals
		Goal LDL <70 if
		  atherosclerotic aneurysm
		  or <100 in others

Tobacco cessation aids: Varenicline (chantix, buproprion, nicotine replacement)	Standard dosing	Smoking cessation

aorta >5.0–5.5 cm as it is possible that these patients will need an intervention at some point in their lifetime.

> **TAKE HOME POINT #2**
>
> Serial follow-up imaging and medical therapy are important aspects in the management of asymptomatic thoracic aortic aneurysms. Early referral to specialty centers in cases of genetically-triggered aneurysms is appropriate.

11.2   ACUTE AORTIC SYNDROMES

11.2.1   Introduction

Acute syndromes of the thoracic aorta include aortic dissection, intramural hematoma and penetrating ulcers. These processes account for an estimated 2.0–3.5 cases per 100,000 person years or 10,000 cases annually in the United States. The estimated mortality is 1–3% per hour after the onset of a dissection with an estimated 40% of patients expiring prior to obtaining medical attention. In those who survive to arrive at a hospital, the mortality ranges from 5–25% in the early perioperative period. The morbidity associated with this syndrome is also significant, thus highlighting the importance of prompt recognition, diagnosis and initiation of appropriate therapy.

11.2.2   Pathophysiology

Acute aortic syndromes involve a distortion or separation of the aortic intima from the remainder of the aortic wall. The mechanism of this injury defines the different types

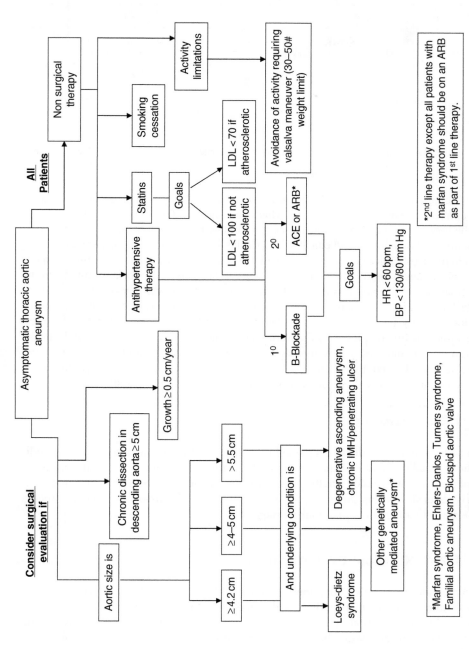

Figure 11.3 Decision-making algorithm for asymptomatic thoracic aortic aneurysm.

145

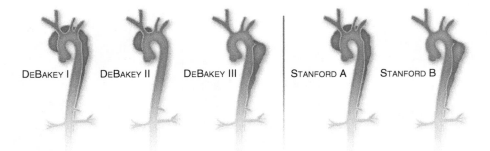

Figure 11.4   Classification schema of acute aortic syndromes. Debakey and Stanford Classification Systems. (See Color plate 11.1).

of acute aortic syndromes. Intramural hematoma is thought to be a consequence of rupture of the medial vaso vasorum which may lead to infarction of the aortic wall and the possible subsequent classic dissection. A penetrating ulcer is likely a precursor of intramural hematomas but can also lead to classic dissection. Erosion of a penetrating atherosclerotic ulcer into the aortic wall can weaken the wall and make rupture more likely. A classic aortic dissection is an acute separation of the aortic intima from the remainder of the aortic wall and this tear can propagate distally or in a retrograde fashion and involve many side branches of the aorta. Patterns of aortic dissection are described by the Debakey system or the Stanford classification system which are outlined in Figure 11.4. The Stanford Classification is used more commonly in the current era. Stanford type A dissection involves the ascending aorta while type B dissection is defined by an intimal tear that does not involve the ascending aorta. Treatment for aortic dissection is driven in large part by these classifications.

11.2.3   Etiology

Factors that can predispose a patient to aortic dissection include many of the conditions listed in Table 11.1 that are associated with thoracic aneurysms and weakening of the aortic wall. Additionally, prior aortic surgery seems to be a predisposing factor. Hypertension is common in all patients who present with dissection, and this process appears to affect more men than women.

11.2.4   Clinical Presentation

Acute aortic dissection commonly presents with acute onset chest or back pain and can mimic many other cardiovascular and pulmonary conditions such as angina, myocardial infarction, pulmonary embolism or pneumonia. Classically, aortic dissection presents with abrupt onset of intense pain – this characteristic may help distinguish dissection from these other conditions. Other symptoms associated with dissection can include arm or leg pain (indicating limb ischemia), severe abdominal pain (indicating mesenteric ischemia), symptoms of a stroke or altered sensorium due to great vessel/cerebrovascular involvement, or congestive heart failure and pulmonary edema due to acute aortic insufficiency.

Patients presenting with dissection may be hypertensive (>70% of cases and more common in Type B dissection), normotensive or hypotensive. Hypotension in the presence of a dissection may suggest that pericardial tamponade is present due to rupture of the aorta into the pericardial space, constituting a surgical emergency. Percutaneous drainage of a pericardial effusion in the setting of acute aortic dissection is contraindicated since it can lead to hemodynamic collapse. Additional exam findings that can be present include a murmur of aortic valve insufficiency, pulmonary rales, pulse differential or diminished pulses in the extremities, and neurologic deficits.

TAKE HOME POINT #3

Aortic dissection mimics many cardiac and pulmonary processes and clinicians should maintain a high index of suspicion in order to facilitate prompt diagnosis.

11.2.5 Evaluation and Diagnostic Studies

An EKG should be performed in all patients to rule out concomitant coronary ischemia, with right coronary artery distribution ischemia due to dissection flap interruption of the ostium of the right coronary artery being the most common mechanism. A CXR should be also performed. This may show a widened mediastinum, displacement of aortic calcification or opacification in the aorto-pulmonary window (Figure 11.1). However, this is rarely diagnostic for acute aortic syndrome and additional imaging is often warranted.

A suggested algorithm for imaging the suspected acute aortic syndrome is shown in Table 11.4. In general, unstable patients should be evaluated by CT (Figure 11.5, Figure 11.6) or transesophageal echocardiography (Figure 11.7) as a first step given their relatively fast acquisition times. MRI can be considered

Table 11.4 Imaging in the Diagnosis of Suspected Acute Aortic Dissection.

	Imaging/diagnostic modality
All patients	EKG and CXR
Stable/chronic	TEE
	CT with contrast or MRI/MRI*
Unstable	TEE
	CT with contrast

*Note: Use of MRI is discouraged in the acute setting due to time of acquisition and physical distance from the patient.

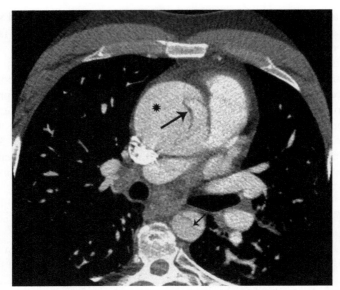

Figure 11.5   CT angiography of a Type A dissection. Note dissection flap (large arrow), in a dilated ascending aorta (*) and continuation of the dissection flap into the descending aorta (small arrow).

in stable patients (Figure 11.8). If the patient is hypotensive or in shock then a surface echo may reveal a pericardial effusion or severe aortic insufficiency. The relative advantages and disadvantages of each of these modalities are shown in Table 11.2. Given that several options for imaging exist, the modality chosen should be based on patient stability and what test is most rapidly available at a particular institution.

11.2.6 Treatment

Type A Dissection

Type A dissection is a surgical emergency. In cases where a Type A dissection has propagated to cause malperfusion of a limb or large branch vessel, some centers have adopted an approach of emergent percutaneous management of the dissection with stenting and/or balloon fenestration to restore perfusion to vital organs prior to definitive operative repair. In either case, emergent cardiac surgical consultation should be obtained. If the dissection involves the proximal aorta and arch, then replacement of the affected segments is performed with a composite graft, with or without replacement of the aortic valve and reimplantation of the coronary arteries. If the dissection extends from the root through the descending aorta then the options for repair typically include replacement of the ascending aorta (with or without the aortic valve) and the proximal arch under hypothermic circulatory arrest. The residual

A

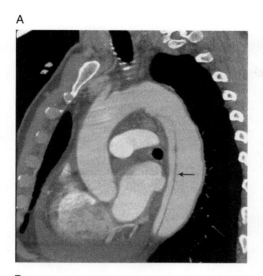

B

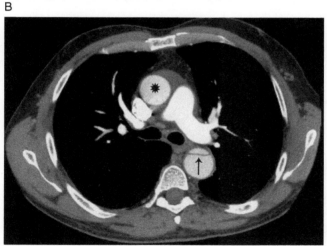

Figure 11.6   **A** Reformatted CT of Type B dissection. Dissection flap (arrow) originates in and propagates down the the descending aorta. **B** CT axial images of Type B dissection. Note dissection flap in the descending aorta (arrow) with an unaffected ascending aorta (*).

dissection is often followed with serial imaging and can be intervened upon at a later time if necessary. Similarly, if an intramural hemorrhage or penetrating ulcer involves the ascending aorta then it is often treated as a Type A dissection and constitutes a surgical emergency.

Prior to operative intervention, care should be given to ensure a secure airway if airway compromise or hypotension is present, and to medically optimize hemodynamics (Table 11.5). These patients should be monitored in the emergency department or intensive care unit setting with intra-arterial monitoring of the blood pressure, if possible. This involves using beta-blockers acutely to decrease ventricular contractile

A

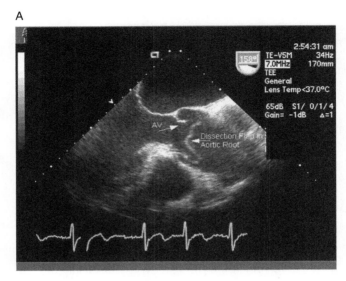

B

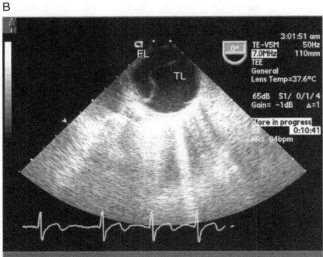

Figure 11.7   **A** TEE of dissection flap in proximal aorta/aortic root in close approximation to aortic valve. **B** TEE of dissection flap in mid descending aorta. FL, false lumen, TL, true lumen.

force if the patient is hyper- or normotensive, with the addition of vasodilators and acute pain control as necessary to reach heart rate and blood pressure targets shown in Table 11.5. Esmolol, an intravenous beta-blocker, is ideally suited as medical therapy due to its immediate onset of action. Calcium channel blockers should only be used in cases of documented severe beta-blocker intolerance. Hypotensive patients with Type A dissection warrant particular surgical urgency to avoid complete hemodynamic collapse.

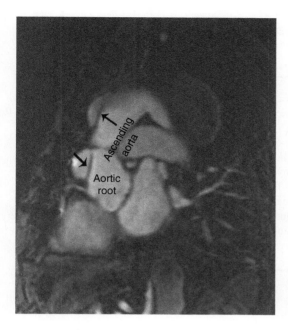

Figure 11.8 MRI of Type A dissection. Dissection flap (arrows) noted in aortic root and ascending aorta.

Table 11.5 Acute Aortic Syndromes: Acute Medical Therapy.

Drug class	Dose	Goal of therapy	Notes
IV B-blocker			
Esmolol	50 mcg/kg/min starting dose, increase to 150 mcg/kg/min to reach goal	HR ≤60 bpm Systolic BP = 100–120 mmHg	Preferred first-line agent
IV Calcium channel blocker			Not preferred, use only if documented severe intolerance to b-blockade
Diltiazem	5–15 mg/hr	Same as above	
IV Vasodilator			Second-line agent if BP goals not met with b-blockade. *Use with a b-blocker to avoid increase in aortic wall sheer stress
Nipride	Initial dose: 0.3 mcg/kg/min – titrate to effect	Systolic BP 100–120 mmHg	Need to monitor cyanide levels. Care to avoid hypotension/malperfusion
Fenoldapam	Initial dose: NEED		Care to avoid hypotension
Pain control	Morphine 2–6 mg IV or Fentanyl 25–100mcg IV. Can be re-dosed as needed	Pain relief	Careful to avoid hypotension

Table 11.6   Chronic/Discharge Therapy in Acute Aortic Syndromes (Non-Operative Cases).

	Drug/drug class	Goals of therapy
First line for hypertension and HR control	B-blockade – oral formulations	BP <120/80 and HR <60
Second line antihypertensive	ACE or ARB	BP <120/80
Third line antihypertensive	Calcium channel blockers (dihydropyridine)	BP 120/80
Can be added if needed for HR control	Non-dihydropyridine calcium channel blockers	HR <60
Lipid lowering therapy	Statins (HMG CoA reductase inhibitors)	Goal of LDL <100 unless documented atherosclerosis then LDL<70

Type B dissection

Uncomplicated Type B dissection or intramural hematoma/penetrating ulcers that do not involve the ascending aorta are often best managed medically given the high morbidity associated with surgical repair. Uncomplicated cases are those that have relatively easily controlled hypertension, prompt resolution of pain and do not involve malperfusion of any vital organs, The initial goals of medical therapy are to decrease the strain on the aortic wall via decreased force of left ventricular contraction. The options for acute medical therapy provided in Table 11.5 should be employed when possible. When stable, patients can be transitioned to chronic oral therapy to optimize blood pressure control. Often more than three medications are required for controlling blood pressure and heart rate. Options for chronic therapy are outlined in Table 11.6.

Indications for percutaneous or surgical intervention in Type B dissection include complications such as refractory pain or hypertension, visceral or peripheral ischemia from malperfusion, or extension of the dissection. Percutaneous intervention may be preferable to open intervention and have improved outcomes in type B dissection but no definitive clinical trials have compared the two approaches.

Pre-discharge imaging should be performed to document for extension of the dissection or aortic enlargement, both of which might prompt earlier intervention. Lifestyle limitations that are discussed in the section above should be reinforced with the patients prior to discharge. Close follow-up with an aortic specialist should be arranged to optimize medical therapy and arrange for follow-up imaging.

TAKE HOME POINT #4

Prompt diagnosis, early medical management and mobilization of surgical teams are keys to the management of acute aortic syndromes.

KEY REFERENCES

ERBEL R, ALFONSO F, BOILEAU C, DIRSCH O, EBER B, HAVERICH A, et al. Diagnosis and management of aortic dissection. Eur Heart J 2001;22(18):1642–1681.

ISSELBACHER EM. Thoracic and abdominal aortic aneurysms. Circulation 2005;111(6):816–828.

NIENABER CA, KISCHE S, SKRIABINA V, INCE H. Noninvasive imaging approaches to evaluate the patient with known or suspected aortic disease. Circ Cardiovasc Imaging 2009;2(6):499–506.

PATEL HJ, DEEB GM. Ascending and arch aorta: pathology, natural history, and treatment. Circulation 2008;118(2):188–195.

TSAI TT, NIENABER CA, EAGLE KA. Acute aortic syndromes. Circulation 2005;112(24):3802–3813.

Chapter 12

Systolic Heart Failure

Shea E. Hogan and Jennifer A. Cowger

12.1 INTRODUCTION

The incidence and prevalence of heart failure (HF) in the US has increased over the past few decades in association with an aging population, an increased prevalence of HF risk factors, and improved survival from coronary artery disease. Due to a lack of consensus regarding the definition of heart failure, as well as non-uniform methods used to determine its presence, an accurate estimate of the problem's magnitude has yet to be determined. HF has been defined as "a complex clinical syndrome that can result from any structural or functional cardiac disorder that impairs the ability of the ventricle to fill with or eject blood." In the case of HF related to decreased left ventricular (LV) systolic function, the heart is unable to eject a blood volume commensurate with physiologic needs. This type of HF is known as systolic HF, and it often results from conditions (infarction, diabetes, viral or toxin exposure) that alter myocardial structure and/or function. While not the focus of this chapter, diastolic LV dysfunction is also often present in patients with systolic HF and the two can be difficult to separate clinically. In this chapter, we use the term HF to discuss the overall syndrome with an emphasis on systolic LV dysfunction will be addressed in Chapter 13.

12.2 INCIDENCE/PREVALENCE

The most recent data from the American Heart Association regarding HF estimate its prevalence to be approximately 5.7 million (3.2 million males and 2.5 million

Inpatient Cardiovascular Medicine, First Edition. Edited by Brahmajee K. Nallamothu and Timir S. Baman.
© 2014 John Wiley & Sons, Inc. Published 2014 by John Wiley & Sons, Inc.

Table 12.1 Annual Rates for New Heart Failure Events Per Age Group.

Age groups	65–74	75–84	85+
White men	15.2 per 1000	31.7 per 1000	65.2 per 1000
Black men	16.9 per 1000	25.5 per 1000	50.6 per 1000
Black women	14.2 per 1000	25.5 per 1000	44 per 1000
White women	8.2 per 1000	19.8 per 1000	45.6 per 1000

females) in adults aged 20 and older. The incidence of HF increases with age but its frequency varies with sex and race (Table 12.1). There are less data regarding the incidence of HF in younger adults, although population-based data suggest that the 5-year risk of HF among white 40-year-olds is 0.1–0.2%, and the lifetime risk for developing HF is one in five.

HF remains one of the most common reasons for hospitalization in the United States, particularly in elderly patients. Hospital discharges for HF increased from 877,000 in 1996 to over 1.1 million in 2006. In contrast, the number of ambulatory visits for HF in 2007 was approximately 3.4 million. The estimated direct and indirect cost of HF in the USA for 2010 is $39.2 billion.

12.3 MORTALITY

While the rate of death after HF onset declined in both sexes by approximately one-third from the 1950s to the 1990s, mortality has not significantly changed over the past two decades. Data from the Framingham Heart Study, which evaluated participants and their offspring, revealed that 80% of males and 70% of females with HF who are younger than 65 will die within eight years. Once HF is diagnosed, females tend to survive longer than males, although less than 15% of females survive more than 8–12 years. The one-year mortality rate after HF diagnosis is estimated at 20%. Patients with heart failure are 6–9 times more likely to die from sudden cardiac arrest compared to the general population.

TAKE HOME POINT #1

HF incidence and prevalence are rising with the aging US population, and its onset is associated with increased mortality and increased medical resource utilization; patients with HF are much more likely than the general population to have sudden cardiac death.

12.4 PATHOPHYSIOLOGY OF LV SYSTOLIC DYSFUNCTION

Cardiac output is the product of stroke volume and heart rate. In LV systolic dysfunction, there is a decrease in myocardial contractility which leads to a decrease in stroke volume, and therefore, cardiac output (Figure 12.1). Associated

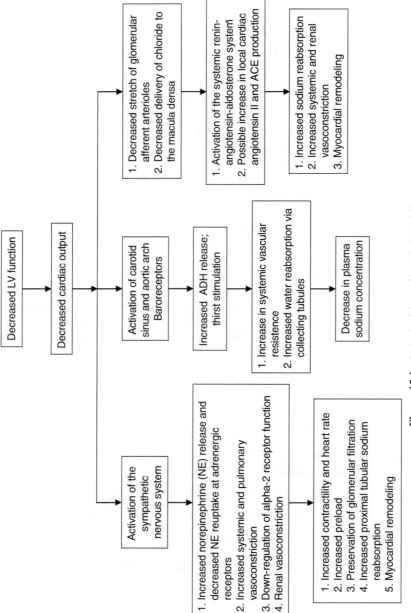

Figure 12.1 Pathophysiology of systolic heart failure.

cardiac remodeling further impairs cardiac function. The body's initial response to decreased cardiac output is increased sympathetic activity which restores cardiac output by increasing heart rate and contractility. Decreased cardiac output also promotes salt and water retention by the kidney via the renin-angiotensin-aldosterone system (RAAS). While these mechanisms initially compensate for the decrease in LV contractility and allow for sufficient end-organ perfusion, they eventually lead to maladaptive consequences including peripheral vasoconstriction, stimulation of myocardial fibrosis, and worsened cardiac remodeling. Adverse cardiac remodeling impairs wall stress and leads to an increase in myocardial oxygen demand. For many, the vicious cycle of RAAS activation and fibrosis leads to end-stage cardiac failure that is recalcitrant to standard medical therapy.

TAKE HOME POINT #2

Systolic heart failure results in cardiac remodeling and impaired myocardial contractility, both of which contribute to decreased cardiac output. Up-regulation of the sympathetic and RAA systems compensates to improve cardiac output initially but over time causes further worsening of heart failure.

12.5 CAUSES AND RISK FACTORS

Hypertension (HTN), diabetes mellitus (DM), and previous myocardial infarction (MI) are the most common risk factors associated with HF in patients with an elevated BMI or a decreased creatinine clearance. Other risk factors include valvular disease, macro- or microvascular coronary artery disease, tobacco use, toxin exposure (alcohol, chemotherapy), viral infection, poorly controlled atrial arrhythmias ("tachycardia-induced cardiomyopathy") and thyroid disease (Table 12.2).

Table 12.2 Risk Factors for the Development of HF.

Hypertension (RR 1.4, PAR 10%)
Coronary heart disease (RR 8.1, overall PAR 62%)
Cigarette smoking (RR 1.6, PAR 17%)
Overweight (RR 1.3, PAR 8%)
Diabetes mellitus (RR 1.9, PAR 3%)
Valvular heart disease (RR 1.5, PAR 2%; this risk factor increases with age)

PAR, Population Attributable Risk (estimates the proportion of cases that could be prevented if the risk factor was eliminated from the population); RR, Relative Risk.

12.6   CLINICAL HISTORY AND PHYSICAL EXAMINATION

Patients with decompensated HF often have a history of worsened dyspnea, fatigue, orthopnea, and PND. Exam often reveals rales, cardiac wheezing, worsened hypoxia or edema (of the legs and/or abdomen), the presence of jugular venous distention, and an S3 on cardiac exam. However, it is important to realize that not all patients with dyspnea and/or volume overload have HF. Other diagnoses that should always be considered include COPD exacerbation, pneumonia, PE, pulmonary hypertension, ischemic heart disease, arrhythmia, liver, and renal disease. Labwork and studies should help elucidate the underlying causative process (although in some cases it may be multifactorial). Brain Naturietic Peptide (BNP) has proven to be useful in distinguishing HF from other potential causes of dyspnea. A level of 400 or greater has a high positive predictive value for HF, whereas a level less than 100 has a high negative predictive value. Levels between 100 and 400 are neither sensitive nor specific for excluding HF. BNP levels tend to be higher in older individuals, women, and those with renal insufficiency; they tend to be lower in obese patients. EKG helps evaluate for evidence of arrhythmia, ischemia, interval infarction, right heart strain, and PE. Chest X-ray may show evidence of HF: cardiomegaly, pulmonary edema, or pleural effusions. Alternatively, it may show evidence of another process such as COPD or pneumonia.

12.7   OUTPATIENT MEDICAL MANAGEMENT

In addition to lifestyle modification and management of underlying etiologies and risk factors, medical therapy improves morbidity and mortality in patients with systolic heart failure. Therapies with proven morbidity and mortality benefit include ACE inhibitors (or ARBs if the former are not tolerated), beta-blockers, aldosterone antagonists, and hydralazine/nitrate combination therapy (Table 12.3). In addition, diuretics and digoxin may be considered for symptom improvement.

TAKE HOME POINT #3

Outpatient management of systolic HF should include treatment of underlying etiologies, patient education on diet, medications and lifestyle modifications, and appropriate medical therapies including ACE inhibitors, beta-blockers, and diuretics. Aldosterone antagonists, CRT, and digoxin should also be considered in appropriate individuals.

12.8   IMPLANTABLE CARIOVERTER-DEFIBRILLATOR (ICD) ± CARDIAC RESYNCHRONIZATION THERAPY

ICD implantation is indicated for primary and secondary prevention of sudden cardiac death in heart failure patients with a history of documented ventricular fibrillation (VF), hemodynamically unstable ventricular tachycardia (VT), VT with syncope, and LVEF less than or equal to 35% with significant HF symptoms. Table 12.4

Table 12.3   Medications Used in HF to Improve Morbidity and Mortality.

ACE inhibitors

Improve morbidity and mortality in all HF classes

Trials: CONSENSUS, SOLVD, XSOLVD, SAVE

May not be as effective in women and African Americans (V-HeFT)

Start with enalapril 2.5 mg bid, captopril 6.25 mg tid, lisinopril 2.5–5 mg daily

Goal enalapril 20 mg bid, captopril 50 mg tid, lisinopril 40 mg daily

Surveillance labs including serum BUN/creatinine and potassium should be checked
   3–7 days after drug initiation, during titration and after goal dose has been reached

Side effects: hypotension, worsened renal function, hyperkalemia, cough, angioedema

Beta-blockers

Carvedilol, metoprolol succinate and bisoprolol have been shown to improve morbidity and
   mortality in patients with NYHA class II–III. There is also evidence that these
   medications may improve morbidity and mortality in NYHA class IV patients

Trials: MERIT-HF; €, £, ¥

Carvedilol may be a better agent in patients with higher BPs, given its peripheral
   vasodilatory effects, while metoprolol succinate may be a better agent for patients with
   lower BPs

Start bisoprolol 1.25 mg daily, metoprolol succinate 12.5–25 mg daily, carvedilol 3.125 mg
   bid

Goal bisoprolol 10 mg daily, metoprolol succinate 200 mg daily, carvedilol 25 mg bid

Start at low dose and titrate up as BP and HR tolerate. While there is no evidence of value
   in aiming for a certain reduction in HR or a goal resting HR, standard practice is to aim
   for resting HRs in the 60s if tolerated

Angiotensin II receptor blockers (ARBs)

Recommended for patients who cannot tolerate ACE inhibitors. Have been shown to
   decrease hospitalization and mortality

Trials: CHARM-Alternative trial

ACC/AHA 2005 Practice Guidelines do not recommend the addition of ARBs to ACE
   inhibitor therapy given the lack of strong evidence and the increased risk of renal
   dysfunction and hyperkalemia

Start candesartan 4 mg daily, losartan 25 mg daily, valsartan bid

Goal candesartan 32 mg daily, losartan 100 mg daily, valsartan 160 mg bid

Similar side effect profile and titration schedule as ACE inhibitors

Aldosterone antagonists (spironolactone and eplerenone)

In patients with NYHA class III or IV HF symptoms or with LV dysfunction early
   after MI.

Patients should have an initial and stable serum creatinine less than 2–2.5 mg/dL. Initial
   sodium potassium should be <5 mEq/dL without a history of severe hyperkalemia

Trials: EPHESUS; Ω

Start spironolactone at 12.5 daily or every other day and eplerenone 25 mg daily

Goal spironolactone 25 mg daily, eplerenone 50 mg daily

(continued)

Table 12.3   Continued.

Consider decreasing or stopping potassium supplementation. The risk of hyperkalemia increases with higher doses of ACE inhibitors and with concurrent use of NSAIDs and COX-2 inhibitors

Side effects: hyperkalemia, worsened renal function, potentiation of other diuretic therapy (with subsequent fluid depletion). Spironolactone may cause gynecomastia

Aspirin

Should be used in patients with known coronary artery disease. No evidence of morbidity or mortality benefit in HF patients without coronary artery disease

Hydralazine plus nitrates

Recommended in African-American patients with moderate-to-severe symptoms already on optimal therapy with ACE inhibitors, beta-blockers and diuretics.

May be added in non-African–American patients with LV systolic function who have persistent HF symptoms despite therapy with ACE inhibitor and beta-blocker

May be used as an alternative to ACE inhibitors or ARBs in symptomatic patients with LVEF <40% when these medications are not tolerated

Trials: V-HeFT I and II

Start hydralazine 25 mg tid and isosorbide dinitrate 20 mg tid with uptitration every two weeks as tolerated

Goal is hydralazine 75 mg tid and isosorbide dinitrate 40 mg tid. There is no direct evidence for isosorbide mononitrate, but this may be used as an alternative to isosorbide dinitrate to improve compliance

Hydralazine can cause a lupus-like syndrome including arthralgias, myalgias, joint swelling, pericarditis/pleuritis, rash, and fever. Medication discontinuation should be strongly considered in this clinical setting

Digoxin

Used to improve symptoms and decrease hospitalization in patients with systolic dysfunction. No mortality benefit has been proven

Recommended in patients with LVEF <40% with NYHA class II, III or IV symptoms despite therapy with ACE inhibitor, beta-blocker and diuretic

Trials: DIG

Subgroup analysis in the DIG trial showed a trend towards increased mortality in women when the serum digoxin level was >1.2 ng/mL (death HR of 1.33 with p = 0.049, see Å for analysis). Renal function and digoxin levels should be monitored regularly.

€: Brophy JM et al. Beta-blockers in congestive heart failure. A Bayesian meta-analysis. Ann Intern Med. 2001; 134(7): 550–560.

£: Packer M et al. The effect of carvedilol on morbidity and mortality in patients with chronic heart failure. NEJM. 1996; 334(21):1349–1355.

¥: Packer M et al. Effect of carvedilol on survival in severe chronic heart failure. NEJM. 2001; 344(22): 1651–1658.

Ω: Pitt B, et al. The effect of spironolactone on morbidity and mortality in patients with severe heart failure. NEJM. 1999; 341:709–717.

Å: Adams KF Jr, et al. Relationship of serum digoxin concentration to mortality and morbidity in women in the digitalis investigation group trial: a retrospective analysis. JACC. 2005; 46(3):497–504.

Table 12.4   ICD Implantation in HF Patients for Primary and Secondary Prevention of Sudden Cardiac Death*.

Primary prevention

Class I recommendations

1. LV dysfunction secondary to ischemia (level of evidence=A)
   a. Patient at least 40 days post-MI with LVEF less than or equal to 35% and NYHA functional class II or III on optimal medical therapy

OR

   b. at least 40 days post-MI, LVEF less than or equal to 30%, and are NYHA functional class I on optimal medical therapy
   c. In patients with nonsustained VT due to prior MI, LVEF less than or equal to 40%, and inducible VF or VT at electrophysiological study (level of evidence=B)
2. LV dysfunction secondary to nonischemic heart disease (level of evidence=B)
   a. EF less than or equal to 35%
   b. NYHA functional class II or III on chronic optimal medical therapy

Class IIa recommendations

1. In patients with unexplained syncope, significant LV dysfunction and nonischemic dilated cardiomyopathy (level of evidence=C)

Class IIb recommendations

1. In patients with nonischemic heart disease (level of evidence=C)
   a. LVEF of less than or equal to 35%
   b. NYHA functional class I receiving chronic optimal medical therapy

Secondary prevention

Class I recommendations

1. In patients who survived ventricular fibrillation or hemodynamically unstable VT after evaluation to determine the cause and exclude any completely reversible cause (level of evidence=A)
2. VT with syncope (level of evidence=A)
   a. LVEF less than or equal to 40%
   b. On chronic optimal medial therapy

---

*All recommendations include the criteria that there is a reasonable expectation of survival with good functional status for more than 1 year.

shows guidelines for ICD implantation in patients with HF. A systemic review published in 2007 found that ICD implantation reduced all-cause mortality in adult patients with LV systolic dysfunction, most of whom had class II or III NYHA symptoms. Among randomized controlled trials this reduction was found to be 20% (largely due to a relative reduction in sudden cardiac death); in observational studies this reduction was found to be 46%.

In patients with advanced HF already on optimal medical therapy, cardiac resynchronization therapy (CRT) in addition to ICD therapy may be implemented. CRT involves placement of an additional lead in the coronary sinus in order to "resynchronize" the heart for more efficient pumping resulting in optimal cardiac function. To qualify, patients must have NYHA class III–IV symptoms, LVEF equal to or less than 35%, and intraventricular conduction delay on EKG (QRS interval >120 msec). Studies have shown a decrease in hospitalizations, an improvement in NYHA functional class and ejection fraction, and a reduction in arrhythmias and mitral regurgitation, in addition to a decrease in mortality with CRT.

While guidelines are useful in determining who may benefit from ICD implantation, the overall health of the patient and his/her long-term projected survival must be taken into consideration. Furthermore, subjects should receive extensive education on the risks and benefits of ICD implantation with the understanding that standard ICD therapy will not improve the quality of life but may impact survival.

TAKE HOME POINT #4

ICDs decrease all-cause mortality and sudden cardiac death in patients with severe LV dysfunction and should be considered in this patient population. Patients who qualify should undergo counseling regarding the risks, benefits and limitations of ICD implantation.

12.9 INPATIENT MEDICAL MANAGEMENT – FLOOR STATUS

After the diagnosis of decompensated heart failure is established, hospitalization is often required (Table 12.5). Once admitted, the patient should have his/her standing weight checked at the same time every day, preferably in the morning after the patient

Table 12.5 Recommendations for Heart Failure Hospitalization.

Hospitalization recommended
1. Evidence of severely decompensated HF (including hypotension, worsened renal function, altered mental status)
2. Dyspnea at rest or increased oxygen requirement
3. Arrhythmias causing hemodynamic instability
4. Acute coronary syndromes

Consider hospitalization
1. Worsened systemic congestion (e.g. weight gain of >5 kg)
2. Signs and/or symptoms of pulmonary congestion
3. Significant electrolyte disturbances
4. Comorbid conditions (e.g. pneumonia, pulmonary embolism, TIA)
5. Repeat ICD firing
6. New diagnosis of HF with evidence of systemic and/or pulmonary congestion

has voided and before he/she has eaten breakfast. Daily weights should be matched against urine output balance to ensure patient compliance with fluid restrictions. Daily symptoms should be assessed and a daily exam should be performed to help determine volume status. Labs (including electrolytes and renal function) should be drawn and reviewed on at least a daily basis. While BNP may be helpful in establishing the diagnosis of HF, repeated levels are unlikely to provide significant benefit over the course of an admission. Similarly, EKG should not be repeated routinely but should be performed if the patient's clinical condition changes. Routine surface echocardiogram is not indicated unless there is reasonable concern about progressive valvular disease (e.g. aortic stenosis) or decreased LV function. Echocardiogram should be deferred until the patient's volume status has improved to attain the most accurate data.

One of the key aspects of inpatient management is identifying and addressing precipitating factors, which can be found in Table 12.6. During this process, diuresis should be started to improve the patient's volume status and symptoms. Intravenous loop diuretics are considered first-line therapy. Standard practice is to start the patient on his/her home dose of oral diuretic but to administer it IV, thereby bypassing issues with reduced oral absorption. Diuretics should be titrated up to achieve sufficient diuresis (standard goal is 1–2 liters net out daily) without causing rapid decreases in intravascular volume causing hypotension and/or worsening renal failure. If intermittent bolus dosing two to three times a day fails to achieve sufficient diuresis then a continuous infusion may be considered. A diuretic primer, such as hydrochlorothiazide, metolazone, or IV diuril, should only be used if patients fail to achieve adequate urine output on higher-dose diuretics.

To improve symptoms of congestion (particularly pulmonary congestion) in patients with adequate blood pressure, afterload reduction is essential. Subjects not requiring ICU monitoring may benefit from IV nitroglycerin or oral afterload reduction. Hydralazine and nitrate combination therapy is often helpful in hypervolemic patients because the short half-life allows discontinuation in the setting of symptomatic hypotension. ACE inhibitors and ARBs can be titrated, although should be done so cautiously during active diuresis. Once the patient is near euvolemia (i.e. improved respiratory status, resolved jugular venous distention and improved abdominal/lower extremity edema), ACE inhibitors, ARBs and aldosterone antagonists should be titrated as tolerated in an effort to reduce RAAS activation. It is no longer standard practice to hold beta-blockers during HF decompensation, except in the setting of severe decompensation. Initiation of beta-blockers prior to discharge has been shown to improve beta-blocker utilization in the outpatient setting without significantly increased risk of serious adverse events.

If a patient does not immediately respond to dieresis, cardiology consultation can be considered.

Prior to discharge, precipitating/exacerbating factors should be addressed (Table 12.6), the patient's fluid status should be near optimal, the transition from an IV to oral diuretic regimen should be complete (ideally the patient should be observed for 24 hours on an oral regimen to ensure adequate urine output), and the patient should be on an appropriate HF medication regimen. Patient and family education should take place during hospitalization, including nutrition/medication counseling

Table 12.6   Precipitating Factors Associated with Decompensated HF.

1. Dietary indiscretion (excessive salt and/or water intake)
2. Medication non-adherence
3. Iatrogenic volume overload (e.g. perioperatively)
4. Progression of underlying cardiac problem
5. Physical/emotional stress
6. Cardiac toxins (alcohol, cocaine, chemotherapy)
7. Arrhythmia (e.g. atrial fibrillation)
8. Persistent RV pacing
9. Poorly controlled hypertension
10. ACS or recent MI
11. Progressive valvular disease
12. Pulmonary disease (e.g. PE, COPD)
13. Anemia
14. Infection
15. Thyroid disorder
16. Medications causing cardiac depression (e.g. nondihydropyridine calcium antagonists, type IA and IC antiarrythmic agents), sodium retention (e.g. NSAIDs) decrease cardiac contractility (anthracyclines, other chemotherapy agents), increased peripheral edema (pioglitazone/rosiglitazone), increased risk of arryhmias (TCAs, theophylline, beta-agonist bronchodilators)

and, if appropriate, tobacco cessation counseling. To reduce the risk of readmission (which is very high in HF), the patient should have close outpatient follow-up (goal 7–10 days following discharge).

12.10 INPATIENT MEDICAL MANAGEMENT – INTENSIVE CARE UNIT STATUS

Cardiology consultation should be obtained for all patients in the Intensive Care Unit (ICU) for HF. ICU transfer should be considered in HF patients with end-organ dysfunction, recurrent arrhythmias, and those needing significant inotrope/vasopressor support or percutaneous cardiac support. Patients should be evaluated for their level of HF decompensation.

In "warm and wet" individuals, perfusion is maintained in the setting of hypervolemia. In addition to diuretic therapy, afterload reduction will often markedly improve symptoms of congestion. IV nitroglycerin or nitroprusside may be considered in this context. Subjects with continuous cardiopulmonary hemodynamic monitoring may demonstrate a marked increase in cardiac output and a reduction in filling pressures and systemic vascular resistance (SVR). Given the potential for associated hypotension, patients on these therapies must have close blood pressure monitoring (usually with arterial line monitoring), and the agents should be decreased or stopped when hypotension (systolic blood pressures <80–85 mmHg) develops – especially in the setting of acidosis or worsening end-organ dysfunction.

Patients on nitroprusside should have thiocyanate levels checked periodically given the potential for this toxicity.

Subjects who are "cold and wet" require prompt intervention aimed at improving perfusion. Often, inotrope, vasopressor, and/or mechanical cardiac support is needed for a brief period to improve renal perfusion before diuresis is undertaken. In these patients, discontinuation of a beta-blocker is warranted. Milrinone and high-dose dobutamine are both first-line agents, but can worsen hypotension in severely-ill patients. Dopamine can be tried, but may augment tachycardia or arrhythmias. Often, percutaneous support (intra-aortic balloon pump, Tandem Heart, Impella) is the best approach to stabilizing a patient who has transplant/LVAD potential. In addition to providing hemodynamic stability, percutaneous support will allow assessment of the potential for end-organ recovery and provide time for completion of a candidacy evaluation.

12.11 INPATIENT MEDICAL MANAGEMENT – INTENSIVE CARE UNIT STATUS WITH TRANSPLANT FOR ASSIST DEVICE CONSIDERATION

Transplant or left ventricular assist device (LVAD) evaluation should ideally be considered in subjects at high risk for death whom are otherwise not in extremis. Outcomes are best in LVAD/transplant candidates referred *early* for intervention. Renal failure, hepatic dysfunction, vasopressor requirement, high-dose or multiple inotrope support, percutaneous mechanical support, and mechanical ventilation markedly increase patient risk for either intervention. A multidisciplinary approach is required during an LVAD/transplant evaluation. Assistance from a transplant/heart failure cardiologist, cardiac surgeon, social worker, nutritionist, and medical consultants (often nephrology) is warranted so that an appropriate care plan can be devised. While selected individuals may be deemed a transplant or LVAD candidate, others may warrant a palliative care/hospice referral.

> **TAKE HOME POINT #5**
>
> Successful inpatient management of decompensated HF includes patient risk stratification, addressing precipitating factors, adjustment of the patient's HF regimen to improve volume status and maintain end-organ function. Critically ill subjects or those with high-risk features warrant evaluation by a HF specialist.

KEY REFERENCES

ACC/AHA/HRS 2008 guidelines for device-based therapy of cardiac rhythm abnormalities. JACC 2008;51(21):e36–e37.

ADAMS K, LINDENFELD J-A, et al. Executive summary: HFSA 2006 comprehensive heart failure practice guideline. JCF 2006;12(1):10–38.

HUNT SA, et al. ACC/AHA 2005 Guideline update for the diagnosis and management of chronic heart failure in the adult: summary article: a report of the American College of Cardiology/American Heart Association Task Force on Practice Guidelines. JACC 2005;46:1116–1143.

Chapter 13

Diastolic Heart Failure

Anubhav Garg and Scott L. Hummel

13.1 INTRODUCTION

Diastolic heart failure patients present with signs and symptoms of heart failure in the setting of normal or near normal left ventricular ejection fraction. Ventricular diastolic dysfunction is the classic etiology for this syndrome, but recent studies indicate that other cardiac and noncardiac factors contribute to this heterogeneous condition. Due to this heterogeneity, diastolic heart failure is now often termed "heart failure with preserved ejection fraction" (HFPEF) or "heart failure with normal ejection fraction" (HFNEF). Despite the increasing prevalence of diastolic heart failure, there are no current evidence-based therapeutic strategies available. Accordingly, hospitalization rates and long-term mortality have not changed in recent years.

TAKE HOME POINT #1

Three conditions need to be satisfied for the diagnosis of diastolic heart failure:

1. Signs and/or symptoms of congestive heart failure
2. Normal or near normal left ventricular ejection fraction, usually defined as greater than 50%
3. Lack of obvious other structural cause for heart failure (i.e. valvular, congenital, pericardial heart disease).

Inpatient Cardiovascular Medicine, First Edition. Edited by Brahmajee K. Nallamothu and Timir S. Baman.
© 2014 John Wiley & Sons, Inc. Published 2014 by John Wiley & Sons, Inc.

13.2   EPIDEMIOLOGY

Diastolic heart failure currently accounts for nearly half of all patients with heart failure. In comparison to systolic heart failure, patients with diastolic heart failure are older, more commonly female, more likely to have hypertension and atrial fibrillation, and less likely to have *previously diagnosed* coronary artery disease. The prevalence of diastolic heart failure increases with age and accounts for more than 50% of the prevalence of heart failure in patients over the age of 70. The mode of death in patients with diastolic heart failure is due to cardiovascular causes in 60% (with sudden death and death from heart failure being the most common), noncardiovascular causes in 30%, and is unknown in the remaining 10%.

13.3   PATHOPHYSIOLOGY

Diastole is composed of four major phases:

1. Isovolumetric relaxation during which time both the mitral and aortic valves are closed
2. Rapid ventricular filling immediately after mitral valve opening
3. Slowed ventricular filling
4. Filling during atrial contraction.

Diastolic function is determined by two major factors: the active process of myocardial relaxation and the passive process of left ventricular elasticity or distensibility. Impairment of either LV diastolic relaxation or distensibility leads to increased pulmonary venous, left atrial, and left ventricular diastolic pressures. This results in a shift in LV filling from early to late diastole with subsequent greater reliance on atrial contraction. Recent studies indicate that "diastolic" heart failure is a heterogeneous condition with multiple additional pathophysiologic mechanisms (e.g. vascular dysfunction, subtle systolic dysfunction, chronotropic incompetence, etc.).

13.4   ETIOLOGIES

Numerous cardiac disorders can result in the development of diastolic dysfunction. The most common underlying etiology of diastolic heart failure is systemic hypertension with associated comorbidities such as diabetes mellitus, chronic kidney disease, coronary artery disease, and atrial arrhythmias likely contributing in many cases. Less common etiologies include hypertrophic cardiomyopathy, infiltrative cardiomyopathy, and restrictive cardiomyopathy. These rarer causes should be considered particularly in patients who do not fit the typical epidemiologic profile, i.e. a younger patient without hypertension. It is important to recognize that patients with normal left ventricular ejection fraction can still have heart failure even without definitive evidence of diastolic dysfunction (Table 13.1). Both clinical history and subsequent diagnostic studies as discussed below are essential for the evaluation of potential etiologies for a patient's diastolic heart failure.

Table 13.1 Etiologies of Heart Failure with Normal Ejection Fraction.

Diastolic heart failure	Hypertension
	Coronary artery disease
	Hypertrophic cardiomyopathy
	Infiltrative cardiomyopathy
	Restrictive cardiomyopathy
Right heart failure	Severe pulmonary hypertension
	Right ventricular infarct
Valvular heart disease	Severe valvular stenosis
	Severe valvular regurgitation
Pericardial disease	Cardiac tamponade
	Constrictive pericarditis
Intracardiac mass	Atrial myxoma
Congenital heart disease	Atrial septal defect
	Ventricular septal defect

TAKE HOME POINT #2

The major etiologies of diastolic heart failure include chronic hypertension and coronary artery disease with less common etiologies including hypertrophic cardiomyopathy, infiltrative cardiomyopathy, and restrictive cardiomyopathy.

13.5 CLINICAL PRESENTATION

The majority of patients with ventricular diastolic dysfunction are asymptomatic and thus, by definition, do not have diastolic heart failure. Several factors, both cardiovascular and noncardiovascular, can potentiate onset of symptoms and subsequently lead to decompensated diastolic heart failure. Such triggers are similar to those for systolic heart failure and include increased salt and water intake, medication noncompliance, tachyarrhythmias, uncontrolled hypertension, acute or chronic renal disease, arrhythmia, and myocardial ischemia. The resulting symptoms of heart failure are similar to those in patients with systolic dysfunction and include dyspnea on exertion, fatigue, and evidence of volume overload such as lower extremity edema and abdominal distention. It is important to recognize that not all patients who are hospitalized with heart failure in the setting of a normal left ventricular ejection fraction necessarily have diastolic heart failure, as these symptoms may instead be caused by valvular heart disease, pericardial disease, congenital heart disease, or intracardiac masses (Table 13.1).

TAKE HOME POINT #3

Patients with diastolic heart failure have clinically similar symptoms to patients with systolic heart failure, including dyspnea on exertion, lower extremity edema, abdominal distention, and fatigue. Findings on examination are also similar and may include jugular venous distention, rales, hepatomegaly, and peripheral edema.

13.6   EVALUATION AND DIAGNOSTIC STUDIES

The diagnosis of diastolic heart failure requires that three conditions are met: (1) signs and/or symptoms of heart failure; (2) preserved left ventricular ejection fraction, usually defined as greater than 50%; and (3) lack of obvious other structural cause (i.e. valvular, congenital, pericardial heart disease). The diagnosis may be obtained by a complete history and physical exam along with a diagnostic evaluation of cardiac structure and function, typically with an echocardiogram. The evaluation of ventricular diastolic function is complex and typically involves special echocardiographic techniques and, rarely, invasive measurements. Currently, there is much controversy about whether definitive evidence of diastolic dysfunction is necessary to make the diagnosis of "diastolic" heart failure.

TAKE HOME POINT #4

The initial evaluation of diastolic heart failure should include a complete history, physical examination, electrocardiogram, chest radiograph, and echocardiogram.

As mentioned above, the initial step to evaluating diastolic heart failure is performing a complete history and physical exam. This is necessary both to evaluate for signs and symptoms of heart failure along with determining potential etiologies for the patient's heart failure. A history of prior hospitalizations for heart failure exacerbation also provides significant prognostic information for both re-hospitalization and death.

Routine laboratory work-up should be performed. Cardiac enzymes can be clinically relevant if the patient presents with signs and symptoms of myocardial ischemia such as angina or rapid onset of heart failure without a clear underlying etiology. The plasma level of B-type natriuretic peptide (BNP) is typically elevated in patients with diastolic heart failure and provides prognostic information. However, a normal BNP level does not rule out diastolic heart failure, and BNP levels cannot be used to differentiate between systolic or diastolic heart failure.

An electrocardiogram should be performed in all patients with diastolic heart failure, and can provide evidence of left ventricular hypertrophy, myocardial ischemia or infarction, and/or arrhythmia to suggest potential etiologies. A chest X-ray can reveal evidence of pulmonary edema or primary pulmonary causes of dyspnea.

All patients with suspected heart failure should have an echocardiogram to distinguish between systolic and diastolic heart failure. An echocardiogram is the most practical routine diagnostic modality to assess cardiac structure and function. Most importantly, it can confirm normal or near normal left ventricular ejection fraction and can evaluate other diagnoses which are associated with signs and symptoms of heart failure and a normal left ventricular ejection fraction (i.e. pericardial disease, valvular disease, intracardiac masses). In addition, echocardiography provides an assessment of left ventricular thickness and mass, left atrial size, and pulmonary artery pressures, all of which are typically elevated in the setting of diastolic heart failure. An echocardiogram may also help to distinguish between different etiologies of diastolic heart failure, which has clinical implications for specific therapies (as discussed in Section 13.8 below).

Specific echocardiographic techniques can provide a comprehensive and noninvasive evaluation of diastolic function. The transmitral Doppler inflow velocity waveform during normal sinus rhythm has two components, the E wave and the A wave, which represent the flow from the left atrium to the left ventricle during diastole. The E wave specifically represents early diastolic filling while the A wave represents left atrial contraction. The E wave velocity is dependent on the pressure gradient across the mitral valve. Transmitral Doppler inflow velocity measurement alone is not sufficient to diagnose diastolic dysfunction as it is very sensitive to left atrial preload and can be misleading with progression of diastolic dysfunction. Tissue Doppler velocity measures the velocity of myocardial motion at the mitral annulus and is less sensitive to left atrial preload, thus providing additional information to

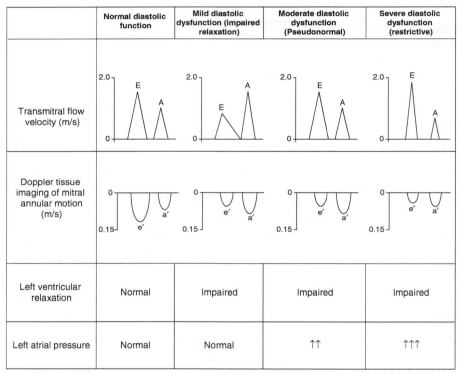

Figure 13.1   Doppler echocardiographic patterns of left ventricular diastolic filling. Mild diastolic dysfunction is characterized by impaired left ventricular relaxation with subsequent decreased transmitral pressure gradient. This results in decreased velocity of early filling with increased velocity with atrial contraction and overall reduced E:A ratio. Moderate diastolic dysfunction is characterized by increased left atrial pressure resulting in normal appearing E-wave velocity and E:A ratio (pseudonormal pattern). With severe diastolic dysfunction, left atrial pressure is markedly increased with subsequent increase in the transmitral pressure gradient above normal, resulting in high E-wave velocity and above normal E:A ratio. Doppler tissue imaging in mild, moderate, or severe diastolic dysfunction reveals reduced mitral annular motion during early filling as compared with during atrial contraction and can help to differentiate pseudonormal diastolic dysfunction from normal diastolic dysfunction.

accurately assess diastolic function (Figure 13.1). Other methods of diastolic function assessment by echocardiography are beyond the scope of this chapter.

Although cardiac catheterization can be used to invasively assess the left ventricular ejection fraction and the presence of diastolic dysfunction, these invasive techniques are impractical given the wide availability and utility of echocardiography. Cardiac catheterization is primarily used when coronary artery disease is suspected as the underlying etiology of the patient's heart failure. Right heart catheterization to assess cardiac output and filling pressures may be useful when the diagnosis of diastolic heart failure is in question, the patient's volume status is unclear, or in the rare instance where endomyocardial biopsy is indicated (e.g. suspicion of infiltrative cardiomyopathy).

13.7 RISK STRATIFICATION

It is important to risk stratify patients presenting with diastolic heart failure. Several variables predict a significantly increased in-hospital mortality rate and can serve as a guide for both in-hospital care as well as the transition to outpatient care. Per the ADHERE registry, BUN >37 mg/dl, systolic BP ≤125 mm Hg, and Cr >2.0 mg/dl are the three most important predictors of mortality but sodium ≤132 mmol/l, age >73 years, presence of dyspnea at rest, and heart rate >78 beats/min are also independent predictors (Table 13.2). A history of prior cardiac hospitalizations is also a strong predictor of both re-hospitalization and overall mortality. In a patient with diastolic heart failure presenting with a high-risk profile, a low threshold for cardiology consultation is warranted.

13.8 TREATMENT

Despite several randomized clinical trials (involving digoxin, beta-blockers, angiotensin converting-enzyme inhibitors, and angiotensin receptor blockers), no specific agents have been shown to improve survival rates in diastolic heart failure. The lack of evidence-based therapeutic strategies may be due to the heterogeneous

Table 13.2   Factors Associated with Increased In-Hospital Mortality Rate.

Systolic BP ≤125 mm Hg
BUN >37
Cr >2.0 mg/dl
History of prior cardiac hospitalizations
Sodium ≤132 mmol/l
Age >73 years
Dyspnea at rest
Heart rate >78 beats/min

nature of the disease and the fact that 30–40% of deaths in this patient population are noncardiovascular in etiology. In the absence of evidence-based therapies, the inpatient approach to diastolic heart failure is threefold: alleviation of the patient's symptoms, treatment of the underlying precipitant for the patient's heart failure, and investigation and treatment of underlying etiologies and comorbid conditions (Table 13.3, Figure 13.2).

TAKE HOME POINT #5

Therapy for diastolic heart failure is largely empiric. There are three main goals of inpatient therapy: alleviation of symptoms, treatment of the precipitant of the heart failure exacerbation, and investigation and treatment of underlying etiologies and comorbid conditions.

Similar to systolic heart failure, patients with diastolic heart failure develop pulmonary venous congestion and peripheral edema due to retention of salt and water. Dietary sodium and fluid restriction (typically 2 grams sodium and 2 liters fluid restriction per 24 hours) along with diuretics remains the mainstay of therapy in these patients to improve volume overload and associated symptoms. Long-term administration of diuretics is usually necessary in these patients. However, it is important to diurese these patients gently since they may be "preload sensitive" and prone to develop hypotension and renal insufficiency with too rapid diuresis. Achieving optimal volume status becomes increasingly more difficult with advancing diastolic heart failure due to the progressively narrowing window between venous congestion and insufficient ventricular preload.

An empiric guide to appropriate use of diuretics is provided in Figure 13.3. First-line therapy typically consists of intravenous loop diuretics. Initially, the patient should be initiated on his/her home diuretic dose in intravenous form. If the patient has good diuretic response within 1–2 hours of diuretic administration, the intravenous dose should be given anywhere from one to three times daily to achieve a standard goal of 1–2 liters net fluid loss per day. If no notable diuretic response is noted within 1–2 hours of diuretic administration, the dosage should be doubled to a maximum of 120 mg intravenous lasix (or equivalent dosing of a different loop diuretic). If, despite the above measures, the patient continues to have limited diuresis, either a diuretic primer such as hydrochlorothiazide, metolazone, or chlorothiazide should be given 30 minutes prior to the intravenous loop diuretic or intravenous bolus of loop diuretic followed by continuous infusion should be considered. If the patient has limited response to diuretic therapy or is noted to have developing hypotension, impending renal failure, or other end organ dysfunction, cardiology and/or nephrology consultation should be considered. Ultrafiltration is sometimes used for volume removal in highly diuretic-resistant patients, although evidence for this approach in diastolic heart failure is limited.

Hypertension contributes to cardiovascular abnormalities found in most patients with diastolic heart failure (i.e. left ventricular hypertrophy and resulting diastolic

Table 13.3 Management Guidelines for Patients with Diastolic Heart Failure.

Goal	Therapy	Suggested medications/referrals
Reduce venous congestion	Salt restriction <2 g/day Fluid restriction <2 L/day Diuretics	Hydrochlorothiazide 12.5–25 mg daily Chlorothiazide 250–1000 mg daily Metolazone 2.5–5 mg daily Furosemide 10–120 mg daily to bid Torsemide 10–200 mg daily Bumetanide 1–4 mg daily to bid
Optimal hypertension control	Antihypertensive agents	Hydrochlorothiazide 12.5–25 mg daily Metoprolol 12.5–200 mg bid Atenolol 12.5–100 mg daily Carvedilol 6.25–25 mg bid Nebivolol 2.5–40 mg daily Amlodipine 2.5–10 mg daily Felodipine 2.5–10 mg daily Lisinopril 2.5–80 mg daily Enalapril 2.5–40 mg daily Candesartan 4–32 mg daily Losartan 25–100 mg daily
Tachyarrhythmia control	Beta blockers Calcium channel blockers Digoxin Cardioversion of atrial fibrillation Atrioventricular nodal ablation with permanent pacemaker	Metoprolol 12.5–200 mg bid Atenolol 12.5–100 mg daily Verapamil 40–120 mg tid Diltiazem 30–90 mg qid Digoxin 0.125–0.25 mg daily Cardiology consultation Cardiology consultation
Treatment of myocardial ischemia	Beta blockers (preferred) Calcium channel blockers Nitrates Percutaneous coronary intervention	Metoprolol 12.5–200 mg bid Atenolol 12.5–100 mg daily Verapamil 40–120 mg tid Diltiazem 30–90 mg qid Isosorbide mononitrate 30–120 mg daily Isosorbide dinitrate 10–40 mg bid to tid Cardiology consultation

dysfunction, vascular stiffness). In addition to its other benefits, blood pressure control reduces left ventricular hypertrophy and may improve ventricular diastolic function over time. If uncontrolled hypertension has precipitated the hospitalization (e.g. hypertensive crisis with pulmonary edema), aggressive blood pressure control may be warranted. Intravenous nitrates can rapidly improve hypertensive pulmonary edema and should be strongly considered in this setting. Many oral antihypertensive agents can take a few weeks to reach full effect. Therefore, rapid up-titration of oral medications in inpatients who are otherwise responding well to therapy is discouraged

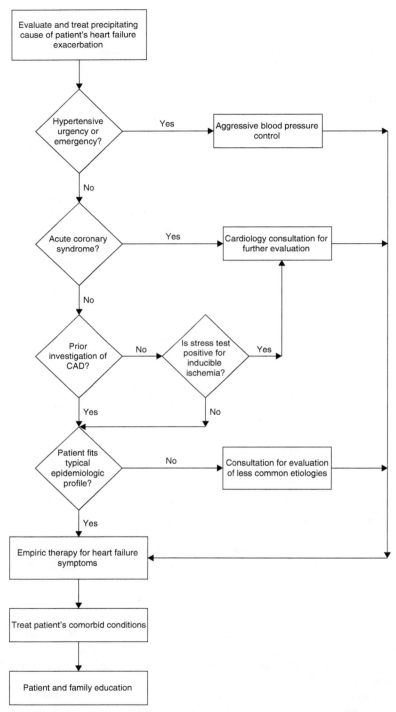

Figure 13.2 Algorithm for inpatient evaluation and treatment of DHF. Treatment of diastolic heart failure is threefold: (1) alleviation of the patient's symptoms; (2) treatment of the precipitant of the heart failure exacerbation; (3) investigation and treatment of underlying etiologies and comorbid conditions. This figure provides a simple algorithm for evaluating and treating diastolic heart failure.

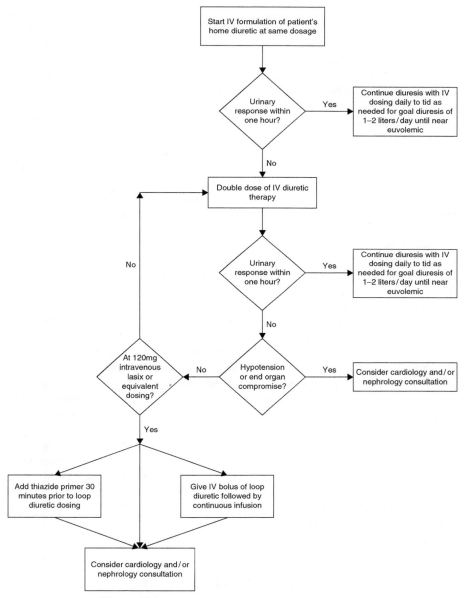

Figure 13.3   Empiric guide to appropriate use of diuretics.

as it may subsequently lead to hypotension and falls, especially in this elderly population of patients. Data are lacking on the choice of specific antihypertensive agents but should be guided by the presence of coexisting conditions such as diabetes mellitus, coronary artery disease, and renal insufficiency (see Chapter 23, Hypertension).

Myocardial ischemia from epicardial coronary artery disease or subendocardial ischemia in the setting of left ventricular hypertrophy can exacerbate diastolic heart failure. In this elderly population with prevalent coronary risk factors, a high index of suspicion for coronary disease is warranted. Any patient without a clear etiology for their diastolic heart failure merits evaluation for coronary artery disease unless its presence would not change management. This may require the assistance of cardiology consultation. It is worth noting that in diastolic heart failure patients with previous myocardial infarction, beta-blockers decrease long-term mortality and can improve anginal symptoms.

Tachyarrhythmias, especially atrial fibrillation, are poorly tolerated in diastolic heart failure due to the shortened time for left ventricular filling and the shift in LV filling from early to late diastole with subsequent reliance on atrial contraction. Thus, in patients with diastolic dysfunction, the development of atrial fibrillation with rapid ventricular response can result in worsening heart failure. It is important to rate control patients who develop atrial fibrillation with beta blockers, nondihydropyridine calcium channel blockers, and/or digoxin. Due to age and comorbidities, most diastolic heart failure patients with atrial fibrillation are at risk of thromboembolic events and should be considered for systemic anticoagulation (see Chapter 20, Atrial Fibrillation and Atrial Flutter). In cases where, despite adequate rate control, patients continue to have significant intolerance of atrial fibrillation, restoration of sinus rhythm may be preferred with cardioversion, antiarrhythmic medication therapy and, in some cases, radiofrequency ablation. Cardiology consultation should be considered in these cases.

Other comorbid conditions should be aggressively sought and treated. Given the high prevalence of obesity, one condition worthy of particular mention is sleep apnea, which contributes to pulmonary hypertension, right heart dysfunction, and atrial arrhythmias. If patients or their family members report a history of frequent snoring, nocturnal apneic spells, morning fatigue, headaches, or daytime somnolence, a sleep study is warranted for further evaluation.

In general, patients should not be discharged home until the precipitating factor for their heart failure exacerbation is addressed, euvolemia or near-euvolemia is achieved, and a stable, effective diuretic regimen is established. Ideally, prior to discharge, the patient should be observed on an oral diuretic regimen for 24 hours to ensure continued and adequate urinary response. Patients sent home before these goals are achieved are at high risk of recurrence of heart failure exacerbation and re-hospitalization.

13.9 TRANSITION TO OUTPATIENT CARE

Limiting re-hospitalization in patients with diastolic heart failure presents a significant challenge. Intensive education about heart failure "self-care measures" and careful coordination of care can improve post-discharge outcomes. Current guidelines recommend that six key components should be addressed in the discharge plan: (1) activity level; (2) dietary restrictions; (3) discharge medications; (4) follow-up appointments; (5) weight monitoring; and (6) what to do if symptoms worsen

Table 13.4 Factors to Address at Hospital Discharge.

Factor to address	Potential interventions
Activity level	Gradual exercise program
	Cardiac rehabilitation
Dietary restrictions	2 g Na restriction, 2 L fluid restriction
	Referral to registered dietician
Discharge medications	List of home medications to continue
	List of home medications to discontinue
	List of new medications to start
	Clear instructions for medication usage
Follow-up appointments	Preferred within 7 days of hospital discharge
	Referral to specialty heart failure clinic
Weight monitoring	Daily weight monitoring
	Instructions on additional dosing of diuretic for weight gain of 2 pounds in one day or 3–5 pounds in 2–3 days
What to do if symptoms worsen	Contact information for PCP/heart failure specialist

(Table 13.4). Dietary sodium restriction is particularly important in this population, and instruction by a registered dietician, either in the hospital or as an outpatient, can be invaluable. Studies have also shown that earlier outpatient follow-up, within seven days of hospital discharge, reduces 30 day re-hospitalization rates. Patients with multiple risk factors for adverse outcomes (see Section 13.7 above) should be considered for follow-up in a specialty heart failure clinic.

TAKE HOME POINT #6

Six key components must be addressed with patient/family at time of hospital discharge: (1) activity level; (2) dietary restrictions; (3) discharge medications; (4) follow-up appointments; (5) weight monitoring; and (6) what to do if symptoms worsen.

KEY REFERENCES

AURIGEMMA GP, et al. Diastolic heart failure. New Engl J Med 2004;351:1097–1105 (classic article).

FONAROW GC, et al. Characteristics, treatments, and outcomes of patients with preserved systolic function hospitalized for heart failure: a report from the OPTIMIZE-HF Registry. J Am Coll Cardiol 2007;50(8):768–777.

JANARDHANAN MD, et al. Therapeutic approaches to diastolic dysfunction. Curr Hypertens Rep 2009;11(4):283–291.

YANCY CW, et al. Clinical presentation, management, and in-hospital outcomes of patients admitted with acute decompensated heart failure with preserved systolic function: a report from the Acute Decompensated Heart Failure National Registry (ADHERE) Database. J Am Coll Cardiol 2006;47(1):76–84.

Chapter 14

Dilated and Restrictive Cardiomyopathy

Brahmajee K. Nallamothu and Timir S. Baman

14.1 INTRODUCTION

Cardiomyopathies are a collection of heterogeneous cardiovascular disorders that directly affect the myocardium, leading to cardiac dysfunction and heart failure. The causes of cardiomyopathy are numerous, and specific etiologies can be difficult for the clinician to determine. They may include infectious etiologies (e.g. viral); genetic, inflammatory or inflammatory processes (e.g. sarcoidosis); toxic agents (e.g. chemotherapeutic drugs, alcohol); metabolic conditions; and storage diseases (e.g. hemochromatosis). Importantly, in order to diagnose cardiomyopathy known cardiovascular insults that may also damage the myocardium must be excluded (e.g. hypertension, valvular heart disease and coronary artery disease).

For hospitalists, the overall management of patients with cardiomyopathy requires a targeted focus on managing acute symptoms related to heart failure (see Chapter 12, Systolic Heart Failure) and determining an individual's long-term risk of complications such as re-hospitalization for recurrent symptoms and sudden death. In this chapter, we focus on dilated and restrictive cardiomyopathies. The next chapter addresses hypertrophic cardiomyopathy, a particular form of cardiomyopathy caused by complex genetic abnormalities in the sarcomere complex.

TAKE HOME POINT #1

To diagnose dilated or restrictive cardiomyopathy, known cardiovascular insults such as hypertension, valvular heart disease, and coronary artery disease must be excluded.

Inpatient Cardiovascular Medicine, First Edition. Edited by Brahmajee K. Nallamothu and Timir S. Baman.
© 2014 John Wiley & Sons, Inc. Published 2014 by John Wiley & Sons, Inc.

14.2   DILATED CARDIOMYOPATHY

14.2.1   Epidemiology and Pathophysiology

Dilated cardiomyopathy is not uncommon. Its prevalence in the general population is estimated to be 1 in 2500 individuals, although this may be an underestimation given the possibility of patients with asymptomatic cardiac dysfunction. Dilated cardiomyopathy arises from a variety of potential etiologies, but its unifying characteristic is myocardial injury that results in significant enlargement of the heart with subsequent ventricular dilatation. Table 14.1 lists several key examples of causes linked to various forms of dilated cardiomyopathy. However, most cases remain idiopathic despite extensive investigations. As with other forms of heart failure, reduced stroke volume from myocardial injury diminishes forward cardiac output, which in turn leads to pulmonary and venous congestion.

TAKE HOME POINT #2

Dilated cardiomyopathy affects 1 in 2500 people worldwide, and its cause is usually idiopathic.

14.2.2   Clinical Characteristics and Evaluation

Patients with dilated cardiomyopathy typically present with classic symptoms of heart failure, including dyspnea on exertion, fatigue, paroxysmal nocturnal dyspnea, and orthopnea. Ascites and peripheral edema are also frequently present and may develop slowly over time. In addition to gathering information about symptoms, a complete history and physical examination should be obtained to look for potential etiologies. The EKG and chest X-ray are usually abnormal in patients with dilated cardiomyopathy, although findings are nonspecific. The EKG may show atrial and ventricular enlargement, conduction defects, atrial and ventricular tachyarrhythmias, and diffuse repolarization changes in the ST and T wave segments. The chest X-ray classically shows an enlarged cardiac silhouette with various degrees of evidence for pulmonary congestion (e.g. interstitial and alveolar edema, pleural effusions).

The echocardiogram is the most critical test in evaluating patients with suspected dilated cardiomyopathy. Findings from the echocardiogram show: (1) significant dilation of the left ventricle (LV) (although it can also involve the right ventricle [RV] and atrial chambers as well); (2) minimal or decreased wall thickness of the LV ventricle; and (3) markedly reduced systolic contraction of the LV as evidenced by a poor ejection fraction (EF) (Figure 14.1). Abnormalities in diastolic function as well as mitral and tricuspid regurgitation that can be detected by Doppler may also exist. Similar findings of LV dilation and systolic dysfunction are often noted on other cardiac imaging studies, such as nuclear scintigraphy and MUGA, cardiac MRI, and cardiac CT. Although these tests may provide additional information (e.g. extent of

Table 14.1   Key Examples of Causes Linked to Dilated Cardiomyopathy.

Etiologies of dilated cardiomyopathy

Idiopathic

Infectious
Coxsackievirus
EBV
HIV
Lyme Disease

Medications
Chemotherapeutic agents (doxorubicin, daunorubicin, cyclophosphamide)
Antiretroviral agents

Toxins
Ethanol
Lead
Amphetamines
Cocaine
Carbon monoxide

Metabolic disorders
Hyperthyroidism
Hypothyroidism
Cushing's disease

Connective tissue disorders
Systemic lupus erythematous
Scleroderma
Sarcoidosis
Autoimmune myocarditis

Others
Peripartum cardiomyopathy
Tachycardia-induced cardiomyopathy
Radiation-induced cardiomyopathy
Duchenne's muscular dystrophy
Hypocalcemia/hypophosphatemia
Carnitine deficiencies

inflammatory or infiltrative processes), their use is typically restricted to specific settings. Cardiac catheterization with coronary angiography, on the other hand, is frequently performed to definitively rule out concomitant coronary artery disease. Right heart catheterization may help guide treatment goals by measuring intracardiac pressures, like the pulmonary capillary wedge pressure, but biopsy of the right ventricle is rarely used as it is unusual for biopsy to change acute or chronic management plans.

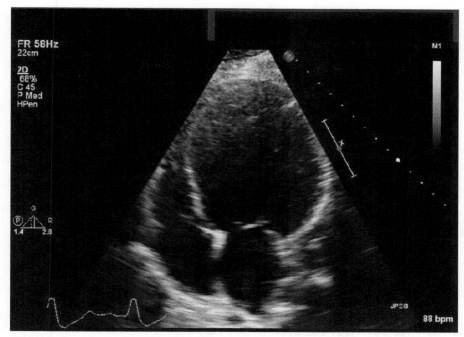

Figure 14.1 Echocardiogram in the apical four chamber view of dilated cardiomyopathy. There is extensive dilatation of the LV with systolic dysfunction.

TAKE HOME POINT #3

The echocardiogram is critical in diagnosing patients with dilated cardiomyopathy given its characteristic appearance of LV dilatation and systolic dysfunction.

A number of additional laboratory studies may be used selectively to identify specific etiologies for dilated cardiomyopathy, but their use is best targeted by information gathered during the history and physical examination. For example, cardiac troponins and CK-MB elevations may be present in some patients with active myocarditis and reflect ongoing necrosis from an infectious or inflammatory process. As in heart failure, the use of serial biomarkers indicative of a fluid overload state, like BNP, can guide treatment in select patients.

14.2.3 Treatment

Consistent with the overall treatment goals for heart failure in general, patients with dilated cardiomyopathy should have therapies instituted for symptom relief and long-term risk reduction. In addition, the identification of any reversible causes should be considered. For example, patients with dilated cardiomyopathy due to a toxic agent (e.g. chemotherapeutic drug) should be counseled to avoid repeated exposure. Other therapies are consistent with the goals of systolic heart failure treatment outlined in Chapter 12 and include ACE inhibitors, ARBs, beta-blockers, aldosterone inhibitors, digitalis, and diuretics. Similarly, the long-term risk of ventricular arrhythmias should prompt consideration for ICD therapies while some patients may benefit from cardiac resynchronization therapy with bi-ventricular pacing. Given their high risk for thromboembolic events, anticoagulation is often used in these patients as well but this frequently depends upon the presence of an LV thrombus on echocardiogram, atrial fibrillation or prior thromboembolic event. In patients with severe or rapidly progressive disease, early consultation with a cardiologist specializing in heart failure may be warranted to consider mechanical assist devices and heart transplantation.

TAKE HOME POINT #4

Treatment for dilated cardiomyopathy should be guided by the general principles for management of heart failure, including diuretics, ACE inhibitors, beta-blockers, and aldosterone inhibitors.

14.3   RESTRICTIVE CARDIOMYOPATHY

14.3.1   Epidemiology and Pathophysiology

The prevalence of restrictive cardiomyopathies is lower than dilated and hypertrophic cardiomyopathies in the general population. The main cause of restrictive cardiomyopathy in Western countries is cardiac amyloidosis, which is due to the deposits of amyloid proteins into the extracellular tissue of the heart. Endomyocardial fibrosis is endemic in certain tropical regions of the world like equatorial Africa and results in fibrosis of the endomyocardium. As in dilated cardiomyopathy, idiopathic forms of restrictive cardiomyopathy have also been linked to genetic defects. Table 14.2 summarizes many conditions responsible for restrictive cardiomyopathy, stratified by myocardial and endomyocardial involvement. The common characteristic unifying this disease process is impairment in ventricular filling due to poor relaxation. For the most part, systolic function of the LV (or RV) remains normal while wall thickness may be normal or enlarged. Restrictive cardiomyopathy should be considered in patients who present with heart failure but normal LV systolic function.

TAKE HOME POINT #5

The most common cause of restrictive cardiomyopathy in Western countries is cardiac amyloidosis.

Table 14.2   Key Examples of Causes Linked to Restrictive Cardiomyopathy.

Etiologies of restrictive cardiomyopathy

Myocardial

Infiltrative
  Amyloidosis
  Sarcoidosis
  Gaucher's disease
  Fatty infiltration

Noninfiltrative
  Idiopathic cardiomyopathy
  Familial cardiomyopathy
  Scleroderma
  Diabetic cardiomyopathy

Storage diseases
  Hemochromatosis
  Glycogen storage disease
  Fabry's disease

Endomyocardial
  Endomyocardial fibrosis
  Hypereosinophillic syndrome
  Carcinoid heart disease
  Radiation

14.3.2 Clinical Characteristics and Evaluation

Patients with restrictive cardiomyopathy also present with classic symptoms of heart failure, including dyspnea on exertion, fatigue, paroxysmal nocturnal dyspnea, orthopnea, ascites and peripheral edema. However, restrictive cardiomyopathy can also be associated with the systemic disorders that lead to infiltrative processes. Gathering information about these systemic disorders, especially amyloidosis and storage diseases, is important. For example, amyloidosis rarely affects the heart in isolation and should be suspected when other symptoms like renal dysfunction with proteinuria, hepatomegaly, and neuropathy are present. As always, a complete history and physical examination should be obtained to look for potential etiologies. The EKG and chest X-ray can be clues for specific disease processes. The EKG may show nonspecific findings like conduction defects, atrial and ventricular tachyarrhythmias, and diffuse repolarization changes in the ST and T wave segments. In cardiac amyloidosis, there is often significant hypertrophy on echocardiography that is accompanied by low voltage on the EKG in the limb leads. The chest X-ray classically shows various degrees of evidence for pulmonary congestion (e.g. interstitial and alveolar edema, pleural effusions) but a normal cardiac silhouette. The

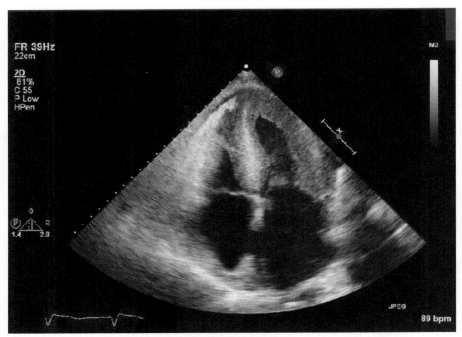

Figure 14.2   Echocardiogram in the apical four chamber view of restricted cardiomyopathy due to cardiac amyloidosis. There is extensive thickening of the LV with a "speckled" pattern noted. Thickening of the RV and biatrial enlargement is also present.

echocardiogram is an important test in evaluating patients for restrictive cardiomyopathy. Findings from the echocardiogram show normal LV systolic function and ejection fraction with restricted diastolic filling (which are covered in Chapter 13). In cardiac amyloidosis, the echocardiogram can reveal a markedly thickened LV wall with a classic "speckled" pattern (Figure 14.2).

A key consideration in evaluating restrictive cardiomyopathy is distinguishing it from constrictive pericarditis given similarities in presentation and the potential for constrictive pericarditis to be treated with surgery. This can be challenging and typically requires cardiac catheterization and additional imaging studies. Findings expected in restrictive cardiomyopathy and constrictive pericarditis are listed in Table 14.3. No technique is entirely reliable but in combination may be useful at predicting those patients who are most likely to benefit from surgical pericardiectomy.

TAKE HOME POINT #6

Restrictive cardiomyopathy must be distinguished from constrtictive pericarditis since both conditions share a number of clinical features.

Table 14.3   Clinical Findings and Imaging Studies for Differentiating Restrictive Cardiomyopathy from Constrictive Pericarditis.

Clinical findings and imaging studies	Restrictive cardiomyopathy	Constrictive pericarditis
History and physical examination	Systemic findings consistent with infiltrative diseases +/– Kussmaul's sign + S3	History of acute pericarditis + Kussmaul's sign + Pericardial knock
Laboratory studies and chest X-ray	BNP usually elevated	BNP can be normal, at or below 100 pg/ml Chest X-ray can show pericardial calcification
Echocardiogram	Increased wall thickness and potentially "speckled" pattern (e.g. amyloidosis) No pericardial thickening Increased inspiratory hepatic vein diastolic flow reversal	Normal wall thickness Possible pericardial thickening Prominent septal "bounce" due to early diastolic filling Increased expiratory hepatic vein diastolic flow reversal
CT/MRI	No pericardial thickening	Pericardial thickening ≥4 mm
Cardiac catheterization	LVEDP>RVEDP by at least 5 mmHg Pulmonary hypertension may be present No ventricular interdependence with concordant LV and RV pressures Endomyocardial biopsy may be abnormal	LVEDP~RVEDP Pulmonary hypertension uncommon Evidence of interventricular interdependence with discordant LV and RV pressures Endomyocardial biopsy is normal

14.3.3   Treatment

As above, patients with restrictive cardiomyopathy should have therapies instituted for symptom relief with diuretics. In addition, a particular focus may be needed to identify specific causes but this will involve the engagement of specialists. For example, patients with amyloidosis and restrictive cardiomyopathy may benefit from chemotherapy although their prognosis typically remains poor. Patients with endomyocardial fibrosis benefit from immunosuppressant agents and valvular surgery when indicated. Treatment of hemochromatosis with iron-chelation therapy is beneficial early on in the course of that disease. The use of pacemakers should be considered in patients with bradyarrhythmias and conduction abnormalities. In select cases, consultation with a cardiologist specializing in heart failure may be warranted to consider mechanical assist devices and heart transplantation.

KEY REFERENCES

Jeffries JL, Towbin JA. Dilated cardiomyopathy. Lancet 2010;375:752–762.
Kushwaha SS, Fallon JT, Fuster V. Restrictive cardiomyopathy. NEJM 1997;336:267–276.
Maron BJ, Towbin JA, Thiene G, et al. Circulation 2006;113:1807–1816.

Chapter 15

Hypertrophic Cardiomyopathy

Sara Saberi and Sharlene Day

15.1 INTRODUCTION

Hypertrophic cardiomyopathy (HCM) is the most common inherited cardiovascular disorder, affecting 1 in 500 individuals worldwide. HCM comprises a wide spectrum of disease severity and is highly heterogeneous in its morphological and physiologic features, clinical presentation, and prognosis. Although most patients with HCM have a normal life expectancy with minimal symptoms, complications such as left ventricular outflow tract (LVOT) obstruction, atrial and ventricular arrhythmias, diastolic dysfunction, stroke and sudden cardiac death (SCD) must be identified early in order to provide optimal clinical care.

> ### TAKE HOME POINT #1
> Hypertrophic cardiomyopathy affects 1 in 500 people worldwide.

15.2 PATHOPHYSIOLOGY

HCM is inherited in an autosomal dominant fashion with a highly variable degree of penetrance. It is primarily the result of mutations in genes encoding cardiac sarcomere proteins. HCM is defined by a hypertrophied, non-dilated left ventricle in the

Inpatient Cardiovascular Medicine, First Edition. Edited by Brahmajee K. Nallamothu and Timir S. Baman.

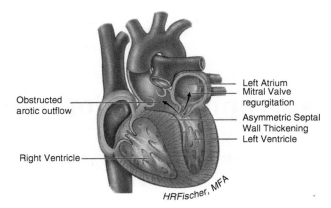

Figure 15.1   Hypertrophic cardiomyopathy with left ventricular outflow tract obstruction. (See Color plate 15.1).

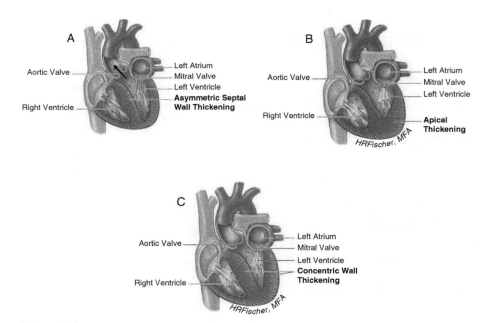

Figure 15.2   Nonobstructive hypertrophic cardiomyopathy. **A** Heart with asymmetric septal wall thickening that is not associated with outflow tract obstruction. **B** Apical hypertrophy. **C** Heart with concentric left ventricular hypertrophy. (See Color plate 15.2).

absence of another cardiac or systemic disease capable of producing the degree of hypertrophy present. It can manifest as negligible (13–15 mm) to significant (>30 mm) hypertrophy and can be associated with LVOT obstruction, as well as varying degrees of fibrosis and myocyte disarray. The hypertrophy is most often asymmetric, preferentially involving the basal intraventricular septum. However, hypertrophy may involve other regions of the intraventricular septum, the left ventricular free walls and/or apex and even the right ventricle. Figures 15.1 and 15.2 demonstrate examples of HCM anatomic variants.

15.3 PATHOPHYSIOLOGY AND CLINICAL MANIFESTATIONS

The clinical manifestations of HCM range from an asymptomatic lifelong course to advanced heart failure refractory to pharmacotherapy. In addition, a subset of the HCM population is at risk for atrial and ventricular tachyarrhythmias. Because of its heterogeneous clinical course and phenotypic expression, as well as its most notorious and devastating complication, sudden cardiac arrest, HCM presents many management dilemmas for practitioners involved in their care.

Dyspnea is a common symptom that typically occurs with exertion and may result from a combination of the following etiologies: (1) high pulmonary venous pressure due to diastolic dysfunction; (2) LV outflow tract obstruction and/or mitral regurgitation; (3) decreased cardiac output due to the low end-diastolic volume of a noncompliant left ventricle; and (4) myocardial ischemia. Angina may occur in the absence of epicardial coronary artery disease and is likely the result of an inability of the coronary microcirculation to meet the demands of the hypertrophied myocardium.

TAKE HOME POINT #2

Patients with HCM may present with variable degrees of dyspnea, angina, lightheadedness, or even syncope and sudden cardiac death.

Those patients with LV outflow tract obstruction characteristically have asymmetric hypertrophy affecting the basal intraventricular septum and resultant systolic anterior motion (SAM) of the mitral valve with varying degrees of mitral regurgitation. In some patients, outflow tract obstruction is present at rest, while in others can be provoked by maneuvers that decrease preload or increase contractility including Valsalva, standing from a squatting position, and exercise (see Chapter 1, Cardiovascular History and Physical Examination). About one-third of patients with HCM have resting obstruction (≥ 30 mmHg), while another one-third have dynamic outflow tract obstruction provoked by exercise. Systolic septal bulging into the LVOT, malposition of the anterior papillary muscle, intrinsic mitral valve abnormalities, drag forces, and hyperdynamic left ventricular contraction (causing the Venturi effect) may contribute to development of an LVOT pressure gradient. Intrinsic abnormalities of the mitral apparatus including leaflet thickening, elongated or redundant leaflets, and anomalous papillary muscle or chordal insertion occur in an estimated 20% of patients with HCM and can also contribute to the severity of mitral regurgitation and increased symptomology.

Table 15.1   Risk Factors for Sudden Cardiac Death (Primary Prevention).

Wall thickness ≥30 mm
Unexplained syncope
Family history of sudden cardiac death in a first-degree relative under the age of 40 years
Spontaneous NSVT (≥3 beats at a rate >120 bpm on 24- or 48-hour ECG monitoring)
Abnormal blood pressure response to exercise (inadequate rise or frank drop in blood pressure) in those <40 years of age

Diastolic dysfunction with preserved ejection fraction is an almost universal feature of the disease resulting from a stiff and noncompliant left ventricle. In patients with and without LVOT obstruction, left ventricular systolic function is generally normal or increased, except in a small subset (<5%) who may develop systolic dysfunction in the so-called "end-stage," leading to significant functional decline.

TAKE HOME POINT #3

All patients with HCM have some degree of diastolic dysfunction which is a significant contributor to dyspnea.

Atrial fibrillation and flutter manifest in approximately 25% of patients with HCM during their lifetime. Patients with HCM may be particularly susceptible to clinical deterioration associated with loss of the atrial "kick" given their noncompliant ventricles.

Patients with HCM must undergo a risk assessment for sudden cardiac death. Overall sudden death rates in the HCM population are currently reported as 1% per year, but there is a wide range of risk. Five major clinical variables (Table 15.1) have been identified as independent risk factors of SCD. The absence of any of the five risk factors has a high negative prognostic value and patients can generally be reassured. The presence of two or more major risk factors carries an annual sudden death risk of ≥3%.

15.4   EVALUATION AND DIAGNOSTIC STUDIES

A meticulous family history is essential to patient management and should focus on details surrounding premature or sudden cardiac deaths of first-degree relatives. There is an important role for genetic counseling in clinical evaluation, diagnosis, patient education, and family support. When a DNA diagnosis is not available, first-degree relatives should undergo regular clinical screening with an electrocardiogram (ECG) and echocardiogram. Consensus guidelines recommend annual screening in children between 12 and 18 years of age and every five years for adults.

Noninvasive risk stratification tests (ECG, echocardiogram, Holter monitoring, exercise testing, and cardiac MRI) usually form part of the clinical evaluation in order to risk stratify for SCD. The majority of patients with HCM have ECGs that show a variety of bizarre findings including T waves abnormalities and left ventricular hypertrophy (Figure 15.3).

Two-dimensional echocardiography is used primarily to quantify the degree and location of hypertrophy, the presence and severity of LVOT obstruction, the degree of SAM and mitral regurgitation, and diastolic dysfunction (Figure 15.4). It is also the most efficient and accessible technique for establishing the diagnosis of HCM. Cardiac MRI is not required in all patients with HCM, but it can be a valuable diagnostic tool in a subset of patients for whom echocardiography is not definitive (Figure 15.5). Cardiac MRIs are becoming widely used in many centers to assess for segmental hypertrophy and the presence of scar tissue which may be a risk factor for SCD (Figure 15.6).

15.5 TREATMENT

Due to the complex interaction of genetic expression and pathophysiology in a relatively young population, we recommend consultation with an experienced center for any patient with a suspected diagnosis of HCM in order to provide a thorough clinical assessment of the patient, as well as all first-degree relatives.

15.5.1 Pharmacologic Therapy

No pharmacologic therapy has been shown to alter the prognosis of HCM; however, medications are useful in relieving symptomatic burden. Figure 15.7 is a schematic summary of the pharmacologic options for management of HCM. When determining how to treat symptoms, it is important to first establish whether patients have LVOT obstruction. Clinicians must be aware that LVOT obstruction worsens with volume depletion, afterload reducing agents such as nitroglycerin and ACE inhibitors, and with augmentation of myocardial contractility with drugs such as digitalis and β-agonists.

β-Adrenergic blockers are first-line therapy in symptomatic HCM patients. Beta-blockers slow the heart rate while prolonging diastole and reducing ventricular filling pressures, thus decreasing exercise-induced outflow obstruction. This class of medication also suppresses arrhythmias and lessens ischemia by reducing myocardial oxygen demand. High doses are often required for these agents to be effective, so clinicians must assess for side effects such as fatigue, poor sleep, impotence, and bradycardia limiting their use. One particular beta-blocker that clinicians should avoid using in patients with LVOT obstruction is carvedilol, as it does have some afterload-reducing properties. Beta-blockers should be titrated slowly until systems of dyspnea are alleviated.

Verapamil can be a suitable alternative when β-blockers are poorly tolerated or ineffective. Verapamil provides most patients with good symptomatic relief and

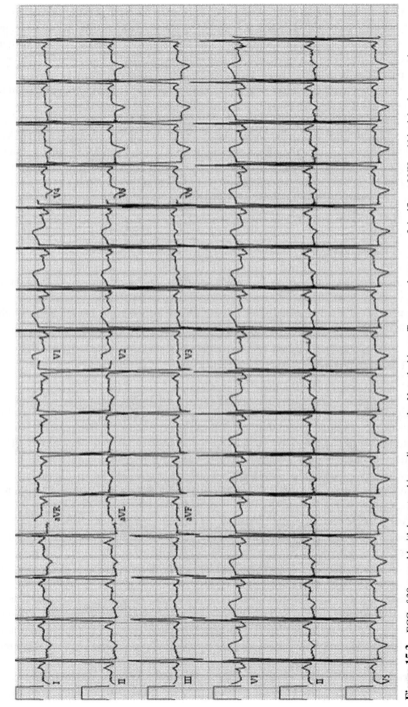

Figure 15.3 ECG of 30 year old with hypertrophic cardiomyopathy. Note the bizarre T waves and presence of significant LVH and biatrial enlargement in a young individual.

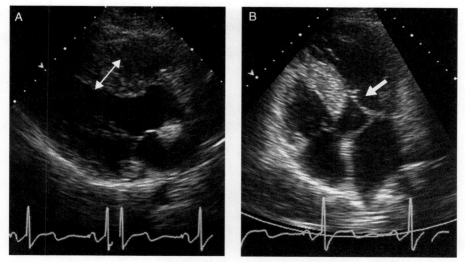

Figure 15.4 Transthoracic echocardiogram in patient with HCM. **A** Asymmetrical septal hypertrophy (thin white double-headed arrow). **B** Systolic anterior motion of the mitral valve (thick white block arrow).

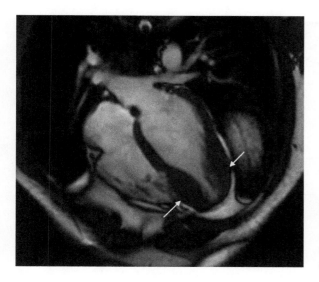

Figure 15.5 Cardiac MRI demonstrating apical hypertrophy (denoted by white arrows) which may not be seen on transthoracic echocardiography.

improved exercise duration. Caution should be exercised in those with elevated LVOT gradients, as its vasodilatory effects may exacerbate outflow tract obstruction.

Disopyramide is a class Ia antiarrhythmic agent that may be used in conjunction with β-blockers or verapamil when a residual gradient is present and symptoms persist. It is effective in reducing LVOT obstruction due to negative inotropic properties. However, anticholinergic side effects and QT prolongation may limit its use.

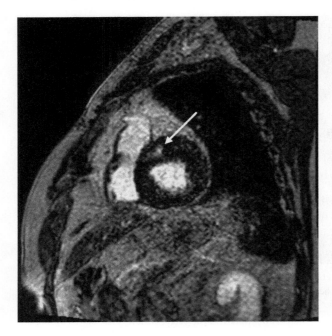

Figure 15.6   Cardiac MRI demonstrating delayed gadolinium enhancement consistent with scar in the anterior septum (block arrow).

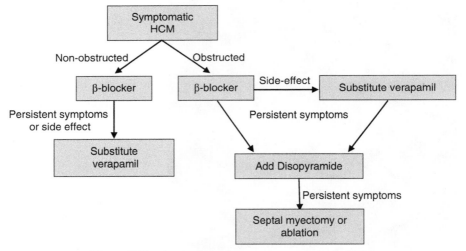

Figure 15.7   An algorithm of management strategies for HCM.

Amiodarone has an important role in maintaining sinus rhythm in patients with paroxysmal atrial fibrillation. Long-term use should include clinical monitoring for adverse effects including evaluation of electrolyte levels, thyroid and liver function, as well as pulmonary function testing. Care should be taken when combining β-blockers, verapamil and amiodarone given their shared negative inotropic effect and risk of potentiating atrioventricular block.

Atrial fibrillation is the most common arrhythmia in HCM and is poorly tolerated. Effective symptom relief may be achieved by rate controlling agents or antiarrhythmic drugs such as disopyramide, sotalol, or amiodarone. Often, invasive measures such as radiofrequency catheter ablation or surgical maze procedures are needed to decrease symptom burden. Anticoagulation with warfarin is recommended for all those with paroxysmal or chronic atrial fibrillation in the absence of a contra-indication regardless of their CHADS2 score.

A subgroup of patients progress toward a dilated, "end-stage" phase character-ized by systolic dysfunction. In the absence of an outflow tract gradient, treatment with standard therapeutics used in the management of chronic ischemic or nonisch-emic systolic heart failure such as diuretics, angiotensin-converting enzyme inhibitors, and angiotensin II blockers can be implemented.

Until recently, antibiotic prophylaxis was recommended in all patients with outflow obstruction or intrinsic mitral valve disease. Although patients with HCM continue to be recognized as high risk, recently updated guidelines suggest that antibiotic prophylaxis is no longer necessary, unless the patient has undergone valvular repair or replacement with prosthetic material. Instead of prophylaxis for dental procedures, maintenance of good oral hygiene is strongly encouraged.

Contrary to common perception, the risk of general anesthesia for noncardiac surgery in patients with HCM is low. Spinal anesthesia may be relatively contraindi-cated in patients with outflow tract gradients as systemic vascular resistance falls. Careful attention to perioperative fluid management, thromboprophylaxis, and vasoactive drugs is paramount.

15.5.2 Invasive Therapy

In patients with significant obstruction (>50 mmHg) who remain severely symptom-atic despite optimal medical therapy, septal reduction procedures can be performed. Septal myectomy is the "gold standard" of treatment and can completely abolish the gradient and improve symptoms in >90% of patients with low complication rates (<1% mortality in high-volume specialty centers). Percutaneous septal ablation, in which alcohol is injected into one of the septal branches of the left anterior descending artery to produce a localized area of necrosis, is an alternative to septal myectomy. Although initial studies have shown this to be effective in relieving symptoms and gradient in selected patients, long-term follow-up data have been lacking thus far and concerns have been raised about the pro-arrhythmic potential of the scar induced by the procedure.

15.5.3   Sudden Cardiac Death Risk Assessment

The presence of two or more major risk factors (see Table 15.1) carries an annual sudden death risk of ≥3% and warrants ICD implantation for primary prevention. The gray area – and a major challenge for clinicians – is the risk stratification of patients with only one risk factor, who comprise about 25% of the HCM population. Data from a recent multicenter ICD registry suggest that the presence of a single risk factor may be sufficient to recommend ICD implantation. It is important to keep in mind, however, that the positive prognostic value of any single risk factor is very low, so the strength of that risk factor has to be weighed against the long-term risks of an implantable device. All patients undergoing risk stratification for SCD should be referred to a cardiologist.

KEY REFERENCES

Fifer MA, Vlahakes GJ. Management of symptoms in hypertrophic cardiomyopathy. Circulation 2008;117(3):429–439.

Ho CY, Seidman CE. A contemporary approach to hypertrophic cardiomyopathy. Circulation 2006;113(24):e858–e862.

Nagueh SF, Mahmarian JJ. Noninvasive cardiac imaging in patients with hypertrophic cardiomyopathy. JACC 2006;48(12):2410–2422.

Chapter 16

Heart Transplantation and Left Ventricular Assist Devices

Nicklaus K. Slocum, Francis D. Pagani, and Keith Aaronson

16.1 HEART TRANSPLANTATION

The increasing incidence of obesity and other cardiovascular risk factors has led to a growing of number of patients developing heart failure. The progressive nature of the heart failure syndrome coupled with advances in its medical, device, and surgical therapy have led to increasing numbers of patients surviving to develop end-stage disease for which conventional treatment is no longer effective. When patients have only limited comorbidities, heart transplantation can be an attractive option as it provides a significant survival benefit and increased quality of life.

When to refer to a cardiologist for transplantation evaluation is a critical aspect of caring for patients with advanced heart failure. In addition, awareness of medical issues specific to the posttransplant patient is important for specialists and generalists alike as a true multidisciplinary approach – cardiologists, cardiothoracic surgeons, infectious disease specialists, primary care physicians, pharmacists, and social workers – is crucial to achieving favorable outcomes following heart transplantation.

16.1.1 Candidacy for Transplantation

As there remains a scarcity of available donor organs, rigorous standardized criteria exist for cardiac transplantation. The United Network of Organ Sharing (UNOS) facilitates organ placement and distribution based on severity of illness, blood type,

Inpatient Cardiovascular Medicine, First Edition. Edited by Brahmajee K. Nallamothu and Timir S. Baman.

Table 16.1   Indications for Cardiac Transplantation.

VO2 ≤12 ml/kg/min
Severe HF requiring continuous inotropes
Progressive heart failure despite maximal medical therapy
Life-threatening ventricular arrhythmias not responsive to medical or ablative maneuvers
Cardiogenic shock (post MI, myocarditis) despite mechanical support
Refractory angina with optimal medical management and no options for revascularization

and geographical location. Prior to transplant listing, a patient must undergo an extensive evaluation to confirm candidacy. Status 1A refers to a transplant candidate who is hospitalized and has a left ventricular assist device (LVAD) or two more inotropic drugs with invasive hemodynamic monitoring with a Swan-Ganz catheter. Status 1B candidates are hospitalized with an LVAD placed for >30 days or continuous inotropic infusion. A candidate who is Status 2 does not meet Status 1A or 1B criteria and is usually stable as an outpatient.

Consideration for cardiac transplantation should be given to patients experiencing disease progression despite maximal therapy including medication, cardiac device therapy including resynchronization (if appropriate), and attempted correction of medical or surgical causes of heart failure. The assessment of prospective recipients requires an individualized evaluation by a team of experienced personnel to identify patients who lack contraindications and will benefit most from cardiac transplantation (Table 16.1).

The ability to estimate survival of the heart failure patient in the absence of transplantation is of great importance in evaluating transplant candidacy. Cardiopulmonary exercise testing, hemodynamic assessment through right heart catheterization, and standardized prognostic scoring are perhaps the most frequently utilized techniques to assess candidacy. Cardiopulmonary exercise testing is part of the transplantation evaluation with measurements of peak exercise oxygen consumption (peak VO_2), anaerobic threshold and ventilatory equivalent for carbon dioxide (VE/VCO_2) each providing valuable prognostic information. Patients on β-blockers with a peak VO_2 ≤12 ml/kg/min and those intolerant of β-blockers with a peak VO_2 ≤14 ml/kg/min should be listed for transplantation in the absence of significant contraindications.

Right heart catheterization is important in assessing transplant candidacy as right heart failure is a potential lethal complication in the early postoperative period. With transplantation, a normal donor right ventricle may be acutely exposed to the chronically elevated pulmonary vascular resistance (PVR, calculated as the difference between mean pulmonary artery pressure and the mean pulmonary artery occlusion ["wedge"] pressure, divided by the cardiac output and measured as Wood Units [WU]) of the recipient due to chronic heart failure. This dramatic increase in afterload leads to right ventricular overload and failure. Patients with PVR <2.5 WU have excellent early post-transplant outcomes compared to a high frequency of right ventricular failure and early postoperative mortality seen in those with higher PVR values. However, patients with PVRs >2.5 WU who respond to intravenous nitroprusside without a reduction in systemic blood pressure had a lower mortality and incidence of right heart failure compared to those with fixed PVR > 2.5 WU. Individuals with elevated pulmonary vascular resistance as the only contraindication to transplantation may be considered for further therapies to allow candidacy. Therapies to decrease chronically elevated PVR include administration of vasodilator medications (e.g. nitroprusside, milrinone or dobutamine) or mechanical therapy with a left ventricular assist device (LVAD).

TAKE HOME POINT #1

Assessment of pulmonary vascular resistance is essential prior to heart transplantation in order to avoid right heart failure and increased mortality.

In addition to these objective measures, candidates must also undergo a thorough evaluation of comorbid conditions and psychosocial health in order to be considered for transplantation. Absolute contraindications are becoming fewer and fewer in the advancing world of cardiac transplantation, although assessing the burden of multiple relative contraindications remains critical to achieving good outcomes. Many patients with concomitant conditions or issues that were once thought too high risk for transplant are now being transplanted successfully in experienced centers. A recent analysis from the Cardiac Transplant Research Database shows that modest improvements in overall transplant survival over the past two decades have occurred despite increased transplant recipient comorbidity and less than ideal organ donors. While physicians will frequently wish to offer transplantation to his or her patient despite substantial comorbidities, the transplant community's societal responsibility to shepherd a limited resource must take precedence as this offers the greatest opportunity to do the most good. For this reason, many centers limit candidacy to patients <70 years of age and BMI <35. Other relative contraindications to transplantation are recognized in a thorough history and physical, and standardized imaging and laboratory testing with subspecialty consultation always required (Table 16.2).

16.1.2   Post-Transplantation Care and Complications

Immunosuppression is required in the transplant recipient to prevent allograft destruction, and is responsible for the longevity that many recipients experience. However, despite their necessity for preventing organ rejection, immunosuppressant medications also lead to significant morbidity and mortality. An extensive description of specific anti-rejection therapy is beyond the scope of this chapter, and questions should be directed to individual transplant centers as protocols vary and treatment is tailored to each patient's risk profile, comorbidities, and subsequent side

Table 16.2   Contraindications to Cardiac Transplant.

Chronic renal insufficiency (Cr >2.5 mg/dL)

Age >70

BMI >35

Peripheral vascular disease: Relative contraindication – Screen patients for AAA, carotid stenoses, and ankle brachial index routinely

Tobacco and substance abuse

Pt may be required to complete formal rehabilitation program prior to listing

Elevated (>4 Woods Units) fixed pulmonary vascular resistance

Active systemic infection

Cancer; history of or current diagnosis

Recent (within 3 months) peptic ulcer disease or gastrointestinal bleed not immediately responsive to therapy or intervention

Recent pulmonary or cerebral infarction

effects. On average, 50% of patients are treated with induction immunosuppressive therapy during the initial post-transplant period. This is followed by lifelong maintenance immunosuppression using a combination of agents. Often this includes "triple therapy" with a combination of a calcineurin inhibitor (i.e. cyclosporine or tacrolimus), a corticosteroid, and an antiproliferative agent (mycophenolate mofetil, sirolimus, everolimus or azathioprine).

Routine cardiac biopsy is an important part of post-transplantation care to detect allograft rejection. If clinically evident, rejection is most commonly heralded by signs and symptoms of congestive heart failure or, less commonly, supraventricular arrhythmias; however, most episodes of cellular rejection are asymptomatic. The presentation of a transplant patient in congestive heart failure is an emergency and should be treated as such with rapid assessment of cardiac function and specialty consultation. The incidence of rejection is highest early after transplantation and decreases substantially over time. In the absence of rejection, the intensity of the immunosuppressive regimen is decreased over time. The schedule of routine surveillance biopsies is correspondingly most intensive in the initial weeks and months following transplantation. Gene expression profiling from peripheral blood mononuclear cells may be used in lieu of biopsies in patients at low risk for cellular rejection.

TAKE HOME POINT #2

A patient with a history of heart transplant who presents with congestive heart failure is an emergency and must undergo immediate evaluation for rejection.

As in any immunocompromised host, opportunistic infections pose a significant challenge to the post-transplant patient (Table 16.3). Cytomegalovirus (CMV) and other herpes family viruses, candida, aspergillus and nocardia are common concerns.

Table 16.3 Prophylaxis of Infection in Heart Transplant Patients.

Medication condition	Prophylaxis agent
Pneumocystis jirovecii (carinii) pneumonia	Trimethoprim-sulfamethoxazole (one single tablet a day or one double-strength tablet 3–7 times a week)
Toxoplasma gondii	Trimethoprim-sulfamethoxazole (one single tablet a day or one double-strength tablet three to seven times a week)
Streptococcus pneumoniae	Pneumococcal vaccination
Influenza	Influenza vaccination
Cytomegalovirus	Acyclovir, ganciclovir, or valacyclovir
Hepatitis B virus	Hepatitis B virus vaccine

In the immediate post-transplant period, recipients are at risk for bacterial infections similar to other cardiac surgery recipients. In the first months following transplant, patients are at highest risk for herpes simplex and oral candida, with CMV becoming more common during months three through six. Post-transplant patients should routinely receive prophylaxis against oral candida, herpes simplex, CMV and Pneumocystis carinii pneumonia (PCP). Consideration must also be taken with regard to specific organisms endemic to the location the recipient is living in and travelling through.

Cardiac allograft vasculopathy (CAV) is one of the leading causes of death in the transplanted patient, especially those surviving greater than five years after transplant. CAV is a progressive arterial narrowing involving the entire coronary vasculature and results from alloimmune response and chronic inflammation. Contrary to the normal progression of coronary disease, CAV is characterized by diffuse narrowing starting in the distal small vessels with progression to the main vessels (Figure 16.1). This smoldering widespread arterial disease is angiographically present in up to 53% of patients greater than 10 years post-transplant. Screening regimens for CAV vary between institutions. Traditionally, centers performed annual coronary angiograms while other centers rely on dobutamine echocardiography especially in recipients with chronic kidney disease. While this is much less sensitive than invasive studies for CAV, negative studies are associated with a very low mortality rate in the following year. The diffuseness of the disease within the coronary arteries makes conventional modalities such as angioplasty and stenting less effective. Currently, treatment is aimed towards decreasing traditional atherosclerosis risk factors including lipid lowering with statin therapy. Pravastatin and simvastatin have been specifically shown to reduce allograft vasculopathy as well as reducing hemodynamically significant rejection and subsequent death. Everolimus and sirolimus have been shown to reduce both the incidence and the progression of CAV. The calcium channel blocker diltiazem may reduce the incidence of CAV when added in the early post-transplant period.

Malignancy is another important complication in the post-transplant period. Neoplasms can be present at the time of transplantation with more aggressive

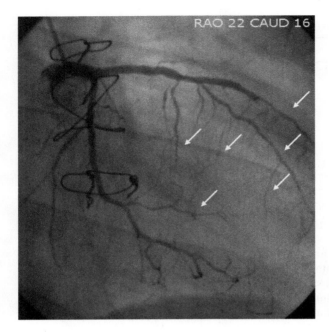

Figure 16.1 Diffuse small vessel disease seen with cardiac transplant vasculopathy (arrows).

proliferation after initiation of immunosuppression or as a result of long-term immunosuppressant therapy. The incidence of skin cancer and lymphomas is particularly elevated in the transplanted population. Hospitalists must be aware that skin abnormalities in transplant patients may be indicative of neoplasm and immediate consultation is necessary.

TAKE HOME POINT #3

Rejection, infection, and malignancy of multiple organs, including skin, are major post-transplantation complications.

16.1.3 Outcomes

Outcomes after cardiac transplantation continue to improve despite the allocation of organs to higher-risk individuals. In current practice, 50% of those transplanted are alive 10 years post-transplant, and if patients survive the first year the average longevity is increased to 13 years. Care for these patients involves the treatment of transplant-specific complications and also treatment of common conditions complicated by transplant status. Hospitalists have a significant role in the longevity of a cardiac transplant patient with early recognition of post-transplant complications.

16.2   VENTRICULAR ASSIST DEVICES

16.2.1   Indication and Utilization

Ventricular assist devices (VAD) are mechanical options for patients with end-stage heart failure. Patients supported with a VAD undergo a marked improvement in quality of life, functional capacity and survival. With improvements in VAD technology and durability, patients are now frequently managed in outpatient settings. While these patients' "medical home" will be in multidisciplinary advanced heart failure/VAD specialty centers, community providers should understand the indications for and basic medical issues arising from VAD therapy.

VADs are a form of support in patients with advanced heart failure and are used to unload the failing ventricle and provide hemodynamic support to other organs. In a small number of patients, VADs can be used as a temporary support system while awaiting recovery. Once recovery occurs, the VAD support is weaned and the device can be explanted. This remains a rare event, but can be seen in patients with acute inflammatory cardiomyopathies or following acute myocardial infarctions. More commonly, VADs are utilized as a "bridge" for patients with decompensated heart failure awaiting transplantation. In these cases, VADs are used as patients await a suitable donor organ or as relative contraindications are treated (such as lowering of PVR). VADs can also be used as "destination" therapy. This treatment modality is for patients with contraindications to transplant as a permanent and palliative procedure. The use of VADs as destination therapy is expected to increase substantially as devices become smaller and more durable.

There are a variety of available devices but the physiologic mechanism is similar in all implanted VADs (Figure 16.2). Blood is removed from the heart through an inflow conduit, pumped or accelerated in some fashion, and returned through an outflow conduit into the aorta or pulmonary artery. The majority of devices currently are placed via a median sternotomy with the pumping chamber positioned intraabdominally, usually in a preperitoneal location. There is a percutaneous driveline that enters through the upper abdominal wall, connecting to a controller (computer) and to a power source. These energy sources may include a power base unit when the patient is at rest or an external "wearable" battery when the patient wishes to be mobile.

Implantation of a VAD is a life-altering transition for a patient with heart failure. An evaluation similar to that described above for a cardiac transplant is in order prior to placement. Programs usually require VAD patients to have one or more adults (usually family members or close friends) trained in VAD troubleshooting, so that a trained adult can be with them 24 hours a day, especially for the first few months of VAD support. It is essential that the patient and these caregivers have a full understanding and independent competence in VAD maintenance and monitoring prior to discharge. Given the much simpler and far less toxic medical regimen and the potentially limitless supply of VADs, it is inevitable that the number of patients on permanent VAD support will vastly outnumber those who receive heart transplants in the near future.

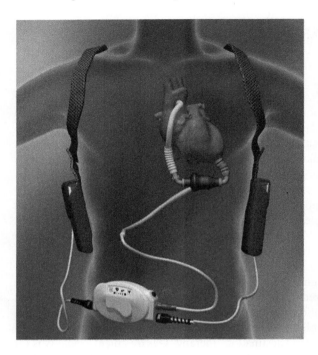

Figure 16.2 Schematic representation of a left ventricular assist device. (See Color plate 16.1).

TAKE HOME POINT #4

VAD patients and their family members receive extensive training on their devices, and can be a resource to health care workers in the acute setting.

16.2.2 Care of the VAD Patient

VAD patients are able to return to an active lifestyle with some important precautions. Patients should be cautioned that they cannot submerge the device, precluding swimming and baths. With time and good care, the skin at the exit site becomes incorporated into the driveline and patients are allowed to shower using an occlusive barrier covering the exit site and external device hardware. They are also not able to participate in contact sports, undergo MRIs, or operate heavy machinery.

VAD patients are at an increased risk of thromboembolism, and most centers treat with warfarin as well as an antiplatelet agent (except for the HeartMate XVE, which requires only the latter). This risk of thromboembolism needs to be weighed against the risk of bleeding as VAD patients are also at an increased risk of gastrointestinal bleeding for multiple reasons.

VAD patients are susceptible to infections – the consequences of which can be devastating. Most infections are related to gram positive organisms and are associated with the driveline site. Often, driveline site infections can be managed with antibiotics but there is a risk of spread of the infection to internal components of the device as well. Strict wound care must be performed by the patient and caregiver on a daily basis to minimize infections.

As a health care worker or emergency responder assisting in the care of a VAD patient, it is important to recognize limitations and obtain consultation from VAD specialists. In many situations, the patient's trained companions can assist health care workers in the acute setting. It is also important to recognize differences in routine therapies when applied to VAD patients. Particular caution needs to be applied when evaluating and treating ventricular arrhythmias. Ventricular arrhythmias occur frequently in VAD patients. These arrhythmias are often better tolerated in patients with VADs though tolerability varies and patients who are symptomatic must be treated. On the other hand, asymptomatic patients with ventricular tachycardia (i.e. those without hemodynamic compromise) do not require immediate cardioversion. CPR should be avoided as chest compressions have been shown to sometimes dislodge the device.

TAKE HOME POINT #5

VAD patients can be PULSELESS (normal) and may experience ventricular arrhythmias. Standard ACLS protocols do not apply and patients should be assessed for symptoms (i.e. hemodynamic compromise) prior to aggressive interventions.

Chapter 17

Syncope

Sanders H. Chae

Syncope is one of the most common causes of hospitalizations in the United States, accounting for up to 3% of visits to the Emergency Room and 6% of hospitalizations annually. Moreover, approximately 40% of individuals will experience a syncopal event during their lifetime. Despite these statistics, it remains a difficult clinical problem to evaluate and manage. Syncope is defined as a sudden, transient loss of consciousness that spontaneously self-terminates and is followed by complete recovery. For the hospitalist, a critical element in managing syncope is to determine whether the cause is cardiovascular in origin, as syncope secondary to cardiovascular disease is a significant predictor of mortality. Hospitalists must be able to ascertain malignant from benign causes of syncope in order to provide immediate therapy for potentially life-threatening conditions.

17.1 PATHOPHYSIOLOGY

The pathophysiology of syncope can be delineated into two major groups: those that result in a transient loss of consciousness due to inadequate cerebral perfusion and those secondary to other conditions. Cardiovascular conditions comprise the majority of conditions related to hypoperfusion while neurologic, metabolic, and psychogenic etiologies encompass the other classification.

Inpatient Cardiovascular Medicine, First Edition. Edited by Brahmajee K Nallamothu and Timir S Baman.

17.2 ETIOLOGIES

The differential diagnosis of syncope can be broad and exhaustive (Table 17.1). A detailed history and physical examination in addition to a 12 lead electrocardiogram and assessment for orthostatic hypotension can accurately assess an etiology for syncope in >65% of patients.

Table 17.1   Differential Diagnosis of Syncope.

Arrhythmias
    Ventricular tachycardia
    Ventricular fibrillation
    Sinus node dysfunction
    Atrio-ventricular conduction disease
    Paroxysmal arrhythmias
    Long QT syndrome
    Brugada syndrome
    Arrhythmogenic right ventricular cardiomyopathy
    Wolfe-Parkinson-White with atrial fibrillation
    Paroxysmal supraventricular tachycardia
Structural Heart Disease with Obstruction to Cardiac Output
    Aortic stenosis
    Hypertrophic obstructive cardiomyopathy
    Other valvular stenotic heart disease
    Atrial myxoma
Other Forms of Structural Heart Disease
    Cardiac ischemia
    Pericardial tamponade
    Pulmonary embolus/severe pulmonary hypertension
    Aortic dissection
Neurocardiogenic Syncope/Vasodepressor Syndrome
    Vasovagal
    Situational (cough, micturition, defecation)
    Carotid sinus syndrome
    Cough syncope
Orthostatic Syndromes
    Dehydration
    Secondary autonomic syndromes (diabetic neuropathy, etc.)
    Primary autonomic failure (Parkinsons, etc.)
    Postural intolerance syndrome (e.g. POTS, rarely)
Cerebrovascular
    Vascular steal syndromes
    Basilar artery insufficiency
    Migraines

TAKE HOME POINT #1

A thorough history and physical examination in addition to simple bedside maneuvers can diagnose the etiology of syncope in the majority of patients.

Furthermore, clinicians should initially concentrate on identifying the presence of structural heart disease such as ischemic heart disease, left ventricular outflow obstruction from hypertrophic obstructive cardiomyopathy or aortic stenosis, congestive heart failure, or other valvular diseases as patients with cardiovascular disease have a higher risk of mortality. Tachyarrhythmias and bradyarrhythmias may also present with an episode of syncope. A history of myocardial infarction or the presence of scar from any etiology renders a patient susceptible to ventricular arrhythmias while bradycardia either from sinus node dysfunction or AV block may account for a syncopal event. Due to significant mortality associated with these disorders, hospitalists should obtain immediate cardiac consultation if a cardiovascular cause of syncope is suspected.

The most common cause of syncope is neurocardiogenic disorders such as vasodepressor syndromes, vasovagal fainting, or carotid sinus hypersensitivity. Neurally-mediated syncope is associated with abnormal blood pressure regulation resulting in hyperperfusion. Although they are generally benign, recurrent episodes of neurocardiogenic syncope can severely limit a patient's quality of life and pose physical threats, particularly if syncope occurs while driving. Orthostatic syncope also accounts for a substantial percentage of syncopal events. Neurological disorders are rarely a cause of syncope.

17.3 CLINICAL PRESENTATION

The clinical presentation of syncope can be challenging because patients invariably present for clinical evaluation after the episode of syncope has occurred. Patients also may not recall the episode well, making the history of symptoms prior to and following the episode critical to making a diagnosis. Any account from a witness of the episode might also be very instructive. A detailed clinical history can often provide clues to the etiology of a syncopal event (Table 17.2). Patients who suffer an episode of neurocardiogenic syncope often describe a prodrome of nausea and lightheadedness. The syncopal episode is frequently followed by a period of fatigue and weakness. Situational episodes of neurocardiogenic syncope during micturition, defecation, prolonged standing, or the sight of blood during venipuncture offer a clearer history.

Arrhythmias will frequently have no prodrome and occur suddenly. Afterwards, patients often report that they are asymptomatic and feel as if they have returned to their baseline. Chest pain, shortness of breath, lower extremity edema, or palpitations should prompt cardiac evaluation to evaluate for acute ischemia or underlying structural heart disease.

Shaking from myoclonic jerks and "seizure-like" activity are nonspecific and do not necessarily indicate neurological disorders. However, focal neurological

Table 17.2   Characteristics of Various Syncopal Etiologies.

Condition	Clinical characteristics
Vasovagal syncope	Precipitating factors such as a emotional situation, fear, crowded environment, coughing, laughing, eating, urinating
	Symptoms of lightheadedness, dizziness, blurriness, nausea prior to syncope
	Associated with prolonged standing
	Symptoms of nausea, vomiting, fatigue post syncope
Orthostatic hypotension	Associated with changes in position
	Recent dehydration or change in diuretic medication
	Chronic conditions such as diabetes, Parkinson's disease, and alcohol abuse
Arrhythmia induced	Associated with palpitations or occurring while at rest or supine
	Previous history of systolic dysfunction, coronary artery disease
	Family history of sudden death at early age or genetic conditions such as long QT syndrome, Brugada syndrome, arrhythmogenic right ventricular dysplasia

findings – auras and post-ictal confusion – may suggest vasospastic migraine disorders or seizure disorders. Cerebrovascular disease in the form of a transient ischemic attack or stroke rarely presents as syncope and will manifest as loss of consciousness only if there is severe bilateral carotid artery or basilar artery insufficiency.

Patient age provides valuable clues to the etiology of syncope. Pediatric and young adult patients most commonly present with neurocardiogenic syncope and primary arrhythmias such as Wolfe-Parkinson-White or long QT syndrome (LQTS). For middle-aged patients, neurocardiogenic syncope remains the most common presentation although acute ischemia should be evaluated. Elderly patients present with neurocardiogenic or orthostatic syncope, however cardiovascular causes such as arrhythmias, valvular disease, and ischemia do become more common. New medications that result in orthostasis may also be a common etiology.

17.4   EVALUATION AND DIAGNOSTIC STUDIES

The workup of syncope should initially focus on history, physical examination, and baseline electocardiogram (ECG) as the presence of structural heart disease can usually be elicited or ruled out on the basis of those three elements. The physical examination will be helpful in diagnosing orthostatic syndromes or structural heart disease. Every patient should have vital signs measured supine and upright to elicit orthostatic hypotension and autonomic syndromes. Orthostatic hypotension is defined as 20 mmHg drop in systolic blood pressure or a 10 mmHg drop in diastolic blood pressure within three minutes of transitioning from a sitting to a standing position. Aortic stenosis and hypertrophic cardiomyopathy can be detected by the presence of systolic murmurs while other cardiomyopathies will present with signs of congestive heart failure. Patients with neurocardiogenic forms of syncope will invariably have a normal physical exam. Carotid sinus hypersensitivity can be diagnosed with syncope or significant sinus slowing during gentle massage of the carotid sinus baroreceptor for 5–10 seconds. Patients with previous history of stroke, transient ischemic attacks, or bruits on auscultation should not undergo this examination.

TAKE HOME POINT #2

Patients with neurocardiogenic syncope often have a normal physical examination.

An ECG should be ordered on every patient presenting with an episode of syncope. Sinus bradycardia, pauses, or 1st degree AV block may suggest sinus node dysfunction while bundle branch block may signify advanced atrioventricular (AV) conduction disease. A delta wave in the QRS complex may reflect the presence of an accessory pathway and Wolff-Parkinson-White syndrome. Brugada syndrome and LQTS have characteristic QRS complexes while T wave inversions in V1–V3 may suggest arrhythmogenic right ventricular cardiomyopathy (ARVC). Ventricular ectopy in a patient with structural heart disease suggests more malignant ventricular arrhythmias.

An initial episode of syncope without an obvious diagnosis by history should be evaluated with longer monitoring, either in the form of inpatient telemetry or Holter monitoring if a cardiovascular cause of syncope is suspected. If episodes of syncope are infrequent, event recorders or implantable loop recorders may be appropriate (Figure 17.1).

Although an echocardiogram is not required in every patient who suffers an episode of syncope, they are frequently performed to exclude structural heart disease in patients who do not have a definitive diagnosis from history, physical exam, and ECG. Echocardiogram should be always ordered when there is a suspicion of structural heart disease. If neurocardiogenic syncope appears to be the most likely diagnosis, head up tilt table testing is almost never indicated in the inpatient setting because the sensitivity and specificity of the test rarely alter the probability of the diagnosis.

Patients with high-risk features associated with syncope should be immediately referred for specialty consultation (Table 17.3).

17.5 TREATMENT

A primary goal in the management of syncope is the prevention of recurrent episodes and mortality reduction. If an evaluation raises the clinical suspicion that tachyarrhythmia has provoked the episode of syncope, referral to an electrophysiologist is appropriate. Patients with structural heart disease and a left ventricular ejection fraction less than or equal to 35% should be referred to an electrophysiologist for implantation of an implantable cardioverter defibrillator (ICD) while patients with a history of myocardial infarction but ejection fraction greater than 35% may be

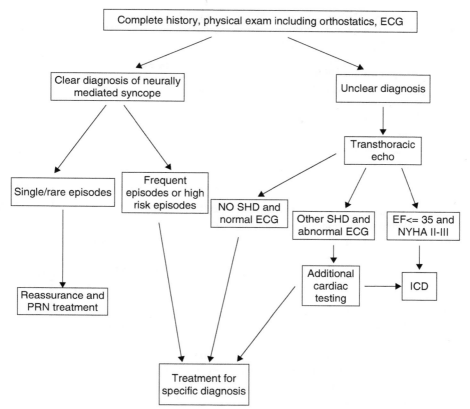

Figure 17.1   Evaluation of syncope. EF, ejection fraction; NYHA, New York Heart Association; SHD, structural heart disease.

considered for electrophysiological study. Patients with symptomatic bradycardia can often benefit from pacemaker placement.

Management of vasovagal syncope can be challenging for the physician and frustrating for the patient (Table 17.4). Physical counter-pressure maneuvers such as leg crossing, lower body muscle tensing, tense hand grip, and squatting are effective in diminishing excess vasodilation that can lead to a drop in central blood pressures. Volume expansion through oral fluid and salt intake should be encouraged although management for patients with hypertension becomes more complex. If these initial maneuvers are unsuccessful in preventing recurrence, referral to a specialist is appropriate.

TAKE HOME POINT #3

Conservative treatment strategies for vasovagal syncope can be beneficial in aborting and preventing syncopal episodes.

Table 17.3 High Risk Features Associated with Syncope.

Chest pain
Shortness of breath
History of cardiac disease
Family history of unexplained sudden cardiac death
Congestive heart failure
Decreased ejection fraction
Frequent premature ventricular complexes
Nonsustained ventricular tachycardia
Severe sinus bradycardia (<50 bpm)
Long QT interval (>450 ms)
Short QT interval (<300 ms)
Epsilon waves or T waves inversions in V1–V3 (suggestive of
  arrhythmogenic right ventricular dysplasia)
Right bundle branch block with ST elevation at T wave inversion in V1–V3
  (suggestive of Brugada syndrome)
Syncope associated with exercise, palpitations, or in supine position

Table 17.4 Treatment Strategies for Vasovagal Syncope.

Physical maneuvers to prevent progression of vasovagal syncope
  Place head between legs with knees up while on floor
  Lie with legs raised higher than heart
  Leg crossing
  Squatting
  Hand grip
  Gluteal clenching
Prevention of vasovagal syncope
  Increased fluid and salt intake
  Compression stockings
  Midodrine 5 mg orally three times a day (efficacy limited)

Patients who suffer an episode of syncope may be subject to restrictions from driving an automobile. In the US, the laws on driving restrictions vary by state. Providers should be aware of the requirements in their own state and are obligated to instruct patients of any restrictions from driving a car if they apply. Individuals who drive commercial vehicles or pilots will likely be subject to more stringent prohibitions.

TAKE HOME POINT #4

Clinicians must be aware of state regulations regarding driving restrictions for patients who have a syncopal episode.

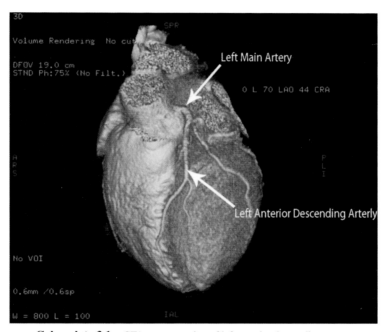

Color plate 3.1 CTA reconstruction of left anterior descending artery.

Inpatient Cardiovascular Medicine, First Edition. Edited by Brahmajee K. Nallamothu and Timir S. Baman.

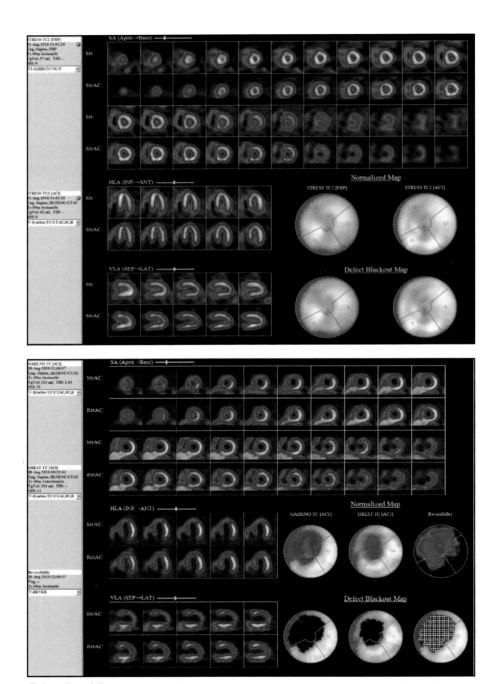

Color plate 4.1 Nuclear stress tests. Top panel demonstrates a normal nuclear stress test (only stress images were acquired). Bottom panel demonstrates an abnormal nuclear stress test with a large anterior, anteroseptal and apical partially reversible defect.

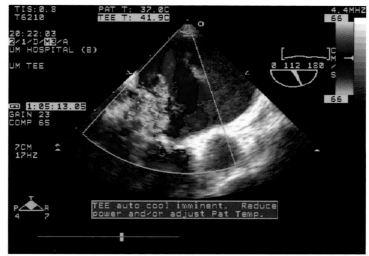

Color plate 8.1 Severe mitral regurgitation.

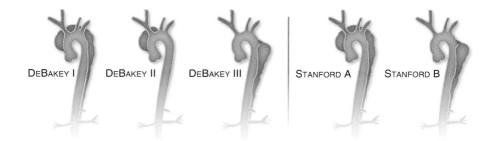

DeBakey I DeBakey II DeBakey III Stanford A Stanford B

Color plate 11.1 Classification schema of acute aortic syndromes. Debakey and Stanford Classification Systems.

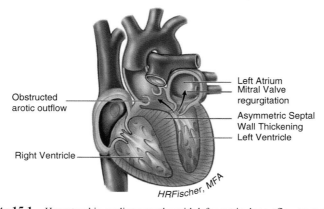

Left Atrium
Mitral Valve regurgitation

Obstructed arotic outflow

Asymmetric Septal Wall Thickening
Left Ventricle

Right Ventricle

HRFischer, MFA

Color plate 15.1 Hypertrophic cardiomyopathy with left ventricular outflow tract obstruction.

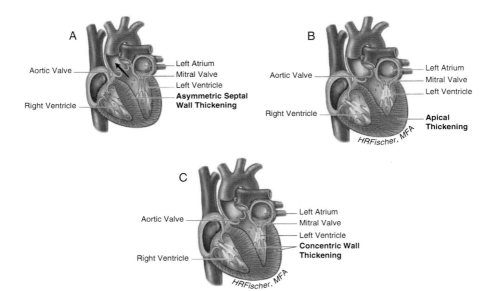

Color plate 15.2 Nonobstructive hypertrophic cardiomyopathy. **A** Heart with asymmetric septal wall thickening that is not associated with outflow tract obstruction. **B** Apical hypertrophy. **C** Heart with concentric left ventricular hypertrophy.

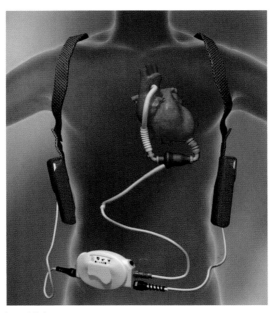

Color plate 16.1 Schematic representation of a left ventricular assist device.

A   B

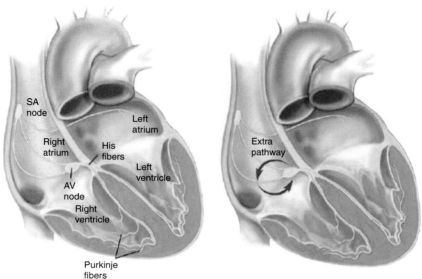

Color plate 18.1   **A** Normal conduction system of the heart. **B** With AVNRT, conduction travels
down the slow pathway of AV node and retrogradely up the bypass tract (fast pathway). (Source: Wang,
PJ and Estes NA. Supraventricular Tachycardia. Circulation 2002: 106: e206–208. Reproduced with
permission of Wolters Kluwer Health)..

Typical AVNRT   AVRT

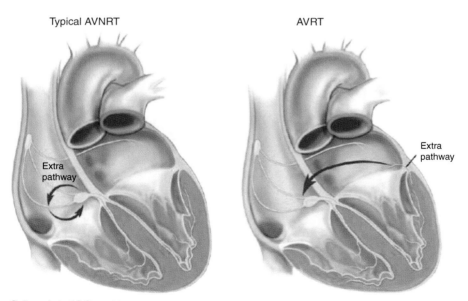

Color plate 18.2   With AVNRT the extra pathway is contained within the AV node as opposed to
AVRT where the accessory pathway involves an atrium and ventricle. (Source: Wang, PJ and Estes NA.
Supraventricular Tachycardia. Circulation 2002: 106: e206–208. Reproduced with permission of Wolters
Kluwer Health).

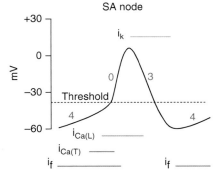

Color plate 21.1 Pacemaker current and ion traffic. (Source: http://www.cvphysiology.com/Arrhythmias/SAN%20action%20potl.gif, with permission from Dr Richard Klabunde).

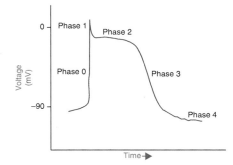

Color plate 21.2 The cardiac action potential (Source: Richard N. Fogoros. Electrophysiologic Testing 5th edition, 2012. Reproduced with permission of John Wiley & Sons Ltd).

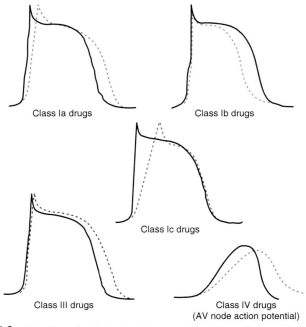

Color plate 21.3 The effect of antiarrhythmic drugs on the cardiac action potential. The solid lines represent the baseline action potential and the dotted lines represent the changes that result in the action potential when various classes of antiarrhythmic drug are given. (Source: Richard N. Fogoros. Electrophysiologic Testing 5th edition, 2012. Reproduced with permission of John Wiley & Sons Ltd).

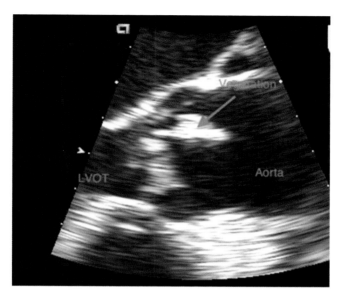

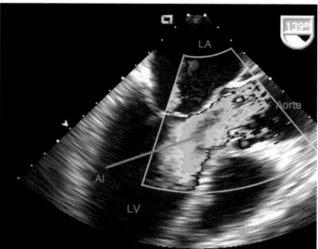

Color plate 25.1 TEE of aortic valve endocarditis with aortic regurgitation. AI, aortic regurgitation; LVOT, left ventricular outflow tract.

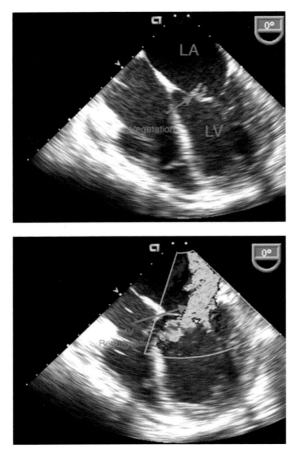

Color plate 25.2 TEE of mitral valve endocarditis with leaflet perforation and mitral regurgitation.

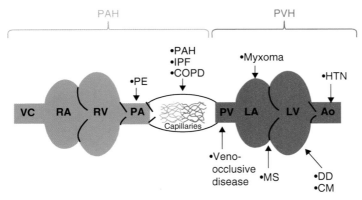

Color plate 27.1 Locations of disease processes resulting in PH. Ao, aorta; CM, cardiomyopathy; COPD, chronic obstructive pulmonary disease; DD, diastolic dysfunction; HTN, hypertension; IPF, interstitial pulmonary fibrosis; LA, left atrium; LV, left ventricle; MS, mitral stenosis; PA, pulmonary artery; PAH, pulmonary arterial hypertension; PE, pulmonary artery; PV, pulmonary vein; RA, right atrium; RV, right ventricle; VC, vena cava.

KEY REFERENCES

BENDITT DG, NGUYEN JT. Syncope: therapeutic approaches. JACC 2009; 53:1741–1751.

FREEMAN R. Neurogenic orthostatic hypotension. New Engl J Med 2008;358:615–624.

GRUBB BP. Neurocardiogenic syncope. New Engl J Med 2005;352:1004–1010.

STRICKBERGER SA, BENSON DW, BIAGGIONI I, et al. AHA/ACCF scientific statement of the evaluation of syncope. JACC 2006;47;473–484.

Chapter 18

Approach to the Patient with a Narrow Complex Tachycardia

Zachary D. Goldberger and Timir S. Baman

18.1 INTRODUCTION

A narrow complex tachycardia is often encountered in the inpatient setting. They are often paroxysmal in nature, do not typically present with hemodynamic compromise, but can cause the patient (and perhaps the physician) considerable distress. A narrow complex tachycardia (QRS duration <120 ms) represents normal activation of the ventricles via the His-Purkinje network. As a general rule, narrow complex tachycardias are supraventricular in origin – that is, they originate from within or above the AV node. However, supraventricular tachycardias (SVTs) can manifest with a narrow or wide QRS complex (see Chapter 19 for a full discussion of wide complex tachycardias). This chapter focuses on the basics of differential diagnosis, mechanisms, electrocardiographic distinction, and treatment of supraventricular narrow complex tachycardias.

18.2 DIFFERENTIAL DIAGNOSIS

The differential diagnosis of narrow complex tachycardias is shown in Table 18.1. This chapter will mainly focus on regular, narrow complex tachycardias that may manifest in a hospitalized patient. Overall, sinus tachycardia is the most common cause of a narrow complex tachycardia and, when present in inpatient settings, the etiology

Inpatient Cardiovascular Medicine, First Edition. Edited by Brahmajee K. Nallamothu and Timir S. Baman.
© 2014 John Wiley & Sons, Inc. Published 2014 by John Wiley & Sons, Inc.

Table 18.1   Narrow Complex Tachycardias.

Narrow complex tachycardias	Rhythm
Sinus tachycardia	Regular
Sinoatrial reentrant tachycardia (uncommon)	Regular
Atrial fibrillation (with a ventricular response >100 bpm)	Irregular
Atrial flutter	Regular or irregular
Atrioventricular nodal reentrant tachycardia (AVNRT)	Regular
Atrioventricular reentrant tachycardia (AVRT)	Regular
Atrial tachycardia	Regular
Multifocal atrial tachycardia	Irregular

Table 18.2   Causes of Sinus Tachycardia.

Pain, anxiety, exertion

Sympathomimetic drugs (e.g. epinephrine, dopamine, tricyclic antidepressants, isoproterenol, cocaine)

Fever, sepsis, infection

Congestive heart failure

Thyrotoxicosis

Pulmonary embolism

Alcohol withdrawal

Hypovolemia (may be caused by conditions such as bleeding, diarrhea, dehydration, pancreatitis)

Inappropriate sinus tachycardia

Note: ectopic atrial tachycardia originating in the high right atrium may mimic sinus tachycardia

needs to be identified as it may herald serious pathology. Sinus tachycardia can be caused by myriad conditions (Table 18.2).

18.3 NOMENCLATURE

When seeing an electrocardiogram (ECG) with a regular, narrow complex tachycardia not felt to be sinus tachycardia, it is not uncommon to say "This patient has SVT." The term "SVT" usually refers to one of the common paroxysmal supraventricular tachycardias (PSVTs): atrioventricular nodal reentrant tachycardia (AVNRT), atrioventricular reentrant tachycardia (AVRT), or atrial tachycardia. However, the general term "SVT" should be avoided as a diagnosis, as it is inaccurate, nonspecific, and may cause confusion. Again, SVT describes a tachycardia that originates within or above the AV node. Atrial fibrillation, atrial flutter, and sinus tachycardia are all, by definition, SVTs. Rather than state that a patient "has SVT," it is more appropriate to describe an ECG as "a regular/irregular, narrow-complex tachycardia at a rate of xx bpm, most likely AVNRT, AVRT, or AT" (Figure 18.1).

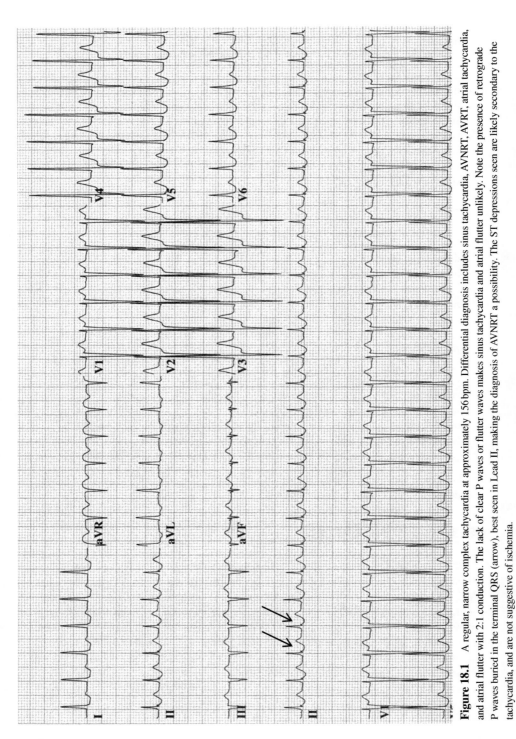

Figure 18.1 A regular, narrow complex tachycardia at approximately 156 bpm. Differential diagnosis includes sinus tachycardia, AVNRT, AVRT, atrial tachycardia, and atrial flutter with 2:1 conduction. The lack of clear P waves or flutter waves makes sinus tachycardia and atrial flutter unlikely. Note the presence of retrograde P waves buried in the terminal QRS (arrow), best seen in Lead II, making the diagnosis of AVNRT a possibility. The ST depressions seen are likely secondary to the tachycardia, and are not suggestive of ischemia.

18.4   ATRIAL FLUTTER WITH 2:1 CONDUCTION

The pathophysiology of atrial flutter is complex, and beyond the scope of this chapter (See Chapter 20). Overall, it is characterized by rapid atrial depolarization generated by an electrical circuit that circles the tricuspid annulus at 300 bpm. However, there is usually 2:1, 3:1, or 4:1 conduction across the AV node. Consequently, the ventricular response is usually some multiple of the flutter rate (in the absence of AV node dysfunction or antiarrhythmic drugs that slow the flutter circuit and AV conduction). For example, 2:1 flutter will usually manifest a ventricular response of 150 bpm; 3:1 flutter will usually manifest a ventricular response of 100 bpm; and 4:1 flutter will have a ventricular response of 75 bpm.

As a rule, whenever a narrow complex tachycardia is seen at a rate of 140–160 bpm, atrial flutter with 2:1 conduction should be suspected. With 2:1 conduction, the classic "saw-tooth" pattern may not be apparent, especially given that there will be only two flutter waves between QRS complexes that are narrowly-spaced (Figure 18.2). Flutter waves are best seen in leads V1 and II, although inspection of all leads is important. In addition, they should be completely uniform and occur at a regular rate, usually at 300 beats/min.

Atrial flutter is often misdiagnosed and overlooked. It may be very difficult to discern atrial flutter from atrial tachycardia with 2:1 conduction (often manifested by digitalis toxicity) (Figure 18.3). The atrial morphology in these two distinct arrhythmias is similar. However, treatment of these two disorders is different – one requiring some combination of anticoagulation, rate-controlling agents, and/or possibly radiofrequency ablation, and the other simply the cessation of digitalis, if toxicity is suspected. This illustrates the importance of a clinical history and medication review when faced with a stable narrow or wide complex tachycardia. In addition, it is important to note that coarse atrial fibrillation may be mistaken for atrial flutter with variable block (Figure 18.4). As above, flutter waves should be uniform in the same lead and occur at a regular rate, even in the presence of variable block.

18.5   PAROXYSMAL SUPRAVENTRICULAR TACHYCARDIAS

The paroxysmal supraventricular tachycardias (PSVTs) include the triad of AVNRT, AVRT, and atrial tachycardia. They are regular, narrow complex tachycardias with a rapid onset and offset, and occur across all age groups. AVNRT and AVRT require the AV node for the initiation and maintenance of the tachycardia, while atrial tachycardia is generated by a rapidly firing ectopic atrial pacemaker in the right or left atrium. These tachyarrhythmias are often difficult to distinguish on the surface 12-lead ECG, but there are certain clues that may help.

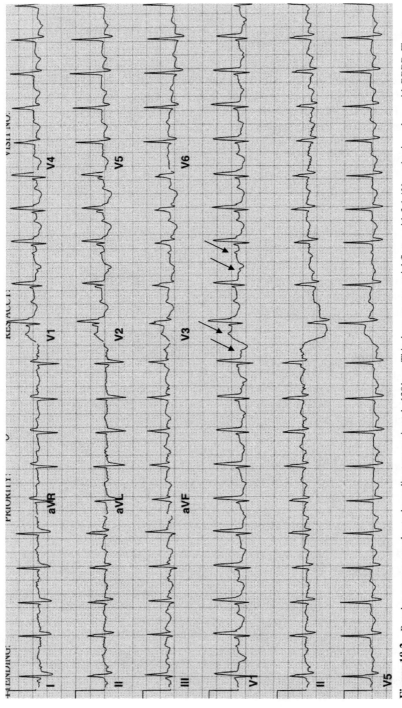

Figure 18.2 Regular, narrow complex tachycardia at approximately 120bpm. This demonstrates atrial flutter with 2:1 AV conduction, along with RBBB. Flutter waves are best seen in lead V1, particularly between the 10th and 11th and 12th and 13th beats, where the rate transiently slows (arrows). The ventricular response is slightly less than expected for 2:1 flutter, which raises the suspicion of the concomitant use of a drug that acts on the AV node (e.g. beta-blocker, calcium-channel blocker, digitalis, amiodarone), often used in patients with atrial flutter.

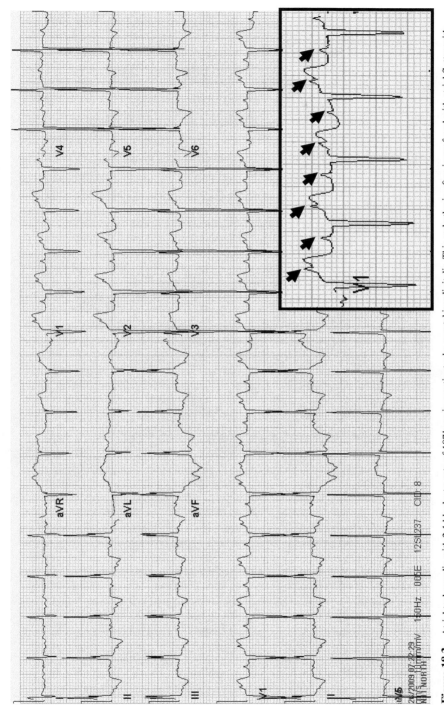

Figure 18.3 Atrial tachycardia with 2:1 block at a rate of 107 bpm in a patient who was taking digitalis. This arrhythmia often is confused with atrial flutter with 2:1 conduction. Ectopic atrial waves at a rate of 214 bpm are best seen in lead V1 (arrows, inset).

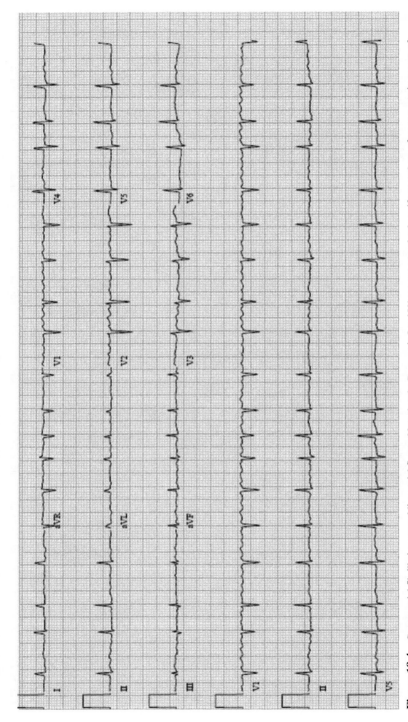

Figure 18.4 Coarse atrial fibrillation resembling atrial flutter. Note that the P waves in Lead V1 are not completely uniform and are often at a rate in excess of 300 bpm. thus excluding atrial flutter.

18.6 MECHANISMS

18.6.1 Atrioventricular Nodal Reentrant Tachycardia (AVNRT)

AVNRT is perhaps the most common of the PSVTs, and the rate is usually 180–200 bpm, but can range from 110–250 bpm. It is often seen in young adults without structural heart disease, 70% of which are women (pregnancy can often be a trigger for AVNRT). Some other triggers of AVNRT include nicotine, stimulants, exercise, or (paradoxically) hypervagotonic states. It is most often manifested by palpitations, although light-headedness and dyspnea can occur. Angina is less common. A sustained episode can theoretically result in syncope but, in general, PSVTs do not manifest with a loss of consciousness – in fact, if syncope is present after an episode of palpitations, ventricular tachycardia should strongly be suspected if coronary disease is present.

A simple diagram of AVNRT is illustrated in Figure 18.5. The AV is comprised of two sets of tissue, the so-called slow and fast pathways. During sinus rhythm, the sinus impulse travels down both the fast and slow pathways. The impulse

A   B

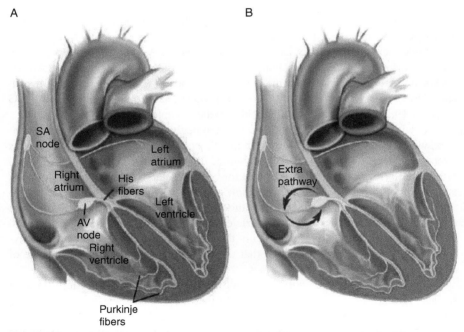

Figure 18.5 **A** Normal conduction system of the heart. **B** With AVNRT, conduction travels down the slow pathway of AV node and retrogradely up the bypass tract (fast pathway). (See Color plate 18.1). (Source: Wang, PJ and Estes NA. Supraventricular Tachycardia. Circulation 2002: 106: e206–208. Reproduced with permission of Wolters Kluwer Health).

that traverses the fast pathway enters the His-bundle prior to the impulse that is traveling down the slow pathway. As such, the slow pathway is rendered refractory and the impulse in that pathway is terminated, while the impulse in the His-bundle depolarizes the ventricles.

One important feature of these pathways is their relative refractory time. The fast pathway has a longer refractory period than the slow pathway. This is important in the initiation of typical AVNRT. A properly and specifically timed premature atrial complex (PAC) enters the AV node, but must travel down the slow pathway, given that the fast pathway (with a longer refractory period) will still be refractory from the prior sinus impulse. By the time the impulse reaches the His-bundle, the fast pathway has recovered, and the impulse will travel both retrogradely up the fast pathway and down the His-bundle into the ventricles. As a consequence, both a QRS complex (from normal His-Purkinje depolarization) and a retrograde P wave (from retrograde, or reverse travel up the AV node into the atria) are often witnessed (Figure 18.1). This circuit then perpetuates itself with subsequent antegrade conduction back down the slow pathway and retrograde conduction up the fast pathway. AVNRT may terminate spontaneously or another PAC may disrupt the cycle.

18.6.2   Atrioventricular Reentrant Tachycardia (AVRT)

AVRT is similar in pathophysiology to AVNRT, with the exception that it incorporates an accessory pathway (bypass tract) located in the ventricle as part of the reentry, rather than having the reentry isolated to the AV node. As an accessory pathway is utilized, it is not surprising that a number of patients who manifest AVRT have Wolff-Parkinson-White (WPW) syndrome, and the presence of a short PR interval, a widened QRS, delta waves, and secondary ST-T wave changes on their baseline ECG (Chapter 19, Approach to the Patient with a Wide Complex Tachycardia).

As with AVNRT, the reentrant circuit often begins with a premature atrial complex, which allows for conduction down the AV node and retrogradely up the bypass tract (Figure 18.6). It is important to recognize that this form of tachycardia – termed orthodromic reentry, due the direction of the circuit – manifests as a narrow complex tachyarrhythmia given that depolarization of the ventricles occurs down the His-Purkinje system. When the direction of the pathway is reversed – termed antidromic reentry – the depolarization of the ventricles occurs down the bypass tract and retrograde activation of the ventricles occurs through the AV node. As such, the tachycardia will be wide complex, given that the ventricles are pre-excited by virtue of depolarization through the bypass tract.

Of note, some patients with AVRT do not manifest the WPW pattern on their surface 12-lead. In this instance, it is likely that there is a concealed bypass tract, meaning that it is only capable of conducting retrogradely. A bypass tract needs to conduct anterogradely in order to manifest the WPW pattern because pre-excitation occurs both by activation of the ventricles normally through the AV node and prematurely over the bypass tract. Of note, some patients may have more than one bypass tract. Localizing the bypass tract by the surface ECG is a useful exercise, but a full discussion is beyond the scope of this chapter.

18.6.3   Atrial Tachycardia

Although the term seems generic, atrial tachycardia usually denotes ectopic (or focal) atrial tachycardia. The mechanism is due to rapid discharge of an ectopic pacemaker within the atria. Of note, atrial tachycardia is usually due to one single site of discharge in the left or right atrium. Experienced electrocardiographers are able to identify where the ectopic focus is by analyzing the morphology of the P wave. Atrial tachycardia can be self-limiting, but also can occur as the predominant rhythm – such instances are termed incessant atrial tachycardia. As opposed to AVNRT and AVRT, which often occur in patients without structural heart disease, atrial tachycardia is more often seen in patients with cardiomyopathy. The atrial rate during atrial tachycardia is usually 130–250 bpm, but can range from 100–300 bpm.

As mentioned above, atrial tachycardia with 2:1 block (Figure 18.3) is a classic ECG manifestation of digitalis toxicity. From a pharmacologic standpoint, the arrhythmia is manifest because digitalis increases the atrial automaticity but also is an AV nodal blocker (2:1 block).

18.7   ELECTROCARDIOGRAPHIC DIAGNOSIS

The most precise means of diagnosing the exact etiology of a PSVT is through intracardiac electrograms obtained during an electrophysiology study. However, the surface 12-lead ECG can be very helpful in determining the likely causes of the arrhythmia in a majority of cases.

18.7.1   Retrograde P Waves

The electrocardiographic difference between AVNRT and AVRT is subtle. As above, the mechanism of both involves reentry within the node (AVNRT) or up a bypass tract (AVRT). AVRT is often suggested by the presence of WPW on the resting ECG. However, some patients with bypass tracts may have other concomitant arrhythmias (i.e. atrial flutter, AVNRT). But common to both AVNRT and AVRT is the presence of retrograde P waves. However, the location of the P wave is slightly different in both arrhythmias (Figure 18.6).

- With AVNRT, the retrograde P wave is buried within or just after the QRS complex as the distance from the node to the atrium is minimal
- With AVRT, the retrograde P wave is more distant from the QRS complex as the distance from the ventricle to the atrium is greater

The reason for this difference stems from the fact that the electrical impulse which reenters the atria after traveling through the AV node has to travel a longer distance in AVRT than in AVNRT. This difference may be on the order of 40–120 ms (1–3 small boxes

Typical AVNRT   AVRT

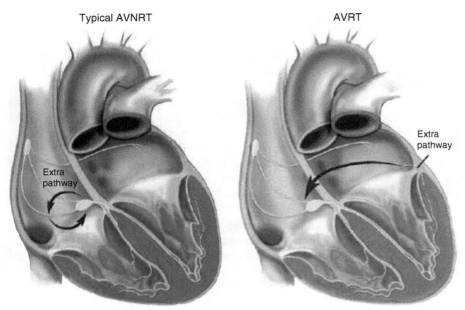

Figure 18.6 With AVNRT the extra pathway is contained within the AV node as opposed to AVRT where the accessory pathway involves an atrium and ventricle. (See Color plate 18.2). (Source: Wang, PJ and Estes NA. Supraventricular Tachycardia. Circulation 2002: 106: e206–208. Reproduced with permission of Wolters Kluwer Health).

on the ECG). Furthermore, the distance the bypass tract is relative to the AV node, and the conduction properties of the bypass tract itself will shorten or lengthen the distance between the QRS complex and the retrograde P wave.

In AVNRT, given the morphology of the retrograde P waves, and their close proximity to the QRS complex (giving the impression of one hybrid complex), one often characterizes the ECG appearance of the QRS-P complex as (1) Pseudo R-prime (R') in V1 and/or (2) pseudo S in the inferior leads (II, III, aVF) (Figure 18.7). This terminology is usually not used with AVRT, given the presence of two discrete entities (a QRS and the P wave). It can be very helpful to have a baseline ECG taken when the patient is in normal sinus rhythm, in which there no pseudo R' or pseudo S complexes present. Shown in Figure 18.8 is a baseline ECG from a patient with WPW who presented with narrow complex tachycardia, likely AVRT. With WPW, it is important not to mistake large voltage or inverted T waves for hypertrophy or ischemia, respectively. These changes often occur in conjunction with the WPW pattern.

P waves that look retrograde may be present in atrial tachycardia and, depending on where the ectopic focus lies, the location may be at a variable distance from the QRS complex. One subtle clue to differentiate atrial tachycardia from AVNRT and AVRT is that there is a "warm up" phase at the onset, in which the rate gradually accelerates before the maximum rate occurs. AVNRT and AVRT typically have a sudden offset and onset without any gradual acceleration (although there may be exceptions to this rule). In addition, an atrial rate that occurs >250 bpm is usually due to atrial tachycardia or atrial flutter; in the latter, there is often 2:1 AV conduction, resulting in a ventricular rate

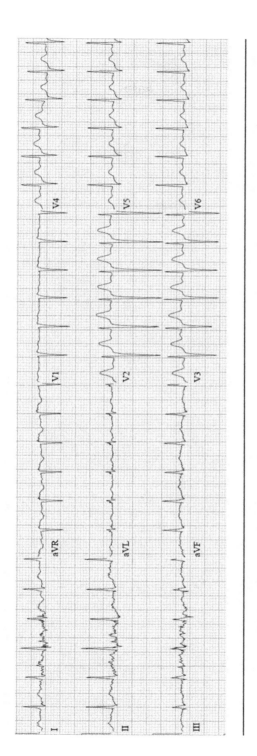

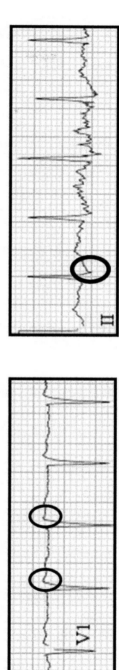

Figure 18.7 AVNRT is shown in the top panel at 144 bpm. What strongly suggests AVNRT is the presence of pseudo R-prime in V1, and pseudo S waves in lead II (bottom panel, leads V1 and II enlarged). These changes are indicative of retrograde P waves traveling up the fast pathway. Baseline artifact is present in lead II.

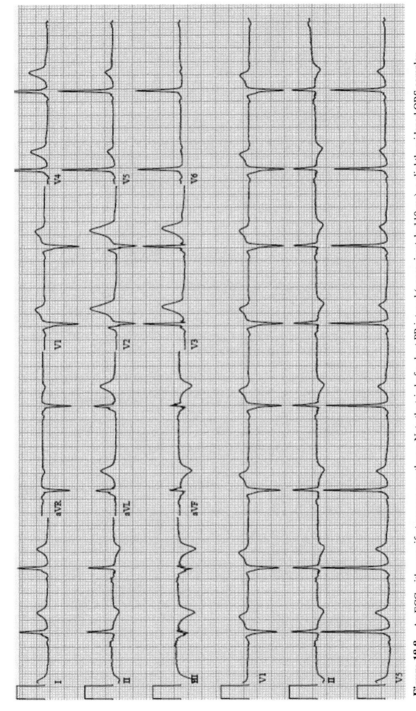

Figure 18.8 An ECG with a manifest accessory pathway. Note the triad of a short PR interval (approximately 110 ms), a slightly widened QRS complex, and a delta wave. Secondary T wave inversions are present, and are not due to ischemia in the context of WPW pattern.

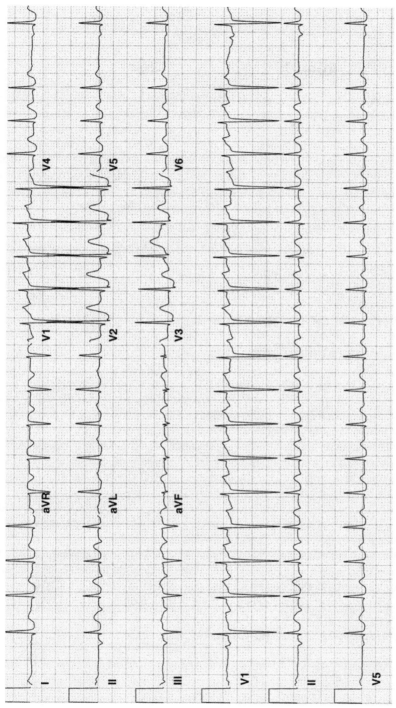

Figure 18.9 Ectopic atrial tachycardia is seen at a rate of approximately 107 bpm. Note the P waves following the initiation and end of the tachycardia – the ectopic focus (negative in Lead II) strongly suggests that this is ectopic atrial tachycardia. There are no flutter waves, nor are there retrograde P waves intimately associated or just after the QRS to suggest reentry.

of 150 bpm in atrial flutter. Finally, if an ectopic rhythm is present on cessation of the tachycardia, atrial tachycardia is highly likely (Figure 18.9).

18.7.2   RP Relationship

There is slightly unusual nomenclature for the PSVTs, that is often helpful in forming a differential diagnosis of PSVTs, termed the RP interval. Clinicians are most accustomed to defining the PR interval (short, as in WPW pattern, and long as in first degree AV block or with hyperthyroidism, see Chapter 2 for a description of normal ECG intervals). The RP interval is defined as the time between the QRS complex and the next visible P wave. A short RP interval is less than half of the interval between contiguous QRS complexes while a long RP interval is greater than half of the interval between QRS complexes. A short RP tachycardia conjures a different differential than a long RP tachycardia:

- Short RP tachycardias: typical AVNRT, AVRT, atrial tachycardia
- Long RP tachycardias: atypical AVNRT, atrial tachycardia, sinus tachycardia

Of note, there are atypical forms of AVNRT and uncommon variations of AVRT that are beyond the scope of this discussion.

18.8   PHYSIOLOGIC DIAGNOSIS

18.8.1   Vagal Maneuvers

As above, the diagnosis of many of the PSVTs centers upon the identification and morphology of the P waves. However, this can be challenging, especially if P waves are not identifiable. In these instances, elucidating the diagnosis may be possible by slowing or terminating the arrhythmia.

The Valsalva maneuver is often the first approach in compliant patients. Straining against a closed glottis, coughing, or compression of the eyes will result in a withdrawal of sympathetic tone. Carotid sinus massage (CSM) works in a similar fashion, and may also be effective, if performed properly. However, bradycardia and hypotension can result from CSM and Valsalva maneuvers. As such, continuous ECG and blood pressure monitoring need to be performed with these vagal maneuvers. Contraindications to CSM do exist, and are listed in Table 18.3.

Vagal maneuvers often slow the AV node. As a result if the tachycardia circuit involves the AV node such as in AVNRT, often times the arrhythmia can be terminated. Such a response would not usually be seen in sinus tachycardia or atrial tachycardia as these arrhythmias does not involved the AV node in the circuit.

18.9   PHARMACOLOGIC DIAGNOSIS

18.9.1   Adenosine

Adenosine is a short-acting ($T_{1/2}$ ~ 8 seconds) intravenous pharmacologic agent that heightens vagal tone, and results in a slowing of the sinus rate and an increase in AV

Table 18.3   Contraindications to Carotid Sinus Massage.

History of stroke or transient ischemic attack (unless recent carotid imaging has
  demonstrated no atheromatous plaque)
Presence of a carotid bruit
Recent myocardial infarction (≤6 months prior)
Ventricular tachyarrhythmia

Table 18.4   Response of Various SVTs to Adenosine.

Narrow complex tachycardia	Adenosine response
Sinus tachycardia	Brief slowing
Atrial flutter (with 2:1 conduction)	Transient slowing of the ventricular rate, increasing AV conduction; serves to clarify presence of flutter waves before tachycardia resumes
AVNRT	Pause with termination of arrhythmia, conversion to sinus rhythm
AVRT	Pause with termination of arrhythmia, conversion to sinus rhythm
Atrial tachycardia	Transient slowing (with possible appearance of ectopic atrial activity) with subsequent resumption of tachycardia

nodal conduction delay. As such, it is an effective means of slowing the ventricular rate. It provides both the diagnosis and/or therapy of several of the PSVTs. It can be given as a 6 mg IV bolus followed by a 20 cc flush; if ineffective, a 12 mg IV bolus can be administered, but this dose should never be repeated more than twice. Administration may cause flushing, palpitations, or chest pain, so patients should be given appropriate warning. It is felt to be contraindicated in cardiac transplant patients, given the heightened risk of asystole.

In a small percentage of patients, adenosine can induce atrial fibrillation. *For this reason, it is dangerous to administer adenosine to patients who are exhibiting WPW with a rapid response*, as the induction of atrial fibrillation with WPW can precipitate 1:1 conduction down the bypass tract. Furthermore, blocking the AV node in a patient exhibiting WPW with rapid atrial fibrillation can lead to unopposed rapid conduction down the accessory pathway, leading to possible degeneration into ventricular fibrillation. However, for most narrow complex tachycardias, it is safe to administer adenosine for the termination of the arrhythmia (if vagal maneuvers are not effective or attempted). Emergency resuscitation equipment should be at the bedside. Continuous blood pressure monitoring and continuous ECG monitoring is critical. Without a continuous ECG, atrial activity in response to adenosine will not be recorded, and the etiology of the arrhythmia will be missed (despite potential termination).

Adenosine should be considered the drug of choice to terminate an arrhythmia strongly suspected to be AVNRT or AVRT, and it can aid in the clarification of atrial flutter with 2:1 conduction. It should not be given to patients with sinus tachycardia. Of note, it is possible for adenosine to have no effect on any of the narrow complex tachycardias. Table 18.4 lists the expected therapeutic responses of adenosine.

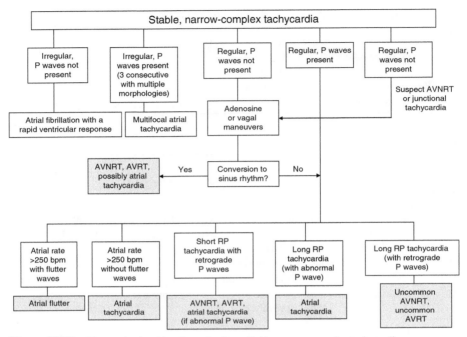

Figure 18.10   Diagnostic algorithm for evaluation of table, narrow complex tachycardia.

18.10 DIAGNOSTIC ALGORITHM

Most narrow complex arrhythmias do not present with hemodynamic instability although, with any degree of tachycardia, the degree of discomfort or hemodynamic instability is case-specific. Unstable rhythms should be quickly recognized and terminated. *With the obvious exception of sinus rhythm, one should never be faulted for terminating any tachyarrhythmia with electrical cardioversion if hemodynamic instability is present.* Figure 18.10 is a step-wise approach that can be used to diagnose a narrow complex tachycardia.

TAKE HOME POINTS

- Narrow complex tachycardia are common, and are often reversible.
- Immediate termination of paroxysmal supraventricular tachycardias (AVNRT, AVRT – the long RP tachycardias) can usually be achieved with carotid sinus massage or IV adenosine.
- IV adenosine can be a diagnostic and therapeutic tool when faced with a regular, narrow complex tachycardia of unclear etiology.
- Atrial tachycardia, atrial flutter, and atrial fibrillation will be transiently slowed, but not terminated, by adenosine or vagal maneuvers. Transient AV block will elucidate the presence of flutter waves, fibrillation waves, or ectopic atrial activity, which will distinguish these rhythms from AVNRT or AVRT.
- Always perform 12-lead monitoring when administering adenosine, and emergency personnel and equipment should be present.

Chapter 19

The Approach to the Patient with a Wide Complex Tachycardia

Zachary D. Goldberger and Timir S. Baman

19.1 INTRODUCTION

The electrocardiographic evaluation of a tachyarrhythmia should begin by deter-mining whether the QRS complex is wide or narrow. Narrow complex tachycardias are usually supraventricular – the initial site of cardiac activation is at or above the atrioventricular (AV) junction as discussed in Chapter 18. Supraventricular tachycar-dias (SVTs) can generate narrow or wide complex QRS complexes; however, when faced with a wide complex tachycardia, clinicians must assume the etiology is ventricular tachycardia (VT) until proven otherwise.

The ability to differentiate between SVT with a wide QRS and VT often pres-ents a diagnostic challenge. This distinction is critical as the treatment for each differs significantly and improper therapy may have potentially lethal conse-quences. As always, a formal cardiology consultation for any arrhythmia, wide complex or otherwise, is always prudent when uncertainties in diagnosis and management arise.

19.2 OVERALL MECHANISMS

A narrow complex tachycardia (QRS duration <120 ms) represents activation of the ventricles via the His-Purkinje network. A widened QRS (≥120 ms) usually represents a ventricular arrhythmia originating below the bifurcation of the bundle

Inpatient Cardiovascular Medicine, First Edition. Edited by Brahmajee K. Nallamothu and Timir S. Baman.
© 2014 John Wiley & Sons, Inc. Published 2014 by John Wiley & Sons, Inc.

of His, or a supraventricular arrhythmia with aberrant ventricular conduction. *Aberrant conduction* is defined as transient bundle branch block due to abnormal conduction to the ventricle, usually caused by conduction when one of the bundles is refractory (see section 19.4).

Numerous mechanisms can be responsible for generating WCTs; however, ventricular tachycardia is the most common etiology (Table 19.1). However, it is always important to first rule out ECG artifact which may be mistakenly misdiagnosed as WCT, since this may lead to unnecessary procedures. Evaluation of the patient when a WCT is seen on telemetry is crucial. Telemetry leads are affected by motion; a rapid, repetitive motion (such as teeth-brushing) may simulate ventricular tachycardia (Figure 19.1). In these instances, the QRS complexes can be "marched out" amidst the artifact. Especially when examining telemetry strips it is imperative to evaluate all leads for artifact.

Other causes of WCTs include Class I antiarrhythmic agents (e.g. procainamide, flecainide) which can cause a rate-related aberrant conduction of an SVT due to a slowing of conduction through the His-Purkinje system. Often overlooked causes of WCTs include marked hyperkalemia, tricyclic antidepressant overdose, or an acute ST elevation myocardial infarction (large ST segment elevations may fuse the peak of the QRS and the T wave, simulating a widened QRS).

Table 19.1   Causes of Wide Complex Tachycardia.

Ventricular tachycardia (80%)
Sinus tachycardia with bundle branch block
SVT with aberrancy due to conduction slowing or bundle branch block
SVT with anterograde conduction over an accessory AV pathway
Ventricular pacing
Electrolyte imbalances such as hyperkalemia
Electrocardiographic artifact
Direct proarrhythmic effect of antiarrhythmic agents

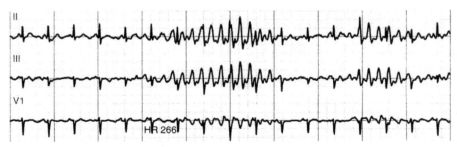

Figure 19.1   Wide complex tachycardia as captured on hospital telemetry. However, upon closer inspection, of all leads this is simply artifact.

19.3   VENTRICULAR TACHYCARDIA

Ventricular tachycardia is the cause of WCT in >80% of patients. Moreover, if faced with a WCT in the setting of a previous myocardial infarction, clinicians can assume the cause is ventricular tachycardia >96% of the time. In general, making an assumption of ventricular tachycardia when uncertainty exists can be a prudent method of treatment. Hemodynamic stability is not an indicator of SVT versus VT and should not be taken into consideration during evaluation.

19.4   SUPRAVENTRICULAR MECHANISMS

With SVT, widening of the QRS complex occurs when conduction in the normal conduction system is slowed or blocked. This condition may be pre-existing, or due to a transient bundle branch block (BBB) (Figure 19.2). A BBB occurring as a result of tachycardia is often referred to as "aberrancy." In this situation, one bundle branch may be ready to conduct another impulse from the atrium; however, the other bundle branch has not fully repolarized, resulting in delayed conduction and a widened beat due to cell-to-cell depolarization.

Aberrancy can occur with any type of supraventricular arrhythmia. The Ashman phenomenon is a unique form of aberrancy classically seen in atrial fibrillation in which a long RR cycle is followed immediately by a short RR cycle, and the second beat of that combination typically shows a right bundle branch block (RBBB) pattern due to refractoriness in that bundle branch. When a WCT occurs in a brief salvo in the setting in atrial fibrillation, Ashman beating should be suspected (Figure 19.3).

With Wolff-Parkinson-White patterns, AV conduction occurs anterogradely over two pathways: the AV node and an accessory pathway (Figure 19.4). The accessory pathway facilitates the maintenance of what are commonly known as AV reentrant (or reciprocating) tachycardias. These tachycardias can manifest with either a narrow or wide complex QRS, depending on which pathway conducts in an anterograde fashion. With orthodromic AV reentrant tachycardia (the most common type), the AV

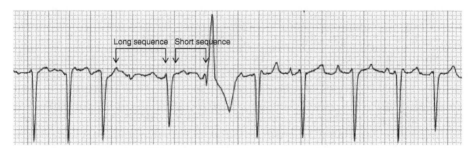

Figure 19.2   Atrial fibrillation with aberrant conduction of one beat. The wide QRS beat occurs as the right bundle is refractory due to the short coupling interval otherwise known as a "long short sequence."

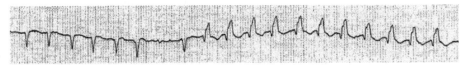

Figure 19.3   Atrial fibrillation with rapid ventricular response at approximately 159 beats/min. Ashman phenomenon is present, with RBBB starting immediately after a short RR cycle.

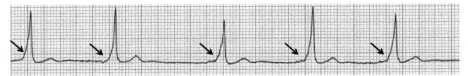

Figure 19.4   A patient with Wolf Parkinson White pattern on ECG. Note the delta wave (arrow) which depicts early ventricular depolarization down the accessory pathway, resulting in a wide QRS and short PR interval.

node conducts anterogradely and the accessory pathway conducts in a retrograde fashion, resulting in a narrow complex tachycardia (unless a BBB is also present). Conversely, if the accessory tract conducts in an anterograde fashion with retrograde conduction occurring over the AV node (antidromic AV reentrant tachycardia), a wide complex pre-excited SVT results which can be difficult to differentiate from VT without an electrophysiology study.

A rapid (>220 bpm) irregular WCT is pathognomonic for pre-excited atrial fibrillation due to a rapidly conducting bypass tract. Patients with WPW who present with atrial fibrillation should not be given AV nodal blocking agents as this can result in excessive ventricular rates and subsequent ventricular fibrillation.

19.5 BENIGN FORMS

It is important to recognize that benign forms of idiopathic VT do exist clinically and are amenable to catheter ablation for symptomatic relief. Ventricular tachycardia arising from the right and left outflow tracts can be commonly seen in young individuals. Recognition of idiopathic VT is important because it is typically seen in patients with structurally normal hearts and, in most cases, is not associated with an increased risk for sudden death. These arrhythmias can be identified by their characteristic 12-lead ECG and clinical presentation. Repetitive monomorphic VT is characterized by salvos of nonsustained VT or paroxysmal sustained VT often triggered by exercise or catecholamines. It typically arises from the right ventricular outflow tract (RVOT). The characteristic 12-lead ECG in RVOT VT is a WCT with a LBBB pattern and tall monophasic R waves in the inferior leads (Figure 19.5), with a transition point (R ≥ S) that occurs late in the precordial leads. In the vast majority of cases, these outflow tract VTs are associated with an excellent prognosis and ablation should be considered.

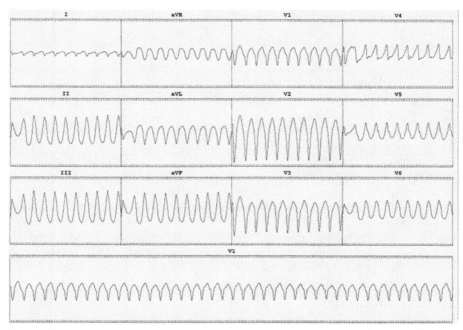

Figure 19.5   Right ventricular outflow tract tachycardia. LBBB pattern is present with tall R waves in leads II, III, aVF.

19.6 DIAGNOSIS

WCTs often arise in, and herald the onset of, an emergent situation. As such, taking a comprehensive history, performing a detailed physical examination, and inspecting prior tracings are often not feasible nor appropriate if the patient is clinically unstable. All clinicians must understand that if a patient has a history of coronary artery disease, VT is the etiology of WCT >98% of the time and emergent evaluation is necessary.

19.6.1 History

Valuable clues to the correct diagnosis begin with a focused history. In the setting of coronary artery disease with previous myocardial infarction, VT is far more likely than SVT. It is always important to identify whether there is concomitant use of anti-arrhythmic (potentially proarrhythmic) medications or other drugs such as tricyclic antidepressants.

Age can be a reliable factor in differentiating SVT from VT. WCT in individuals >35 years old is likely to be due to VT with a positive predictive value (PPV) of 85% while WCT due to SVT in a patient <35 years of age has a PPV of 70%. In addition, presenting symptoms (e.g. palpitations, light-headedness, chest pain) are not specific to any particular mechanism of tachycardia – they can appear both in VT and SVTs. Of note, SVTs rarely present with syncope. *Of utmost importance, hemodynamic stability does not rule out VT.*

19.6.2 Physical Examination

The physical examination may be helpful, especially if AV dissociation is present (strongly suggesting VT). However, less than 50% of cases of VT are associated with AV dissociation and only a subset of these are unambiguously apparent by surface ECG or physical exam. When AV dissociation is present, intermittently prominent (cannon) A waves in the jugular venous pressure waveform (reflecting simultaneous atrial and ventricular contraction) can be seen. Other suggested findings including variability of beat-to-beat blood pressure, suggest AV dissociation, but these criteria are less specific than intermittent cannon A waves. Often these subtle physical examination findings are hard to detect (especially in a loud setting such as the Emergency Department), even by an experienced examiner. A patient with WCT and a sternotomy scar likely has coronary disease thus making VT a highly probable diagnosis.

19.6.3 Imaging

Evaluation of the chest radiograph can also be helpful as cardiomegaly or evidence of prior cardiac surgery may favor the diagnosis of VT implying underlying structural heart disease. The presence of a defibrillator in a patient with WCT may be suggestive of VT that is below the detection rate. Transthoracic echocardiography may show prior scarring or segmental wall motion abnormalities indicative of prior MI. Whenever possible, clinicians should utilize clues that favor a diagnosis of coronary disease, thus making the diagnosis of VT more likely than SVT. The presence of a cardiomyopathy with depressed ejection fraction can also suggest an ischemic substrate for VT. Cardiac MRI is becoming increasingly more utilized to evaluate for the presence of infiltrative cardiomyopathies (e.g. amyloidosis, sarcoidosis), arrhythmogenic right ventricular dysplasia, and myocardial scarring.

19.6.4 Electrocardiography

While the history, physical exam, and additional data may provide clues to the presence of VT, a systematic and thoughtful analysis of the 12-lead ECG is the cornerstone of the diagnosis of a WCT in a hemodynamically-stable patient. Inspection of prior ECGs while identifying the rate, regularity, evidence of AV dissociation, and QRS duration in addition to morphology will usually help to discern the cause of a WCT.

One must be careful to evaluate the full 12-lead ECG since a WCT can generate an apparently narrow QRS in a single lead. This possibility is one of the factors that limit the accuracy of tachycardia diagnosis on a telemetry tracing or monitor. Prior ECGs can be quite helpful, especially when the patient was in sinus rhythm. Evidence

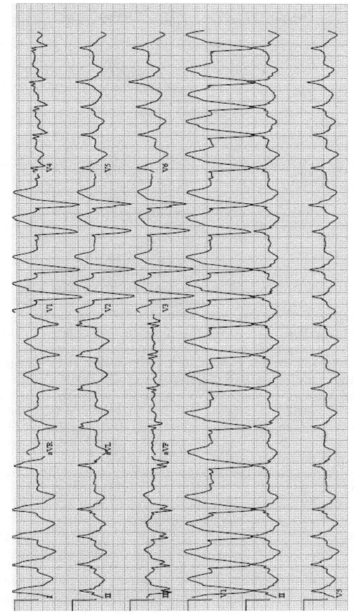

Figure 19.6 Wide complex tachycardia secondary to atrial fibrillation with rapid ventricular response and left bundle branch block. Note the irregularly irregular rhythm, the hallmark of atrial fibrillation.

237

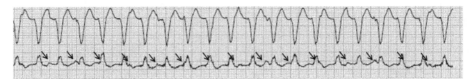

Figure 19.7   AV dissociation present thus making the diagnosis of VT likely. AV dissociation is a result of asynchronous activation of the ventricles and atrium. As the ventricular rate is greater than the atrial rate, the origin of the WCT is occurring from ventricular myocardium – hence VT is the diagnosis. Arrows denote atrial activity. Subtle changes in the WCT (top strip) can also been seen directly above the arrows denoting P waves.

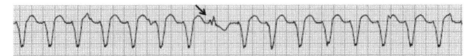

Figure 19.8   A fusion beat is present, thus making the diagnosis of VT likely. The fusion beat is a result of simultaneous activation of the ventricular myocardium by an atrial impulse and the ventricles.

of a pre-existing BBB, prior ST elevation myocardial infarction, a change in axis, or prior evidence of overt Wolff-Parkinson-White pattern can greatly help in the diagnosis.

Rate is not usually a useful criterion, as either SVT or VT may occur over a wide range of heart rates. Regularity is a more useful feature. Paroxysmal SVT and atrial flutter with 2:1 conduction are usually very regular. A grossly irregular WCT is likely atrial fibrillation with aberrancy/pre-existing bundle branch block (Figure 19.6) or atrial fibrillation with conduction over an accessory pathway. However, irregular VT cannot be excluded. Polymorphic VT and torsade de pointes should also be considered in the setting of an irregular WCT and can usually be diagnosed by the characteristic variations in QRS morphology and long underlying QT interval. These arrhythmias, however, when sustained, are not well-tolerated hemodynamically and usually require immediate intervention.

A QRS width >160 ms has been shown to be a strong predictor of VT. However, SVT with aberrancy (especially in the presence of class I antiarrhythmic agents) and pre-excitation can sometimes generate QRS durations >160 ms as well. VT arising from the intraventricular septum may have a QRS duration <140 ms.

As noted, with rare exceptions, the presence of AV dissociation is diagnostic of VT (Figure 19.7). When there is underlying sinus rhythm with AV dissociation, fusion and capture beats may be seen on the ECG. A fusion beat is the result of simultaneous activation of the ventricular myocardium from one impulse generated in the atrium (conducted via the His-Purkinje system) and one from the ventricles as part of the VT (Figure 19.8). A true capture beat has the morphology of a normal sinus QRS complex, originating solely from the right atrium, conducting down the His-Purkinje system and is also diagnostic of VT. When all QRS complexes in the precordial leads

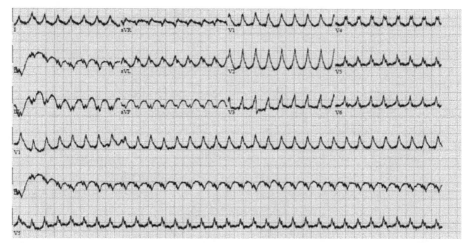

Figure 19.9   Ventricular tachycardia at approximately 200 bpm with positive precordial concordance.

Table 19.2   ECG Criteria to Rapidly Diagnose Ventricular Tachycardia*.

AV dissociation
Fusion beats
Capture beats
QRS >160 ms if LBBB
QRS >140 ms if RBBB
Right superior (northwest) axis
Positive or negative concordance in V1–V6

*Note that lack of these features does not exclude VT.

are either upright or downgoing (positive or negative concordance, respectively), VT is strongly suggested (Figure 19.9). Utilizing these quick and easy methods of determining VT from SVT can prove valuable in clinical decision making (Table 19.2).

Determining whether the arrhythmia represents VT with a BBB morphology versus SVT with aberrancy is challenging. Examination of bundle branch morphologies can provide further assistance in deterring the cause of WCT.

19.6.5   Diagnostic Algorithms

Brugada et al. combined and simplified criteria for RBBB- and LLLB-like WCTs based on four criteria applied in a step-wise algorithm to differentiate VT from SVT (Figure 19.10). By evaluating 554 tachycardias with a widened QRS and confirmation with an electrophysiologic study, they found their algorithm had a sensitivity of 98.7% and a specificity of 96.5% in distinguishing VT from SVT. The

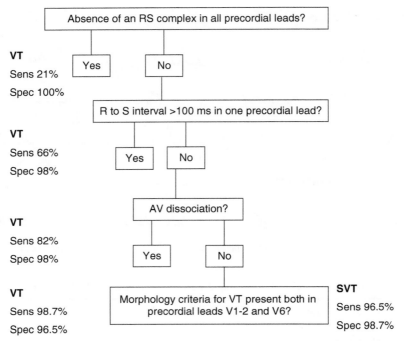

VT
Sens 21%
Spec 100%

VT
Sens 66%
Spec 98%

VT
Sens 82%
Spec 98%

VT
Sens 98.7%
Spec 96.5%

SVT
Sens 96.5%
Spec 98.7%

Figure 19.10 Algorithm designed to distinguish VT from SVT (Source: Adapted from Brugada P et al. 1991. Reproduced with permission of Wolters Kluwer Health).

absence of an RS complex in all precordial leads or an RS complex interval of >100 ms is easily recognizable and highly specific for the diagnosis of VT. If the RS complex is <100 ms, AV dissociation must be evaluated. If AV dissociation is present, VT is highly likely; if absent, then specific morphology criteria in leads V_1, V_2, and V_6 must be present to diagnose VT as described above.

While widely cited, the Brugada study has important limitations. Most notably, the authors excluded patients who were on antiarrhythmic agents – as such, it is not appropriate to apply their parameters to patients receiving antiarrhythmics. Class Ic agents (e.g. flecainide, propafenone) are sometimes used treat recurrent, paroxysmal atrial fibrillation and not only are these drugs potentially proarrhythmic, but some patients with atrial fibrillation treated with Class Ic agents can develop atrial flutter with 1:1 conduction down the AV node. In that situation, the mechanism of the WCT will be difficult to discern. Additionally, the investigators did not take into account patients with pre-excitation syndromes whose ECGs would strongly suggest VT as the mechanism for their WCT were they entered into the algorithm. It is also uncertain how the algorithm performed in patients with idiopathic ventricular tachycardia.

TAKE HOME POINTS

- The first diagnosis to consider when faced with a wide-complex tachycardia is VT. The etiology is ventricular tachycardia (VT) until proved otherwise.
- VT is much more likely with a history of ischemic heart disease (prior MI, history of CABG).
- Rate, QRS width, and age are not reliable criterion for diagnosis.
- Hemodynamic instability does not rule out a supraventricular origin.
- Immediate termination of a wide-complex termination with electrical cardioversion/defibrillation is necessary with hemodynamic instability. Antiarrhythmic therapy should be reserved for prohylaxis, or the presence of a stable wide-complex tachycardia.
- Algorithms do exist for differentiating a wide-complex tachycardia from a supraventricular versus ventricular origin. However, they do have limitations, and should be used in conjunction with the history, physical, and other data.

KEY REFERENCES

AKHTAR M. Electrophysiologic bases for wide QRS complex tachycardia. Pacing Clin Electrophysiol 1983;6:81–98.

BRADY WJ, SKILES J. Wide QRS complex tachycardia: ECG differential diagnosis. Am J Emerg Med 1999;17:376–381.

BRUGADA P, BRUGADA J, MONT L, SMEETS J, ANDRIES EW. A new approach to the differential diagnosis of a regular tachycardia with a wide QRS complex. Circulation 1991;83:1649–1659.

GOLDBERGER ZD, RHO RW, PAGE RL. Approach to the diagnosis and initial management of the stable adult patient with a wide complex tachycardia. Am J Cardiol 2008;101:1456–1466.

KINDWALL KE, BROWN J, JOSEPHSON ME. Electrocardiographic criteria for ventricular tachycardia in wide complex left bundle branch block morphology tachycardias. Am J Cardiol 1988;61:1279–1283.

LERMAN BB, STEIN KM, MARKOWITZ SM. Idiopathic right ventricular outflow tract tachycardia: a clinical approach. Pacing Clin Electrophysiol 1996;19:2120–2137.

Chapter 20

Atrial Fibrillation and Atrial Flutter

Sanjaya Gupta and Hakan Oral

20.1 INTRODUCTION

Atrial fibrillation is the most common arrhythmia in the United States, affecting 2.5 million adults with the majority of these patients over the age of 65. The prevalence of atrial fibrillation is expected to increase to an estimated 15.9 million affected adults by the year 2050. In addition to its effects upon quality of life, atrial fibrillation also is an independent risk factor for the development of stroke and heart disease – two leading causes of mortality in the United States. Moreover, atrial fibrillation is associated with numerous comorbidities including hypertension, coronary artery disease, heart failure, and valvular heart disease. Consequently, patients with atrial fibrillation have higher mortality rates than those in sinus rhythm. The cost of direct care of patients with atrial fibrillation of all ages is estimated to be $6.65 billion annually. However, if one includes the cost of caring for all atrial fibrillation-related complications, this annual cost to Medicare alone is an estimated $15.7 billion annually. The majority of this cost is attributed to hospitalizations due to rapid ventricular response, congestive heart failure, and stroke.

Atrial flutter has some very similar characteristics to atrial fibrillation; however, it is a distinct disease entity. It is less common than atrial fibrillation, with an estimated prevalence of 70,000 people for atrial flutter and 190,000 people for both coexistent atrial flutter and atrial fibrillation. Overall, the management of atrial flutter is very similar to atrial fibrillation; however, this review highlights important differences as well as similarities.

Inpatient Cardiovascular Medicine, First Edition. Edited by Brahmajee K. Nallamothu and Timir S. Baman.

20.2 PATHOPHYSIOLOGY

The underlying pathophysiology of atrial fibrillation differs from that of atrial flutter and it is multifactorial in nature. Atrial fibrillation is a multifactorial *micro*-reentrant phenomenon whereby localized regions of myocardium are automatically excited to produce a rapid and irregular atrial depolarization (Figure 20.1). The majority of cases of paroxysmal atrial fibrillation appear to originate in the left atrium from foci within the pulmonary veins. It is thought that the intersection of atrial myocardium with fibrous tissue within the pulmonary veins predisposes some patients to develop the micro-reentrant arrhythmias that cause atrial fibrillation. However, as paroxysmal atrial fibrillation progresses to become persistent atrial fibrillation, there is remodeling of the left atrium and atrial fibrillation foci develop within the atria itself. Whilst a tremendous amount has been discovered about the etiology of atrial fibrillation, much of the underlying pathogenesis behind atrial fibrillation still remains unclear.

Atrial flutter, in contrast, is a *macro*-reentrant arrhythmia that originates from either the left or right atrium. In atrial flutter, the arrhythmia appears to follow a circular tract within the atria such that the myocardium that lies within this tract is continually undergoing sequential depolarization and repolarization (Figure 20.1).

TAKE HOME POINT #1

Atrial fibrillation is a micro-reentrant arrhythmia that usually involves the left atrium and pulmonary veins while typical atrial flutter is a macro-reentrant arrhythmia that involves the cavo-tricuspid isthmus.

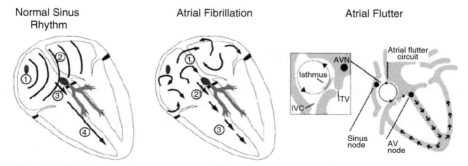

Figure 20.1   Atrial fibrillation and atrial flutter pathogenesis. (Source: Waktare J. Circulation 2002; 106:14–16 and Boyer M, Koplan BA. Circulation 2005; 112:e334–336. Reproduced with permission of Wolters Kluwer Health).

20.3 ETIOLOGY

The most common predisposing factor for the development of atrial fibrillation is structural heart disease. Mitral valvular regurgitation, congenital heart disease, heart failure/cardiomyopathy, hypertrophic cardiomyopathy and diastolic dysfunction can all lead to atrial fibrillation by causing increased atrial pressure or atrial stretch. This, in turn, leads to left atrial enlargement. Atrial fibrillation can also occur secondary to other disease processes that cause generalized inflammation of the myocardium, such as hyperthyroidism, sepsis, and myocarditis. Other risk factors for the development of atrial fibrillation include obesity, metabolic syndrome, older age, obstructive sleep apnea and other cardiopulmonary disease such as pulmonary embolus and chronic obstructive pulmonary disease (COPD). In addition, atrial fibrillation is a common arrhythmia after cardiac surgery due to the resultant hyper-inflammatory state. Atrial fibrillation can occur in the absence of structural heart disease, in which case it is referred to as "lone" atrial fibrillation. This typically occurs in younger males and it carries a favorable prognosis.

TAKE HOME POINT #2

Risk factors of atrial fibrillation involve clinical conditions that cause left atrial dilatation or hyperinflammatory states.

Atrial flutter can be divided into typical or atypical atrial flutter. Typical atrial flutter occurs in the right atrium; it moves in a counterclockwise direction and involves a tract that passes through the cavo-triscuspid isthmus. While it shares some of the etiologic factors with atrial fibrillation, it is frequently idiopathic. In contrast, atypical atrial flutter is either a right atrial flutter that moves in a clockwise direction or a left-sided atrial flutter. Left atrial flutters are most common after a previous left atrial radiofrequency ablation procedure, MAZE procedure, or previous mitral valve surgery. In this situation, the myocardial scars from previous ablations or surgical suture lines create an anatomical substrate around which the flutter can move in a circular fashion.

20.4 CLINICAL PRESENTATION

The initial clinical presentations of atrial fibrillation and atrial flutter can range from asymptomatic to markedly symptomatic. To a large degree, whether or not a patient is symptomatic depends upon the ventricular rate associated with the atrial arrhythmia. Patients with a rapid ventricular response (>100 beats per minute) will often complain of dyspnea, exercise intolerance, fatigue and the sensation of rapid palpitations. If the rapid ventricular response has been present for a prolonged period of time, the patient may develop a tachycardia-mediated cardiomyopathy and their initial presentation may mimic that of newly-diagnosed congestive heart failure. However, many

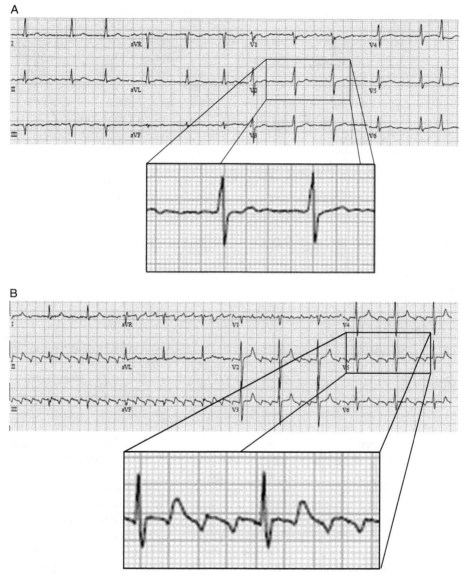

Figure 20.2 **A** Electrocardiogram of atrial fibrillation. **B** Electrocardiogram of typical atrial flutter. Note the regular uniform P waves.

patients with atrial fibrillation are often asymptomatic or minimally symptomatic at diagnosis. These patients' only complaint may be that of generalized fatigue which they may have attributed to some other cause. Approximately 50% of patients with atrial fibrillation state that they are asymptomatic; however, a large percentage of the population relay an increase in functional capacity post cardioversion when in normal rhythm. Thus, many patients do not realize that atrial fibrillation limits their functionality until they are in a normal rhythm.

Upon physical examination, patients with atrial fibrillation and atrial flutter are often noted to have a rapid and irregular pulse. Cardiac auscultation is classically notable for an "irregularly irregular" heartbeat. Atrial flutter can have a regular or a "regularly irregular" heartbeat. An electrocardiogram confirms the diagnosis of atrial fibrillation or atrial flutter (Figure 20.2). Atrial fibrillation is characterized by a lack of evidence of organized atrial activity. There are no clear p waves seen on the ECG. The ventricular response is variable and irregular due to the chaotic nature of atrial depolarizations. In contrast, atrial flutter has a "sawtooth" pattern of the atrial flutter waves that range from 250–350 beats per minute. The ventricular response typically occurs in a pattern of 2:1 or 3:1 conduction from the flutter waves. As compared to atrial flutter, atrial fibrillation appears more disorganized on the electrocardiogram.

20.5 EVALUATION AND DIAGNOSTIC STUDIES

The initial evaluation of a patient with atrial flutter or atrial fibrillation should proceed in a systematic fashion. The first step is to assess the patient and determine whether or not he/she is hemodynamically stable or unstable. A patient with atrial flutter or atrial fibrillation that has associated hypotension, angina or evidence of ongoing myocardial ischemia, dyspnea or other symptoms of decompensated heart failure is considered to be unstable and treatment should be geared towards restoring sinus rhythm via cardioversion. Most commonly, this is accomplished by giving the patient intravenous sedation and then performing a synchronized DC cardioversion. In these patients, the risk of a potential thromboembolic event is outweighed by the immediate risk posed by the unstable nature of the arrhythmia.

If the patient is hemodynamically stable, or once sinus rhythm is achieved through cardioversion, then a search for etiologic factors is the next logical step. A detailed history should focus on elucidating symptoms of heart failure, hyperthyroidism, and sleep apnea as these are all conditions associated with the development of atrial fibrillation and atrial flutter. Since anticoagulation will also be part of the initial management of atrial flutter and atrial fibrillation, it is important to assess for any historical elements that may indicate a contraindication to anticoagulation, such as recent stroke, intracranial mass, major surgical procedure, or gastrointestinal bleed requiring blood transfusion. With elderly patients, an assessment of their fall risk and consequent risk for intracranial bleed if anticoagulated should also be taken into consideration. For patients with suspected atrial flutter, additional historical elements that should be considered are a previous history of atrial ablation procedure and/or cardiac surgery.

In terms of diagnostic studies, the initial test should be a 12-lead electrocardiogram to confirm the diagnosis of atrial flutter or atrial fibrillation. Initial laboratory investigations should include serum thyroid stimulating hormone (TSH) level, a B-type natriuretic peptide (BNP), and a coagulation profile (PT, PTT and INR) to establish a baseline for initiation of anticoagulation. An echocardiogram should also be performed to evaluate for the presence of structural heart disease. This is important for both an etiologic as well as prognostic evaluation. A patient with a cardiomyopathy or valvular heart disease has a higher incidence of secondary atrial arrhythmias than patients without these structural abnormalities. Treatment should also address the underlying cause for the cardiomyopathy or valvular heart disease in addition to treatment of the arrhythmia itself. If patients have a newly-discovered non-ischemic cardiomyopathy that cannot be attributed to any other condition (e.g. infiltrative disease, viral infection, familial dilated cardiomyopathy, etc.) then consideration should be given for a tachycardia-mediated cardiomyopathy that may be the result of a prolonged period of uncontrolled atrial fibrillation. For these patients, maintenance of sinus rhythm and/or aggressive rate control will be of paramount importance. Atrial fibrillation also carries a more ominous prognosis for patients with a previous history of stroke/transient ischemic attack or congestive heart failure.

20.6 TREATMENT

The initial treatment strategy for new onset atrial fibrillation and atrial flutter should proceed in a stepwise fashion (Figure 20.3). As discussed above, the initial step is assessment of hemodynamic stability and the need for immediate cardioversion. If the patient is considered hemodynamically stable, then the next step is geared towards stabilization of the ventricular rate. This is accomplished by intravenous infusions of beta-blocker or calcium channel blocker medications. The dose of the infusion should be titrated to bring the ventricular rate below 90 beats per minute without inducing systemic hypotension. The addition of digoxin, via a loading dose regimen, may be helpful as an adjunct to help achieve rate control without causing additional hypotension. Alternatively, an intravenous antiarrhythmic medication, such as amiodarone, can also be used as an adjunct to help achieve rate control. However, this medication also increases the potential for pharmacologic cardioversion and, therefore, increasing risk for a thromboembolic event if the arrhythmia has been present for greater than 48 hours.

Along with ventricular rate stabilization, an initial therapeutic approach to new onset atrial fibrillation or flutter should include initiation of anticoagulation to prevent/or minimize the formation of atrial thrombi. This can be achieved via initiation of a weight-based anticoagulation regimen of either intravenous heparin or low-molecular weight heparins. Concurrently, the patient should be initiated on oral warfarin with a goal to achieve an INR between 2.0 and 3.0. Once the INR reaches 2.0, the heparin or low-molecular weight heparin can be discontinued.

Once the ventricular rate is controlled and therapeutic anticoagulation has been achieved, the next step in the management of atrial fibrillation and atrial flutter is to attempt to restore sinus rhythm. Some patients may spontaneously revert to sinus once the ventricular rate is controlled, especially if an antiarrhythmic is utilized to help control the rate. However, the majority of patients admitted to hospital will still be in atrial fibrillation after 24 hours. The most common method to restore sinus rhythm is a synchronized DC cardioversion; however, pharmacologic cardioversion is a reasonable alternative in select patients. Regardless of the method of cardioversion

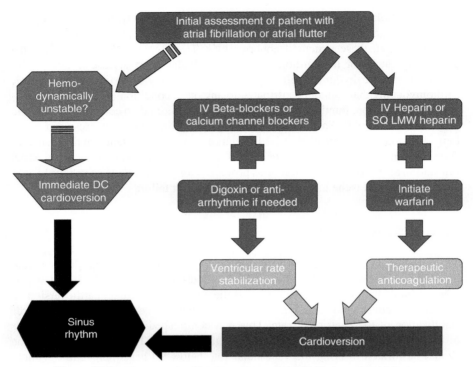

Figure 20.3   Treatment algorithm for new onset atrial fibrillation and atrial flutter.

chosen, it is important to determine the likelihood of atrial thrombus formation. It is well accepted that atrial thrombus formation occurs after approximately 48 hours of atrial fibrillation. Therefore, it is safe to proceed directly to a cardioversion if the onset of atrial fibrillation or atrial flutter can be documented to have occurred within 48 hours. However, rare is the patient for which this situation occurs. Most patients who present to the hospital in atrial fibrillation are not monitored prior to their arrival. While some patients can describe a precise onset of their symptoms, it is impossible to know if the patient had atrial fibrillation for a longer period of time and only became symptomatic once the ventricular rate became rapid. It is important to note that patients who can be documented to be in atrial fibrillation for less than 48 hours do not require anticoagulation after a cardioversion unless their CHADS2 score dictates so.

Therefore, many patients with atrial fibrillation or atrial flutter must undergo a trans-esophageal echocardiogram to rule out the presence of left atrial thrombus. The vast majority of atrial thrombi occur in the left atrial appendage and this cannot be adequately visualized on a trans-thoracic echocardiogram. In patients who had esophageal strictures or cannot be adequately sedated to undergo a trans-esophageal echocardiogram, a cardiac CT scan with contrast or a cardiac MRI can also assess for the presence of left atrial thrombi. If none of these imaging modalities are

Table 20.1   Anticoagulation in Atrial Fibrillation: The CHADS$_2$ Score.

Clinical parameter	Points
Congestive heart failure	1
Hypertension	1
Age >75	1
Diabetes	1
Stroke or TIA	2

Table 20.2   Risk of Stroke and Proposed Treatment Based on CHADS$_2$ Score.

CHADS$_2$ score	Adjusted annual stroke rate (1.9%)	Proposed anticoagulation
0	1.9	Aspirin 325 mg daily
1	2.8	Aspirin 325 mg daily or Coumadin or novel anticoagulant
2	4.0	Coumadin or novel anticoagulant
3	5.9	Coumadin or novel anticoagulant
4	8.5	Coumadin or novel anticoagulant
5	12.5	Coumadin or novel anticoagulant
6	18.2	Coumadin or novel anticoagulant

available, then the patient can be anticoagulated with warfarin for a period of six weeks and then undergo a cardioversion. During this period of anticoagulation, patients must have a documented therapeutic INR for a minimum of four consecutive weeks prior to the cardioversion. Once the cardioversion has been completed, all patients should be anticoagulated for the following six weeks due to a high risk of atrial thrombi formation in the post-cardioversion period. Whether or not a patient needs to be anticoagulated for a period longer than six weeks post-cardioversion depends upon their relative risk of thromboembolic events. Each patient should be risk stratified utilizing the CHADS$_2$ scoring system which assigns points based upon clinical risk factors for thromboembolism (Tables 20.1 and 20.2). If the total score is 0, then anticoagulation with a daily full-strength aspirin is appropriate. If the total score is greater than 1, warfarin is recommended. If the total score is 1, then therapy should be individualized to a given patient scenario. In order to further assist clinicians in determining an adequate anticoagulation regimen, the CHA$_2$DS$_2$-VASc Score has been developed to decrease those patients categorized as indeterminate, i.e. CHADS$_2$ score of 1 (Tables 20.3 and 20.4). Of note, dabigatran, rivaroxaban, and apixaban are recently-approved oral direct thrombin inhibitors that can be used instead of warfarin for patients with nonvalvular atrial fibrillation.

Table 20.3   Anticoagulation in Atrial Fibrillation: The CHA$_2$DS$_2$-VASc Score.

Clinical parameter	Points
Congestive heart failure or ejection fraction <40%	1
Hypertension	1
Age >75	2
Diabetes	1
Stroke, TIA, or thromboemboli	2
Vascular disease	1
Age 65–74	1
Female	1

Table 20.4   Risk of Stroke and Proposed Treatment Based on CHA$_2$DS$_2$-VASc Score.

CHA$_2$DS$_2$-VASc score	Adjusted annual stroke rate (1.9%)	Proposed anticoagulation
0	0	Aspirin 325 mg daily
1	1.3	Aspirin 325 mg daily or Coumadin or novel anticoagulant
2	2.2	Coumadin or novel anticoagulant
3	3.2	Coumadin or novel anticoagulant
4	4.0	Coumadin or novel anticoagulant
5	6.7	Coumadin or novel anticoagulant
6	9.8	Coumadin or novel anticoagulant
7	9.6	Coumadin or novel anticoagulant
8	6.7	Coumadin or novel anticoagulant
9	15.2	Coumadin or novel anticoagulant

TAKE HOME POINT #3

All patients who undergo either pharmacologic or electrical cardioversion must have documented therapeutic INR for a minimum of four consecutive weeks or a transesophageal echocardiogram to rule out left atrial thrombus. Moreover, these patients must have a therapeutic INR or heparin therapy during the cardioversion and for six weeks thereafter.

A cardioversion is typically performed by initially placing defibrillator patches in either the anterior/posterior configuration or the right upper chest/left lower ribs configuration. The patient should have an empty stomach for at least six hours and should be sedated to a level of moderate or deep sedation. If available, an anesthesia

Table 20.5   Antiarrhythmic Medication Dosages and Side Effects.

Drug	Daily dosage	Potential adverse effects
Amiodarone	100–400 mg	Photosensitivity, pulmonary toxicity, polyneuropathy, GI upset, bradycardia, torsades de pointes (rare), hepatic toxicity, thyroid dysfunction
Disopyramide	400–750 mg	Torsades de pointes, HF, glaucoma, urinary retention, dry mouth
Dofetilide	500–1000 mcg	Torsades de pointes
Flecainide	200–300 mg	Ventricular tachycardia, congestive HF, enhanced AV nodal conduction
Procainamide	1000–4000 mg	Torsades de pointes, lupus-like syndrome, GI symptoms
Propafenone	450–900 mg	Ventricular tachycardia, congestive HF, enhanced AV nodal conduction
Quinidine	600–1500 mg	Torsades de pointes, GI upset, enhanced AV nodal conduction
Sotalol	240–320 mg	Torsades de pointes, HF, bradycardia, exacerbation of lung disease

Adapted from Fuster V. et al. ACC/AHA/ESC 2006 guidelines for the management of patients with atrial fibrillation–executive summary: a report of the American College of Cardiology/American Heart Association Task Force on Practice Guidelines and the European Society of Cardiology Committee for Practice Guidelines (Writing Committee to Revise the 2001 Guidelines for the Management of Patients With Atrial Fibrillation). J Am Coll Cardiol 2006;**48**(4): 854–906.

provider should be utilized for patient safety and comfort. A biphasic defibrillator with an initial setting of 200 J to be delivered synchronized to the QRS is the preferred method. Once adequate level of sedation is confirmed, the patient is shocked and then observed for a period of time. Occasionally post-conversion bradycardia is observed that requires temporary pacing or atropine. If the shock is not successful then a second shock should be performed once an adequate level of sedation is confirmed. Doses up to 360 J can be utilized and care should be taken to ensure that the synchronized mode is turned on before each shock. If two successive shocks have not worked, it is unlikely that a third shock will work. For patients that have failed a high voltage shock, intravenous ibutilide can be used to lower the defibrillation threshold and increase the probability of success for a subsequent shock. If there is immediate return of atrial fibrillation (IRAF) after a shock, then the patient should be loaded with an antiarrhythmic and should return for an elective cardioversion after steady-state levels of the drug have been achieved. Some patients are refractory to cardioversion, even with antiarrhythmic medications, and the goal of therapy for these patients is to provide ventricular rate control and therapeutic anticoagulation.

    If the cardioversion is successful, the patient should be discharged on an oral regimen of a calcium channel blocker or beta-blocker that will provide some level of rate control should the atrial fibrillation or atrial flutter recur. If therapeutic INR has not been achieved, the low-molecular weight heparins can be self-administered by the patient at home until a therapeutic INR is achieved. If digoxin or an antiarrhythmic medication is used, the patient should undergo appropriate surveillance for side effects and, if applicable, appropriate follow-up testing (Table 20.5 as well as see Chapter 21.). Each patient should follow up with a cardiologist as an outpatient for long-term management of atrial fibrillation or atrial flutter.

Management of the patient with recurrent admissions of atrial fibrillation and atrial flutter is similar to that of the management of the acute onset of these arrhythmias. That is, in each recurrent admission the patient should have the ventricular rate stabilized and level of anticoagulation confirmed. An attempt should be made to restore sinus rhythm via cardioversion and a decision to employ trans-esophageal echocardiogram is identical to that described above. However, if a patient has recurrent admissions with atrial fibrillation or atrial flutter, particularly if they have failed antiarrhythmic therapy, then consideration should be given for a catheter-based ablation procedure. These patients can be referred to a cardiac electrophysiologist as an outpatient. If a patient is not a candidate for an ablation, then a strategy to optimize rate control with beta-blocker or calcium channel medications is appropriate. If a patient continues to have persistent episodes of rapid ventricular rates despite adequate rate control agents, then an AV node ablation coupled with a pacemaker implantation can be considered for those patients who failed all other options.

TAKE HOME POINT #4

If patients are truly asymptomatic and have well controlled rates, then repetitive attempts to restore normal sinus rhythm are not necessary. Repeat cardioversions and radiofrequency catheter ablation should be reserved for patients who are moderately symptomatic despite medical therapy.

KEY REFERENCES

FUSTER V, RYDÉN LE, CANNOM DS, CRIJNS HJ, CURTIS AB, et al.; American College of Cardiology/ American Heart Association Task Force on Practice Guidelines; European Society of Cardiology Committee for Practice Guidelines; European Heart Rhythm Association; Heart Rhythm Society. ACC/ AHA/ESC 2006 Guidelines for the management of patients with atrial fibrillation: a report of the American College of Cardiology/American Heart Association Task Force on Practice Guidelines and the European Society of Cardiology Committee for Practice Guidelines (Writing Committee to Revise the 2001 Guidelines for the Management of Patients With Atrial Fibrillation): developed in collaboration with the European Heart Rhythm Association and the Heart Rhythm Society. Circulation 2006;114(7):e257–354.

GAGE BF, WATERMAN AD, SHANNON W, BOECHLER M, RICH MW, RADFORD MJ. Validation of clinical classification schemes for predicting stroke: results from the National Registry of Atrial Fibrillation. JAMA 2001;285(22):2864–2870.

PAGE RL. Newly diagnosed atrial fibrillation. N Engl J Med 2004;351(23):2408–2416.

Chapter 21

Antiarrhythmic Drug Therapy

Sanjaya Gupta and Thomas C. Crawford

21.1 INTRODUCTION

The use of pharmacologic therapy for the treatment of cardiovascular arrhythmias dates back hundreds of years. However, it remains a source of much concern and confusion for both noncardiologists and cardiologists alike. While there are a multitude of pharmacologic agents, relatively few are used in clinical practice. Antiarrhythmic medications have various mechanisms of action, dosages, drug interactions, adverse effects, and contraindications. The aim of this chapter is to summarize the usage of these agents and to provide a simplified construct for their usage. However, initiation of any antiarrhythmic drug therapy should be performed under the guidance of cardiology consultation.

21.2 PHARMACOLOGY

The Vaughan-Williams system of classification divides antiarrhythmic agents according to their mechanism of action (Table 21.1). In order to best understand the pharmacology of these drugs, it is useful to review the basics of the cardiac action potential.

The cardiac action potential originates within specialized cells of the sino-atrial node. These pacemaker cells have a continuous influx of sodium ions (Na^+), termed "funny current" or If, which is perpetually raising the voltage of the pacemaker cells until it reaches a threshold for depolarization. Once it reaches this threshold, there is

Inpatient Cardiovascular Medicine, First Edition. Edited by Brahmajee K. Nallamothu and Timir S. Baman.

Table 21.1   Vaughan-Williams Classification of Antiarrhythmic Drugs.

Class	Mechanism	Repolarization effects	Example
Ia	Moderate Na^+ blockade	Prolongation of repolarization	Quinidine
Ib	Mild Na^+ blockade	Shorten repolarization	Lidocaine
Ic	Marked Na^+ blockade	No change in repolarization	Flecainide
II	Decrease phase 4 slope in pacemaker cells	Prolongation of repolarization at AV node	Propranolol
III	Repolarizing K^+ current	Marked prolongation of repolarization	Amiodarone
IV	AV nodal $Ca2^+$ block	Prolongation of repolarization at AV node	Verapamil

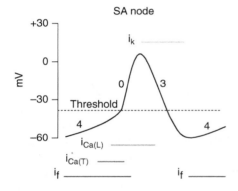

Figure 21.1   Pacemaker current and ion traffic. (See Color plate 21.1). (Source: http://www.cvphysiology.com/Arrhythmias/SAN%20action%20potl.gif, with permission from Dr Richard Klabunde).

rapid influx of calcium through voltage-gated calcium channels. This is immediately followed by rapid potassium efflux through specific ion channels, which serves to repolarize the cell membrane and bring the voltage below the threshold for activation (Figure 21.1). Once the cardiac action potential originates within the pacemaker cells, it is conducted through the atria to the AV node, the His bundle and the Purkinje cells and then the remainder of the myocardium.

This conduction process follows five phases of depolarization and repolarization (Figure 21.2). The resting membrane potential is set by phase 4. When the action potential reaches the cell, it raises the resting membrane potential until it reaches a threshold potential that opens voltage gated sodium (Na^+) channels. The rapid influx of sodium ions causes a rapid depolarization that characterizes phase 0. This is immediately followed by phase 1 that is governed by potassium efflux. This is subsequently followed by phase 2, which consists of a balance between calcium ion (Ca^{2+}) influx and potassium ion (K^+) efflux. Therefore, phase 2 creates a plateau phase that effectively prolongs the action potential. In the myocardium, this is important as it allows sufficient time for calcium influx to bind to the contractile elements and initiate myocardial contraction. Finally, phase 3 of the action potential is caused by potassium ion (K^+) efflux, which returns the membrane potential back to its resting state.

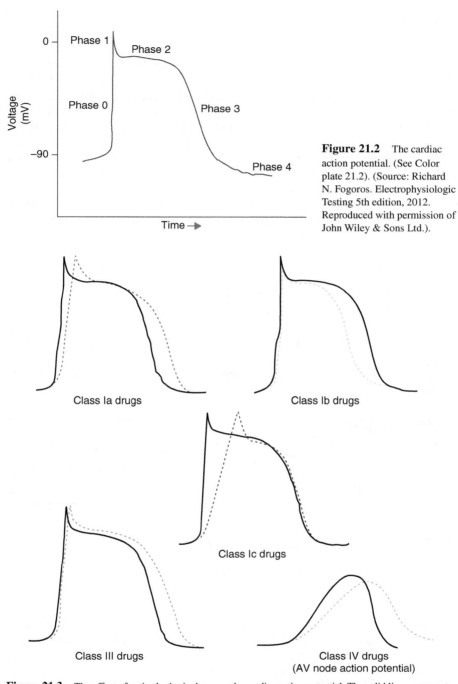

Figure 21.2 The cardiac action potential. (See Color plate 21.2). (Source: Richard N. Fogoros. Electrophysiologic Testing 5th edition, 2012. Reproduced with permission of John Wiley & Sons Ltd.).

Figure 21.3 The effect of antiarrhythmic drugs on the cardiac action potential. The solid lines represent the baseline action potential and the dotted lines represent the changes that result in the action potential when various classes of antiarrhythmic drug are given. (See Color plate 21.3). (Source: Richard N. Fogoros. Electrophysiologic Testing 5th edition, 2012. Reproduced with permission of John Wiley & Sons Ltd.).

255

The Vaughan-Williams classification system groups antiarrhythmic drugs into four classes based upon which phase of the action potential is altered (Table 21.1). Class I agents mostly influence sodium channels. This class is further subdivided into three subclasses based upon the degree of sodium channel blockade that these agents produce (Figure 21.3). Class IA agents produce moderate sodium channel blockade, which causes slow phase 0 conduction and prolongs repolarization. Examples of agents in this class are quinidine, disopyramide and procainamide. Class IB agents produce mild sodium channel blockade, which shortens repolarization and has little effect on phase 0 depolarization in normal tissues. However, in abnormal tissue, this causes depressed phase 0 conduction. Examples of agents in this class are lidocaine and mexiletine. The IC agents produce marked sodium channel blockade, which causes a significant depression of phase 0 conduction but only a slight effect upon repolarization. Examples of agents in this class are flecainide and propafenone.

Class II agents produce sympatholytic, anti-ischemic, and anti-fibrillatory effects. Beta-blockers, such as propranolol and metoprolol, are the prototypical agents for this class.

Class III agents produce prolonged repolarization via potassium channel blockade. The typical agents for this class are sotalol and amiodarone. Both of these agents also have actions in other classes – sotalol is also a beta-blocker and amiodarone has properties of each of the four classes of antiarrhythmics. Dofetilide is an antiarrhythmic with pure class III properties.

Finally, the Class IV agents are calcium channel blockers, such as verapamil and diltiazem.

TAKE HOME POINT #1

Antiarrhythmic agents are categorized by mechanism of action. Class I agents are sodium channel blockers, Class II agents are beta-blockers, Class III are mostly potassium channel blockers, and Class IV are calcium channel blockers.

21.3   DISEASE-SPECIFIC THERAPY

21.3.1   Ventricular Tachycardia

Many studies have examined the efficacy of antiarrhythmic medications on ventricular tachycardia and sudden cardiac death. Large randomized controlled clinical trials have shown limited efficacy of antiarrhythmic therapy utilizing the endpoint of sudden cardiac death. Beta-blockers are a notable exception, in which case multiple trials in patients with a spectrum of cardiovascular conditions, including ventricular tachycardia, showed improved survival. Beta blockade is effective in preventing sudden cardiac death (SCD) and ventricular fibrillation (VF), but less so in suppressing spontaneous ectopy or monomorphic ventricular tachycardia (VT). Consequently, antiarrhythmic medication is used as adjunctive therapy to implantable cardioverter defibrillator (ICD) and/or catheter-based ablation procedures in most patients with structural heart disease.

Table 21.2 Major Side Effects and Recommended Monitoring for Patients on Amiodarone.

Side effect	Monitoring/precautions
Hyperthyroidism/hypothyroidism	Thyroid functions tests at baseline and every 6 months
Abnormal liver enzymes[1]	Liver function tests at baseline and every 6 months
Pulmonary toxicity symptoms including cough, fever, dyspnea	Pulmonary function tests with the diffusing capacity at baseline with yearly chest X-ray
Corneal deposits/optic neuropathy	Eye examination at baseline with repeat examinations as needed
Conduction abnormalities including prolonged QT	ECG at baseline and yearly
Photosensitivity to UV light	Avoid sunlight and use sunscreen
Blue-gray skin discoloration	Reduce dose or discontinue medication

[1]Defined as AST or ALT elevation ≥2x upper limit of reference range.

The usage of antiarrhythmic medication must be governed by careful consideration of the risks versus the benefits of therapy. Many agents have significant toxicities and/or the potential for proarrhythmic consequences. Consequently, beta-blockers are the most appropriate initial agent, as the incidence of side effects is low and there is potential for mortality reduction, especially in patients with concomitant coronary artery disease or heart failure. Class III agents amiodarone and sotalol have been shown to reduce appropriate ICD therapies. These drugs act to suppress ventricular tachycardia (VT) by causing prolonged repolarization that increases the wavelength of the reentrant arrhythmia. Amiodarone, in particular, has multiple mechanisms of action that span all four antiarrhythmic classes. As such, it can be used for a broad variety of arrhythmias. However, amiodarone can cause significant extracardiac toxicities, particularly to the lungs, liver, thyroid, and skin. The likelihood of development of toxicity is directly related to the dosage of the medication and the length of therapy. Therefore, amiodarone necessitates periodic surveillance testing to monitor for the development of toxicities that would prompt discontinuation of the medication (Table 21.2).

Sotalol is also effective in suppression of ventricular arrhythmias by prolonging repolarization and, compared to amiodarone, it has significantly fewer side effects and toxicities. The disadvantage of sotalol is the greater risk of potential proarrhythmia related to QT prolongation. Proarrhythmia may occur in 2–4% of patients taking sotalol. Genetic predisposition, female gender, renal dysfunction, excessive dosages or interactions with other medications are common causes for proarrhythmic effect of sotalol. In addition, sotalol should be avoided in patients with severely depressed left ventricular function and/or decompensated heart failure, as it may be associated with heart failure exacerbation. Sotalol may be indicated in a patient with normal renal function and only a mild reduction in left ventricular function. Conversely, amiodarone therapy would be more appropriate for an older patient with significant left ventricular dysfunction and normal baseline lung, liver and thyroid function.

In the inpatient setting, antiarrhythmic therapy is often directed towards acute management of recurrent ventricular arrhythmias. Intravenous amiodarone as a bolus followed by a continuous infusion is a common initial management strategy. If ventricular tachycardia or fibrillation recur, lidocaine may be added as a bolus followed by continuous intravenous infusion. Electrolyte abnormalities should be corrected, particularly hypomagnesiemia or hypokalemia to a goal of 2.0 meq/dl and 4.0 meq/dl, respectively. A rapid search for the underlying cardiac abnormality should be pursued. Once the patient is stabilized, the intravenous amiodarone can be converted to an oral formulation. Various loading dosing regimens are used for amiodarone; however, 400 mg 2–3 times a day during the first week of therapy is appropriate for most cases of ventricular tachycardia. Regardless of the schedule chosen, amiodarone load continues until the patient has received a total cumulative dosage of 10 g, at which point the medication is considered to be at a steady state level. After this, a dosage of 400 mg daily is sufficient for suppression of most ventricular arrhythmias. After a period of clinical stability, doses of amiodarone may be reduced further to keep the likelihood of toxicity as low as possible.

Intravenous lidocaine is a useful adjunct to inpatient treatment of patients with ventricular arrhythmia, especially in the setting of ischemic cardiomyopathy. Lidocaine administration requires monitoring of signs and symptoms of toxicity such as delirium, tremor, nausea/vomiting, or seizures in addition to daily serum levels. Lidocaine levels may be higher in patients with congestive heart failure and renal dysfunction, and caution should be exercised during the administration of this drug in such patients. If lidocaine is effective in the initial management of ventricular tachycardia, it can be substituted with oral mexiletine.

Patients with VT/VF refractory to amiodarone and lidocaine are at high risk for mortality. Three or more separate episodes of VT/VF within a 24-hour period define electrical storm. If amiodarone and lidocaine are ineffective in suppressing electrical storm, deep sedation and pharmacologic autonomic blockade may be helpful.

TAKE HOME POINT #2

Amiodarone and procainamide are first-line agents for acute stabilization for ventricular tachycardia, followed by lidocaine. For chronic ventricular tachycardia, beta-blockers are commonly used, followed by amiodarone, sotalol or mexiletine.

21.4 ATRIAL FIBRILLATION AND ATRIAL FLUTTER

Antiarrhythmic agents are suited for maintenance of sinus rhythm in patients with paroxysmal atrial fibrillation and flutter. Benefits of maintaining sinus rhythm include symptom reduction and improvement in exercise capacity. It remains unclear if maintenance of sinus rhythm is associated with reduction in thromboembolism, heart failure, or death. If symptomatic, patients with persistent atrial fibrillation usually require a cardioversion; antiarrhythmic agents may be initiated before or after cardioversion and aid in maintenance of sinus rhythm in the post-conversion period. The choice of appropriate antiarrhythmic agent is dictated by the patient's comorbidities (Table 21.3). For a patient with a structurally normal heart (i.e. normal left and right ventricular size and function and no substantial left ventricular hypertrophy), the antiarrhythmic drugs of choice are flecainide, propafenone, sotalol, or dofetilide. In patients at risk for coronary artery disease, a stress test to rule out significant coronary

Table 21.3   Choice of Antiarrhythmic Agents in Atrial Fibrillation/Flutter.

Tier	Normal heart	Hypertension with LVH	Heart failure	CAD with normal EF	Renal failure
First line	Flecainide, Propafenone, Sotalol	Dronedarone	Dofetilide, Amiodarone	Sotalol	Amiodarone, Dronedarone
Second line	Dronedarone, Procainamide	Dofetilide, Amiodarone		Dronedarone, Dofetilide	Propafenone
Avoid		Flecainide, Propafenone	Flecainide, Propafenone, Dronedarone	Flecainide, Propafenone	Sotalol, Procainamide, Dofetilide

artery disease may be performed when propafenone or flecainide are considered. In addition, either beta-blockers or calcium channel blockers are prescribed in order to avoid paradoxical tachycardia due to 1:1 conduction. For patients with coronary artery disease and no significant left ventricular dysfunction, sotalol may be preferred due to its beta-blocker properties. However, for patients with hypertension and left ventricular hypertrophy, the agents of choice are dronedarone or amiodarone. Finally, patients with congestive heart failure should be treated with dofetilide or amiodarone, as these drugs do not increase mortality in heart failure. Dronedarone should not be administered to patients with depressed ventricular function and recent heart failure decompensation or New York Heart Association class IV heart failure, as it is associated with significantly higher mortality over placebo in this group of patients.

Inpatient initiation of sotalol is advisable, while 3-day hospitalization on telemetry is mandated by the Food and Drug Administration for dofetilide initiation due to concern for proarrhythmia, especially torsades de pointes. Important drug–drug interactions preclude co-administration of defetilide with cimetidine, hydrochlorothiazide, ketoconazole, megestrol, prochlorperazine, trimethoprim, or verapamil. The risk of proarrhythmia is related to the length of the depolarization phase of the action potential. Dofetilide should not be used in patients with QTc greater than 440 msec (500 msec in patients with ventricular conduction abnormalities). The corrected QT should be measured two hours after each dose of medication and if there is an increase of 15% above baseline or the corrected QT exceeds 500 msec, the dosage of the medications should be decreased. Potassium and magnesium levels should also be monitored during the hospitalization and electrolyte supplementation should be given to keep potassium levels greater than 4.0 meq/dl and magnesium levels greater than 2.0 meq/dl. In addition, the patient should discontinue any other QT-prolonging medications. Dofetilide is available only to hospitals and prescribers who have received appropriate dofetilide dosing and treatment initiation education.

Pharmacologic cardioversion is an alternative to direct current cardioversion for atrial fibrillation termination. The agent of choice is ibutilide, which is an intravenous class III agent. Prior to infusing ibutilide, the standard precautions should be undertaken to ensure that the absence of a left atrial thrombus, either by transesophageal echocardiogram or by the documentation of weekly therapeutic INR levels for at least three consecutive weeks. Of note, pharmacologic cardioversion carries the similar risk of thromboembolism as electrical cardioversion. The typical dose of ibutilide is 1 mg infused slowly over the course of 10 minutes. It may take up to 30 minutes for the drug to take effect. If no rhythm conversion is achieved, then another 1 mg intravenous dose can be repeated. The success rate for pharmacologic cardioversion is 40–50%. Ibutilide may also increase the efficacy of electrical cardioversion. After the drug is infused, the patient must remain on telemetry for several hours due to a 4% incidence of ventricular tachycardia or ventricular fibrillation in patients who receive ibutilide. This medication should be avoided in patients with a known cardiomyopathy with an ejection fraction less than 30% due to an increased risk of polymorphic ventricular tachycardia. Other contraindications to ibutilide administration include previous adverse reaction, ischemic heart disease and a corrected QT greater than 500 msec.

TAKE HOME POINT #3

Choice of antiarrhythmic agents for atrial fibrillation/flutter depends upon a patient's comorbidities. For patients with lone atrial fibrillation, the first line drugs are flecainide, propafenone, or sotalol. For heart failure patients, the drugs of choice are amiodarone and dofetilide. Patients with coronary artery disease and atrial fibrillation may be managed with sotalol due to its beta-blocking effects.

21.5 SUPRAVENTRICULAR TACHYCARDIA

Antiarrhythmic agents may be used for acute management of patients with supraventricular tachycardia. Intravenous adenosine is most commonly used due to its ability to cause a transient block in the AV node, thus treating AV nodal reentry or AV reentry. Adenosine can be useful in the diagnosis of atrial tachycardia as this arrhythmia will persist and P waves will be visualized in the setting of AV block. Prior to administration of adenosine, it is important to determine if there is any evidence of ventricular pre-excitation via an accessory pathway, as would be present in Wolf-Parkinson-White syndrome. Administration of adenosine, calcium channel blockers, or beta-blockers may result in conduction blockade through the AV node and preferentially allow conduction down the accessory pathway. Adenosine administration may result in AF in 12% of patients. In the setting of a rapid atrial fibrillation or atrial tachycardia, facilitation of 1:1 AV conduction down the pathway may precipitate ventricular fibrillation or ventricular tachycardia. Thus, adenosine administration should always be performed with an external defibrillator and crash cart readily accessible. Adenosine should not be used in patients who have severe bronchospastic disease.

Despite these caveats, adenosine administration is generally safe and very widely used. Due to adenosine's extremely short half-life, rapid infusion of medication and flush is essential. The proper method to administer adenosine is to connect a syringe with 6, 12 or 18 mg of the medication to a stopcock and connect another 20 cc syringe of flush to be given immediately after adenosine injection. A 12-lead ECG rhythm strip should be running continuously during adenosine infusion. The

Table 21.4 Common Antirrhythmic Agents with Class, Dosage, Common Usage, Major Side Effects and Drug Interactions.

Agent	Class	Daily dose	Best used for	Avoid use in	Major side effects	Drug interactions
Quinidine	IA	600–1500 mg	Refractory atrial and ventricular arrhythmias	Pts with QT prolonged >500 msec	Proarrhythmia, diarrhea, rash, thrombocytopenia, hemolytic anemia, c inchonism, orthostatic hypotension	Increases levels of warfarin, heparin, digoxin. Amiodarone and Verapamil increase quinidine levels.
Procainamide	IA	1000–4000 mg	Refractory atrial and ventricular arrhythmias	Pts with QT prolonged >500 msec, Renal failure	Rash, fever, agranulocytosis, hemolytic anemia, lupus syndrome, Raynaud's phenomenon, cholestatic jaundice	Amiodarone increases procainamide levels, concomintant use of class III agents can cause proarrhythmia.
Disopyramide	IA	400–750 mg	Refractory atrial and ventricular arrhythmias	Pts with LV dysfunction	Dry mouth, blurred vision, constipation, nausea, vomiting, rash, cholestatic jaundice, agranulocytosis, glaucoma	Phenobarbital, rifampin, phenytoin decrease plasma levels
Lidocaine	IB	1–4 mg/min(IV)	Ventricular arrhythmias (as combination agent)		Slurred speech, altered consciousness, seizures, altered consciousness,	Propranolol and metoprolol increase levels up to 80%; phenobarbital decreases levels
Mexiletine	IB	450–600 mg	Ventricular arrhythmias (as combination agent)		Tremor, blurred vision, confusion, ataxia, nausea, vomiting	Phenytoin, phenbarbital, rifampin increase metabolism of mexiletine
Flecainide	IC	200–300 mg	Atrial arrhythmia for pts without CAD	Pts with CAD, low EF, LVH	Proarrhythmia, blurred vision, headache, ataxia, 1:1 AV conduction	Increases digoxin levels by 25%; flecainide levels increased by amiodarone and cimetidine

(Continued)

Table 21.4 (Continued).

Agent	Class	Daily dose	Best used for	Avoid use in	Major side effects	Drug interactions
Propafenone	IC	450–900 mg	Refractory atrial and ventricular arrhythmias	Pts with CAD, low Ef, LVH	Nausea, dizziness, metallic taste, blurred vision, paresthesia, constipation, increased LFT, asthma exacerbation, conduction abnormalties	Digoxin, warfarin, propranolol, metoprolol, disopyramide, theophylline levels increased
Amiodarone	III	100–400 mg	Atrial and ventricular arrhythmias	Pts with thyroid, liver or lung dysfunction	Pulmonary fibrosis, hypo- or hyperthyroidism, corneal deposits, increased LFT, photosensitivity with discoloration of the skin, tremor, ataxia	Increases digoxin, warfarin, cyclosporine levels
Sotalol	III	240–320 mg	Atrial and ventricular arrhythmias	Recent HF, Recent MI, prolonged QT	Fatigue, QT lengthening causing proarrhythmia, wheezing in patients with reactive airway disease, worsened heart failure	Concomitant use of beta-blockers or calcium channel blockers may exacerbate effects
Dofetilide	III	500–1000 mcg	Atrial arrhythmias	Renal failure, prolonged QT	Proarrhythmia, palpitations/ syncope	Cimetidine, verapamil, fluconazole, trimethoprim increase dofetilide levels
Dronedarone	III	800 mg	Atrial arrhythmias	Recent HF	Fatigue, GI discomfort	Increases digoxin levels
Ibutilide	III	1 mg (IV only)	Atrial arrhythmias	Renal failure, prolonged QT	Proarrhythmia	Cautious use with other QT prolonging agents on board

patient should be warned that the medication may cause transient flushing and dyspnea. If the patient fails to convert with an IV antiarrhythmic or becomes hemodynamically unstable, then DC cardioversion is appropriate.

Patients with SVT who are candidates for catheter ablation can be managed with beta-blockers until the procedure. For patients who are not ablation candidates or do not desire an ablation, a beta-blocker and/or a class IC antiarrhythmic (flecainide, propafenone) can be used in the absence of coronary artery disease or substantial left ventricular hypertrophy. Table 21.4 provides a summary of the essential information needed to utilize many of the commonly-prescribed antiarrhythmic medications.

21.6 SUMMARY

Despite the success of ablation therapy, antiarrhythmic agents are an important component of initial as well as chronic management of many arrhythmias. Selecting the appropriate agent depends upon an understanding of the agent's mechanism of action, side effects, and drug interactions, as well as the patient's comorbidities. The risks and benefits of antiarrhythmic drugs are important considerations. All antiarrhythmic drug therapy should be initiated under the guidance of an experienced cardiologist.

TAKE HOME POINT #4

Adenosine is the drug of choice for initial management of supraventricular tachycardia. Outpatient management of patients with supraventricular tachycardia awaiting ablation should be accomplished by beta-blockers.

KEY REFERENCES

BLOMSTROM-LUNDQVIST C et al. ACC/AHA/ESC guidelines for the management of patients with supraventricular arrhythmias – executive summary: a report of the American College of Cardiology/American Heart Association Task Force on Practice Guidelines and the European Society of Cardiology Committee for Practice Guidelines (Writing Committee to Develop Guidelines for the Management of Patients with Supraventricular Arrhythmias) developed in collaboration with NASPE-Heart Rhythm Society. J Am Coll Cardiol 2003;42(8):1493–1531.

CAMM AJ et al. Guidelines for the management of atrial fibrillation: the Task Force for the Management of Atrial Fibrillation of the European Society of Cardiology (ESC). Europace 2010;12(10):1360–1420.

OPIE LH, GERSH, BJ. eds. *Drugs for the heart*, 6th ed. 2005. Elsevier-Saunders: Philadelphia, PA. p.437.

ZIPES DP et al. ACC/AHA/ESC 2006 guidelines for management of patients with ventricular arrhythmias and the prevention of sudden cardiac death: a report of the American College of Cardiology/American Heart Association Task Force and the European Society of Cardiology Committee for Practice Guidelines (Writing Committee to Develop Guidelines for Management of Patients with Ventricular Arrhythmias and the Prevention of Sudden Cardiac Death). J Am Coll Cardiol 2006;48(5):e247–e346.

Chapter 22

Cardiac Pacemakers and Implantable Defibrillators

Karl J. Ilg

22.1 BACKGROUND

The history of implantable devices designed to treat cardiac rhythm disturbances dates back several decades. Tremendous advancements have been made in transistor, lead, and battery technology in recent years. A pacemaker implanted today can have a lifespan of 5–10 years, depending on the amount of pacing that is required of the pulse generator. Furthermore, simple implantable devices are no longer only treating heart block or bradycardia. Cardiac rhythm management with device therapy now also includes aiding in the management of congestive heart failure with devices designed to restore electrical and mechanical left ventricular synchrony (cardiac resynchronization therapy also known as biventricular devices) as well as the prevention of sudden cardiac death with the implantation of implantable cardioverter-defibrillators (ICDs).

The internist or hospitalist is likely to encounter patients with implantable devices, and should be familiar with the indications to place such devices, as well as how to manage issues that might ultimately arise. The purpose of this chapter is to:

1. Provide the internist with a description of the components of implantable cardiac devices
2. Provide familiarity with the indications and contraindications for the implantation of pacemakers, ICDs, and biventricular devices

Inpatient Cardiovascular Medicine, First Edition. Edited by Brahmajee K. Nallamothu and Timir S. Baman.

3. Review the pre-implantation testing that will be beneficial to the implanting electrophysiologist
4. Review early post-implant care
5. Discuss the evaluation of a previously implanted device.

22.2   COMPONENTS OF A PACEMAKER OR ICD

Understanding the differences in the features and components of pacemakers and ICD systems that can be evaluated by history, physical examination, and radiographic appearance is of great clinical importance. Not only will it help the hospitalist target possible abnormalities with the device, but it will also provide some additional insight into the patient's past medical history, as well as allow for a more informed discussion with an electrophysiologist when an abnormality is suspected.

As mentioned earlier, the first implanted devices were pacemakers that were used to treat bradycardia resulting from disease of the sino-atrial (SA) node or the atrio-ventricular (AV) node. The basic components of these early devices have been carried through to the modern pacemaker (Figure 22.1), ICD, and biventricular device. A pulse generator, consisting of the power source and circuitry, is located in a site remote from the heart, usually in the left anterior chest wall inferior to the clavicle

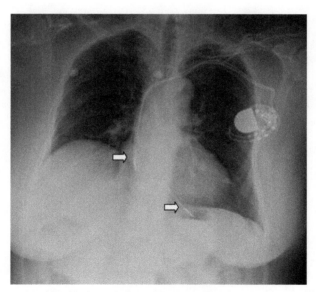

Figure 22.1   PA chest film showing the standard appearance of a dual-chamber pacemaker. Note the pulse generator overlying the left chest wall with the redundant portion of two leads coiling in the device pocket before entering the vasculature at the subclavian vein. The leads extend to overly the right atrium and right ventricle. The leads are uniform in diameter and radiodensity throughout their length. Arrows indicate insertion sites of leads into right atrium and ventricle.

(though in some circumstances the pulse generator can be located in the right chest or in the abdominal wall). Modern pacemakers are often so small and thin that they are difficult to palpate in many patients. The lead(s) are placed into the vasculature at this site and extend to the chamber(s) of the heart, where they are held in place by either an active fixation mechanism (a helical mechanism which burrows into the myocardium) or by passive fixation (barbs or fins which become ensnared in the irregularities in the chambers of the heart).

Implantable cardioverter-defibrillators (ICDs) are similarly designed, though the pulse generator tends to be larger owing to the need for the increased size of the power source. Most often, the pulse generator produces a noticeable and easily palpable protrusion on the chest wall. These devices may be single-chamber, dual chamber, or part of a biventricular pacing system. They can be identified radiographically by the presence of one or more coils on the lead which extends into the right ventricle. The coiled appears as a "notched" or "rippled" portion of the lead which is thicker and more radiodense than the remaining portion of the lead (Figure 22.2).

Biventricular devices also tend to have larger pulse generators. The additional size is necessary to accommodate the power source as well as a requisite increase in the amount of circuitry. These devices are designed not only to defibrillate a patient

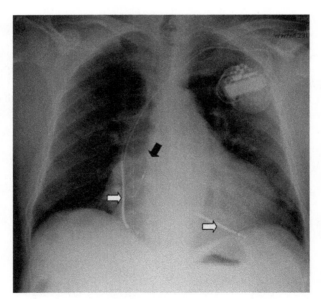

Figure 22.2   PA chest film showing the usual appearance of a dual-chamber ICD system. Note the pulse generator in the left chest wall, with leads entering the vasculature and coursing to a position overlying the right atrium and right ventricle. Note that the atrial (pacing) lead is of smaller diameter than the ventricular (ICD) lead (black arrow). Note also the appearance of the coils (white arrows) on the ventricular lead (superior vena cava and right ventricle).

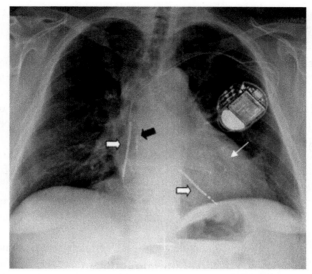

Figure 22.3   PA chest film showing the appearance of a biventricular pacemaker system. Note the pulse generator with three leads exiting the header. The right ventricular (ICD) lead can be identified by the presence of the coils on the lead and the slightly larger diameter (block white arrows). The right atrial lead has an intermediate diameter (block black arrow). The coronary sinus lead has the smallest diameter, and can be seen coursing through the coronary sinus to a location in a lateral branch on the left ventricular free wall (thin white arrow).

if necessary but also to deliver pacing stimuli as frequently as possible. The additional lead tends to be of smaller diameter, and achieves its location preferably on the lateral wall of the left ventricle by exiting the right atrium through the coronary sinus, extending posteriorly around the left ventricle (Figure 22.3) and then into a lateral venous branch where it is held in place by the shape of the lead tip and the tortuosity of the venous branch.

All of these devices are capable of transcutaneous transmission of data. This is done in the hospital or cardiology/electrophysiology clinic with a device analyzer. These computers are manufacturer-specific, and can provide information about battery status, pacemaker/ICD parameters, and lead diagnostic information, as well as events programmed to be monitored or treated by the device.

TAKE HOME POINT #1

Pacemakers, ICDs, and biventricular devices have unique features which can allow for identification by physical examination and chest radiography. Device lead variation from typical locations may be of clinical importance when troubleshooting.

22.3 INDICATIONS FOR THE IMPLANTATION OF PACEMAKERS AND ICDS

This section addresses the indications for the various forms of cardiac device therapy. It is intended to provide a brief overview rather than a detailed discussion, so that the hospitalist may begin to formulate a plan of care even before a cardiologist or electrophysiologist become involved. A much more detailed description of the indications for and contraindications to pacemaker or ICD implantation can be found in the most recent guidelines.

In general, pacemakers are designed to supply a pacing stimulus to a chamber of the heart where the native conduction system has failed to supply a sufficient pacing stimulus of its own. As such, they are implanted for acquired or congenital disorders affecting the cardiac conduction system producing a heart rate that is not sufficient. This can result from disorders of the SA node (Table 22.1), the AV node (Table 22.2), or a combination thereof.

Despite the effects of carotid sinus syndrome and neurocardiogenic syncope on both the sinus and AV node, pacemaker implantation is often not helpful. Pacemaker implantation is indicated for recurrent syncope due to spontaneously occurring carotid sinus stimulation that induces ventricular asystole of more than three seconds. Pacemaker implantation is not indicated for hypersensitive cardioinhibitory response to carotid sinus stimulation without symptoms or with vague symptoms, or for situational vasovagal syncope in which avoidance behavior is effective and preferred.

Implantable cardioverter-defibrillators (ICDs) are designed primarily to treat ventricular tachyarrhythmias, though all ICDs do possess pacing capabilities. As such, they are indicated in patients who have a history of ventricular tachycardia or ventricular fibrillation, or who are at high risk for developing these potentially lethal

Table 22.1   Pacing Indications and Contraindications for Sinus Node Dysfunction.

	Pacing indications for sinus node dysfunction
Indications	Symptomatic sinus node dysfunction, including sinus pauses of more than 3 seconds in the awake patient
	Symptomatic chronotropic incompetence
	Symptomatic bradycardia resulting from essential pharmacotherapy (beta blockers post-MI)
Contraindications	Asymptomatic sinus node dysfunction
	Sinus node dysfunction when symptoms suggestive of bradycardia are documented in the absence of bradycardia
	Sinus node dysfunction due to non-essential pharmacotherapy

Table 22.2   Pacing Indications and Contraindications for AV Node Dysfunction.

	Pacing indications for AV node dysfunction
Indications	Third-degree and advanced second-degree block associated with bradycardia resulting in symptoms
	Third-degree and advanced second-degree block associated with arrhythmias requiring medications producing symptomatic bradycardia
	Third-degree and advanced second-degree block in a patient who is asymptomatic in sinus rhythm who has a period of asystole greater than 3 seconds, or a ventricular escape rate less than 40 beats per minute
	Third-degree and advanced second-degree block in a patient who is asymptomatic in atrial fibrillation with bradycardia with a pause of greater than 5 seconds
	Second-degree block with associated symptomatic bradycardia
	Advanced second-degree or third-degree block associated with neuromuscular disease (myotonic dystrophy, Erb dystrophy, peroneal muscular atrophy, etc.)
Contraindications	Asymptomatic first-degree AV block
	Asymptomatic Type I second-degree (Wenkebach) AV block
	Any AV block which is transient and not likely to recur (Lyme disease, drug toxicity, transient increases in vagal tone)

Table 22.3   Implantable Defibrillator Indications and Contraindications.

	Indications for ICD implantation
Indications	Patients who are survivors of cardiac arrest (VT or VF) after evaluation and treatment of reversible cause
	Patients with structural heart disease and spontaneous VT
	Patients with prior MI, LVEF ≤35%, with Class II–III CHF who are at least 40 days post-MI
	Patients with non-ischemic cardiomyopathy, with LVEF ≤35% and Class II–III CHF
Contraindications	Patients with incessant VT or VF
	Patients who do not have a reasonable expectation of survival with acceptable functional class for at least one year (even if they meet criteria otherwise)
	Patients with drug-refractory Class IV CHF who are not candidates for transplantation or biventricular pacing
	Patients with VT or VF due to a completely reversible disorder in the absence of structural heart disease
	Patients who have VT or VF amenable to surgical or catheter-based ablation (outflow tract VT, Wolff-Parkinson-White syndrome)

Table 22.4   Indications and Contraindications of Biventricular Pacing/Cardiac Resynchronization.

	Biventricular pacing/cardiac resynchronization
Indications	LVEF ≤35%, QRS duration >120 ms, and Class II–IV CHF despite optimal medical therapy LVEF ≤35, Class I–II CHF despite optimal medical therapy who are undergoing pacemaker or ICD implant for other reasons, who have anticipated need for frequent ventricular pacing
Contraindications	Patients whose functional status and life expectancy are limited predominantly by chronic noncardiac conditions Patients with reduced LVEF (>35%) in the absence of other indications for pacing

rhythm disturbances. Common indications and contraindications for ICD implantation are listed in Table 22.3. Those patients who meet criteria for ICD implantation and have a QRS duration >120 ms may obtain benefit from an implantable defibrillator with cardiac resynchronization therapy, i.e. placement of a biventricular ICD with a coronary sinus lead (Table 22.4). These devices have been studied and shown to be of benefit in the treatment of New York Heart Class II, III or IV heart failure in a patient on optimal medical therapy due to either ischemic and non-ischemic processes. Benefits of cardiac resynchronization provided by these devices include improved exercise tolerance, improvement in NYHA functional class, improved quality of life, and survival benefit.

22.3.1   Pre-Implantation Evaluation

As seen in the previous section, a majority of the indications for pacemaker implant rely on the temporal correlation of bradycardia or heart block with symptoms. For this reason, telemetry recordings, surface EKG during exercise, or Holter monitor recordings are very helpful to the implanting physician, as are pre-hospital or emergency department rhythm strips showing periods of bradycardia, pause, or asystole which can be correlated with symptoms. At the very least, a current resting surface EKG should be reviewed.

Regarding ICDs and biventricular devices, documentation of any rhythm disturbance (bradycardia or tachycardia) should also be a priority. A recent estimation of LV systolic function with echocardiogram, ventriculogram, or nuclear study will help to identify patients who may be at high risk for sudden death and would benefit from ICD implantation. In addition to the knowledge of LV function, QRS morphology and duration as seen on the surface EKG will also potentially identify patients who may benefit not only from ICD implantation but resynchronization therapy as well. An evaluation for significant coronary artery disease will not only identify patients who may have recovery of LV function with revascularization, but also may impact the implanting electrophysiologist's decision as to whether or not to "test the ICD," i.e. induce ventricular fibrillation during implantation to ensure that the device can adequately sense and treat ventricular fibrillation.

Finally, regardless of which type of device might be implanted, the patient needs to be treated optimally in order to reduce risk of these invasive procedures. This includes ensuring that the patient is close to euvolemia and able to lie supine for several hours, metabolic conditions are addressed (glycemic control, renal dysfunction), and there is no fever or active bloodstream infection.

The issue of anticoagulation with warfarin and/or heparin deserves special mention. As device implantation is an invasive procedure with inherent bleeding risk (particularly pocket hematoma), the implanting electrophysiologist will need to be made aware of the degree of anticoagulation. The current trend is moving towards device implantation on therapeutic anticoagulation, so as to avoid the fluctuations in partial thromboplastin time which can accompany heparin product administration. The implanting physician will need to make perioperative anticoagulation decisions based on the patient's history.

TAKE HOME POINT #2

Ensuring documentation of rhythm disturbance is of utmost importance (telemetry strip, EKG, Holter monitor) when assessing candidates for devices therapies. Evaluation of LV systolic function and for reversible myocardial ischemia should be obtained within a reasonable timeframe.

22.4 POST-IMPLANTATION CARE

It is important to understand that most often device implantation (pacemaker, ICD, or biventricular device) is performed as a scheduled procedure that will require inpatient observation overnight with discharge the following morning. The purpose of overnight observation is to monitor heart rate and rhythm, allow for recovery from sedation, provide early wound assessment, monitor newly-implanted lead stability, and evaluate for acute procedural complications. These goals are accomplished by telemetry monitoring overnight, chest radiography, device interrogation, and physical examination on the first postoperative day. Complications that may arise in the post-implantation period are listed in Table 22.5.

Table 22.5   Complications in the Post-Implant Setting.

Related to vascular access (arterial puncture, pneumothorax, hematoma)
Infection
Lead dislodgement
Phrenic nerve stimulation
Arrhythmia
Myocardial or coronary sinus perforation
Pocket pain

In the days to weeks after device implantation, the patient will be followed by the implanting electrophysiologist to evaluate the wound and lead stability. The use of post-implantation antibiotics is typically determined in consultation with the electrophysiologist.

TAKE HOME POINT #3

Most often, device implantation can be accomplished with discharge the following day. Postoperative chest radiography serves the following purposes: (1) A portable chest film immediately following the procedure is used to evaluate for pneumothorax if axillary or subclavian access has been used. (2) Postero-anterior and lateral chest radiographs will usually be obtained 24 hours following implantation to evaluate lead stability and placement in addition to the late recurrence of pneumothorax.

22.5   EVALUATION OF AN EXISTING DEVICE

When caring for a patient with an implanted cardiac device, the clinical history is of utmost importance in follow-up care. Weakness, poor exercise tolerance, fatigue, palpitations, and syncope may alert the hospitalist to consider pacemaker or ICD malfunction or inadequate programming. When an abnormality is suspected, the 12-lead ECG, chest radiography, and ultimately device interrogation will add to the clinical history during patient evaluation. Rhythm strips from cardiac telemetry monitors can be used to raise the suspicion of pacemaker malfunction; however, these monitors often use electronic filters that can significantly alter (hide altogether or introduce what appears to be) pacing artifact. For this reason, the 12-lead ECG is preferred. Patients who are pacing with a nonbiventricular device will always have a left bundle branch morphology in lead V1. Clinicians must keep in mind that, if a patient's intrinsic rhythm is greater than the lower pacing limit of the device, pacing will be inhibited.

TAKE HOME POINT #4

When a pacemaker or ICD malfunction is suspected, the clinical history and chest radiography are of great importance in focusing evaluation. Cardiac telemetry units often mask pacemaker artifact, making the use of the 12-lead ECG or prolonged 12-lead rhythm strip more useful when attempting to diagnose device malfunction.

In general, pacemaker malfunctions can be grouped as abnormalities in "sensing" versus "pacing." Abnormalities in sensing can be further characterized as "undersensing" and "oversensing" (Table 22.6 and Table 22.7). Undersensing occurs when the device is not able to "see" electrical activity that is present which will result in inappropriate and unnecessary overpacing. Oversensing occurs when the device is "seeing" inappropriate signals resulting from electrical activity that is not functional or physiologic, which will usually result in inappropriate inhibition of pacing.

Table 22.6   Causes of Pacemaker Undersensing.

Lead related (lead migration, dislodgement, or fracture)
Lead/myocardium interface fibrosis or maturation
Infarction at lead tip
Electrolyte abnormality
Medication effect
Rhythm change (atrial fibrillation/flutter, new bundle branch block)

Table 22.7   Causes of Pacemaker Oversensing.

Inappropriate sensing of P, R, or T waves
Inappropriate sensing of pacing artifact
Loose set screw
Lead fracture
Skeletal muscle signals
Electromagnetic interference (EMI) such as arc welding

Abnormalities in pacing can be divided into problems with failure of the device to capture, failure of the device to provide a pacing stimulus, or pacing too frequently. Failure to capture the myocardium (a pacing artifact without a following P wave or QRS complex) may be due to the pulse generator (battery depletion, loose set screw), the lead (migration, fracture), or the lead/myocardium interface (fibrosis or maturation, medication effect, electrolyte abnormalities). An example of failure to capture can be seen in Figure 22.4. A failure of the device to provide a pacing stimulus where one is needed or expected is almost uniformly due to oversensing.

One instance which results in inappropriate rapid pacing is pacemaker-mediated tachycardia (PMT) also known as "endless loop tachycardia." This occurs when a PVC is conducted retrograde through the AV node with resultant depolarization of the atria. This event causes an appropriate sensing of the atrial event and resultant ventricular pacing with the paced impulse again causing retrograde conduction through the AV node. This phenomenon can cause ventricular pacing at or near the upper programmed limit for the device (120 or 130 beats per minute, in most cases). The circuit requires intact retrograde AV node conduction and a dual-chamber device. The ECG (Figure 22.5) will show characteristic inverted P waves and ventricular paced beats occurring at a fixed rate. Most new devices have special algorithms to detect and treat PMT; however, the keen hospitalist will suspect the diagnosis in the correct clinical setting.

A simplified algorithm for the evaluation of an implanted pacemaker is shown in Figure 22.6. It should be noted that the algorithm makes use of a magnet in several instances. The application of a magnet (which can usually be found on crash carts or in the intensive care unit) over the pulse-generator has differing effects on pacemakers and ICDs. In pacemakers, a magnet will close a reed switch that will result in

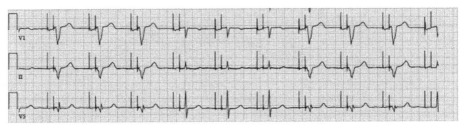

Figure 22.4 Failure to capture. Note that this is a dual-chamber pacing system that is delivering pacing stimuli to both the atrium and the ventricle. There are discernible P waves after each atrial pacing stimulus, suggesting that the atrial lead is pacing appropriately. The QRS complex, however, has two different morphologies. The first 3 beats have a short pacing artifact-to-QRS complex, which is of a left bundle branch block morphology (indicating capture of the myocardium). However, the next 3 beats have a longer pacing artifact-to-QRS complex and the QRS is narrow and not of LBBB morphology (suggesting the ventricular lead has failed to capture the myocardium and the resulting narrow QRS results from the native conduction sustem).

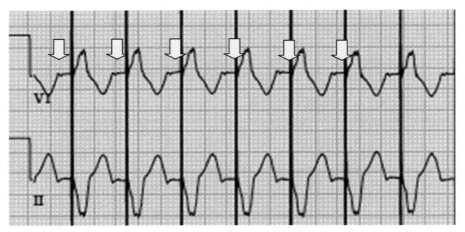

Figure 22.5 Pacemaker-mediated tachycardia. Note that the surface ECG shows ventricular pacing (pacing artifact prior to QRS complex, which has a right bundle-branch block morphology suggesting right ventricular pacing) at 120 beats per minute. Also note the inverted P-waves, resulting from retrograde AV conduction (block arrows).

asynchronous (VOO or DOO) pacing at rates which are manufacturer-specific and will change with battery voltage. Previously-programmed pacing mode and rate will resume when the magnet is removed.

Magnet placement over the pulse generator of an ICD (single or dual-chamber, or biventricular device) will result in inhibition of tachycardia detection. It will not change programmed pacing parameters. As such, placement of a magnet over an ICD system will prevent a patient from receiving a therapy, inappropriate or not. This may be useful in the patient receiving inappropriate therapies for oversensing, lead

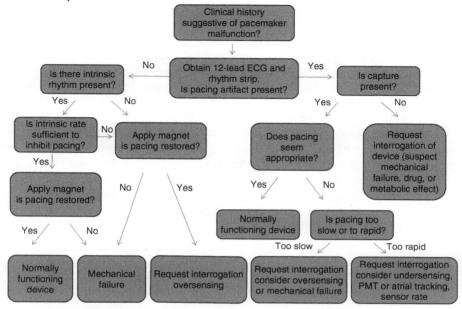

Figure 22.6 Decision tree for the evaluation of suspected pacemaker malfunction.

fracture, atrial fibrillation, or supraventricular tachycardia, but should only be done when the diagnosis is clear or when an external defibrillator has been applied to the patient and under the guidance of a cardiologist.

Finally, implanted cardiac devices are capable of transcutaneous transmission of data, and can be interrogated with manufacturer-specific analyzers. Device interrogation can prove helpful in diagnosing the cause of pacemaker or ICD malfunction when there are still questions after the above steps have been taken. Interrogation provides insight into pacing mode, battery status, lead performance, and episodes of arrhythmia and/or therapy. As the analyzers used to interrogate devices are manufacturer-specific, a knowledge of what device and the manufacturer of the device should be obtained so that proper equipment can be made available.

TAKE HOME POINT #5

Placement of a magnet over a pacemaker results in temporary changes to the pacing mode and rate, resulting in asynchronous pacing. Removal of the magnet will return normal pacing. Placement of a magnet over an ICD will result in the cessation of tachycardia detection and therapies (appropriate or not). This should be done only when the patient is closely monitored with an external defibrillator in place, and typically under the guidance of a cardiologist.

22.6   PERIOPERATIVE MANAGEMENT

The care of the patient with an implanted cardiac device in the perioperative setting deserves special mention. Electromagnetic interference can be caused by the use of electrocautery, possibly resulting in inappropriate oversensing in the atrium (with resultant rapid ventricular pacing), or ventricle (resulting in the inhibition of ventricular pacing from a pacemaker, or the inappropriate "detection" of ventricular tachycardia or fibrillation resulting in therapy from an ICD).

It should be noted that most modern devices are relatively unaffected by electrocautery as long as a bipolar configurataion is utilized with short bursts of cautery. As mentioned above, the application of a magnet over the pulse generator of a pacemaker will result in asynchronous pacing which will not be disrupted by cautery. Intraoperative application of a magnet over an ICD will disable the device from detecting such inappropriate "noise," thus preventing ICD therapy. In both cases, preoperative device function will be resumed when the magnet is removed.

TAKE HOME POINT #6

Most surgical procedures can be safely performed on patients with implanted cardiac devices, as long as care is taken to ensure continuous cardiac monitoring, and to minimize the use of long bursts of electrocautery in close proximity to the device. Application of a magnet over a pacemaker pulse generator will result in asynchronous pacing, which will be unaffected by even prolonged use of cautery near the device. Similarly, application of a magnet over an ICD will temporarily inhibit an ICD therapy.

KEY REFERENCES

EPSTEIN AE et al. ACC/AHA/HRS 2008 guidelines for device-based therapy of cardiac rhythm abnormalities: a report of the American College of Cardiology/American Heart Association Task Force on Practice Guidelines (Writing Committee to Revise the ACC/AHA/NASPE 2002 Guideline Update for Implantation of Cardiac Pacemakers and Antiarrhythmia Devices) developed in collaboration with the American Association for Thoracic Surgery and Society of Thoracic Surgeons. J Am Coll Cardiol 2008;51(21):e1–e62.

KASZALA K, HUIZAR JF, ELLENBOGEN KA. Contemporary pacemakers: what the primary care physician needs to know. Mayo Clinic Proceedings 2008;83(10):1170–1186.

Chapter 23

Hypertension

Sascha N. Goonewardena and Fareed U. Khaja

23.1 INTRODUCTION

Hypertension is a complex disease modified by both environmental and genetic factors. It is the most common chronic disease in developed nations, affecting up to 25% of all adults. Studies have demonstrated a significant relationship between levels of blood pressure (BP) and risk for cardiovascular events. Because of this relationship, inadequate BP control is one of the most common causes of death worldwide, being responsible for 62% of cerebrovascular disease and 49% of ischemic heart disease as well as an estimated 7.1 million deaths per year. Although the management of hypertension is predominately a long-term concern, it is important for the hospitalist to understand it given the high prevalence of hypertension among inpatients and the need to treat patients admitted with urgent hypertensive crises and emergencies. This chapter addresses both these specific issues in the broader context of hypertension management.

TAKE HOME POINT #1

Hospitalists have to be aware of both the long-term management of hypertension as well as its acute treatment in inpatients.

Inpatient Cardiovascular Medicine, First Edition. Edited by Brahmajee K. Nallamothu and Timir S. Baman.
© 2014 John Wiley & Sons, Inc. Published 2014 by John Wiley & Sons, Inc.

23.2 ASSOCIATION WITH CARDIOVASCULAR OUTCOMES

The association between BP and cardiovascular disease (CVD) is continuous across multiple patient populations. The more elevated a patient's BP, the greater the risk for heart attack, stroke, and kidney disease. The Seventh Report of the Joint National Committee on Prevention, Detection, Evaluation, and Treatment of High Blood Pressure (JNC VII) released in 2003, categorized hypertension into four primary categories to increase the awareness of high blood pressure and to stratify and help guide therapeutics (Table 23.1).

While antihypertensive trials have shown some variability in the degree of benefit, almost all have demonstrated some clinical benefits of treating hypertension with regards to outcomes including heart attack, stroke, and heart failure. On average, antihypertensive therapy has been associated with reductions in the incidence of heart attack by 25–30%, stroke by 35–40%, and heart failure by more than 50%.

TAKE HOME POINT #2

The risk of CVD beginning at 115/75 mmHg doubles with each increment of 20/10 mmHg; individuals who are normotensive at age 55 have a 90% lifetime risk for developing hypertension.

23.3 EVALUATION

High blood pressure management can be broadly divided into three components (Figure 23.1): identification; diagnostic work-up (including risk factor assessment and secondary cause evaluation); and treatment. Although the identification of patients with high blood pressure has been a national objective for years, most patients with elevated blood pressures are unaware of their condition. Additionally, much of the existing literature on hypertension is focused on therapeutics; as the incidence and prevalence continue to grow, much research is needed to evaluate resource allocation and

Table 23.1   Classification and Management of Blood Pressure for Adults*.

BP classification	SBP mmHg*	DBP mmHg*	Lifestyle modification	Initial drug therapy
Normal	<120	and <80	Encourage	No antihypertensive indicated
Prehypertension	120–139	or 80–89	Yes	No antihypertensive indicated
Stage 1 Hypertension	140–159	or 90–99	Yes	Thiazide diuretics. May consider ACEI, ARB, CCB, BB, or combination
Stage 2 Hypertension	>160	or >100	Yes	Two drug combination for most

*Treatment determined by hightest BP category.
ACEI, angiotensin converting eznyme inhibitor; ARB, angiotensin receptor blocker;
BB, beta-blocker; CCB, calcium channel blocker.

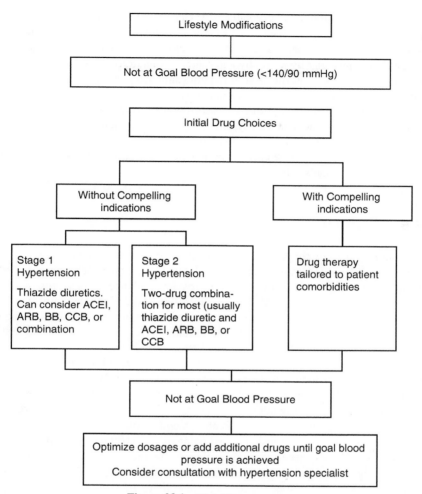

Figure 23.1   High BP management.

management strategies. As patient demographics and risk factors change, appropriate management strategies that consider not just efficacy but compliance and comorbidities are crucial components to better optimizing the care for patients with hypertension.

23.4 DIAGNOSIS

Hypertension is defined as a blood pressure of 140/90 mmHg or higher and is typically diagnosed in the outpatient clinics, in the patient's home using ambulatory blood pressure monitoring (ABPM), or through patient self-assessment. Typical ambulatory monitors are programmed to take readings every 15 to 30 minutes throughout the day and night without disruption of the patient's daily activities. In a clinic setting, blood pressure readings can be recorded using standard electronic units or manually using blood pressure cuffs. Care should be taken to ensure that the patient is comfortable, typically resting for five minutes prior to measurement. Several studies suggest that ABPM is more closely correlated with target organ damage (left ventricular hypertrophy and renal dysfunction) compared to traditional office measurements. Classification of hypertension category should be based on an average of two or more blood pressure readings.

Almost 33% of patients with increased blood pressure in the office may have normal pressure at home. One can assume that if daytime blood pressures out of the office are below 130/80 and there is no evidence of end organ disease due to hypertension, the patient has "white coat" hypertension secondary to the adrenergic surge of being in a physician's office.

23.5 WORKUP

The diagnostic strategy for patients with documented hypertension includes a workup for other typical cardiovascular risk factors (Table 23.2), identifiable causes of hypertension (Table 23.3), and to evaluate systems for evidence of end-organ damage (Table 23.4). Specifically, the physical examination should include confirmation of elevated BPs in the contralateral arm, fundoscopic examination, calculation of body mass index (BMI), auscultation of heart and lungs with a focus on signs suggestive of vascular abnormalities (bruits, abdominal masses, and peripheral pulses), and neurologic assessment. Standard laboratory tests obtained before initiation of antihypertensive therapies include: electrocardiogram (ECG); urinalysis; basic metabolic profile; lipid panel; thyroid stimulating hormone; and blood glucose. More extensive laboratory tests are generally not indicated unless a secondary cause of hypertension is suspected or the patient is resistant to pharmacotherapies.

If the diagnosis of hypertension is first being made in patients under the age of 20 or greater than 60 or resistant to medical therapy, secondary causes of hypertension should be sought more aggressively. Resistant hypertension is defined as blood pressure that remains above goal despite the use of three or more different classes of antihypertensive agents. Primary aldosteronism should be considered in those with hypertension and any of the following characteristics: (1) unexplained hypokalemia; (2) hypokalemia secondary to diuretics but not responding to treatment; (3) family history of mineralcorticoid excess; (4) highly resistant hypertension; or (5) adrenal mass noted on imaging study. A diagnosis of primary aldosteronism can obtained with a plasma aldosterone level >15 ng/dl in the setting of a low renin level. Renovascular hypertension can occur as a result of secondarily elevated renin levels in the presence of renal artery stenosis. A diagnosis can be confirmed by renal angiogram (Figure 23.2), ultrasound and magnetic resonance arteriography imaging studies. Finally, pheochromocytomas are catecholamine-producing tumors that result in hypertension and nonspecific symptoms such as palpitations, diaphoresis, headaches, and anxiety. Additionally, many common medications can interfere with blood pressure control, mimicking resistant hypertension. Some common examples include NSAIDS, decongestants, stimulants, alcohol, oral contraceptives, and herbal compounds such as ephedra.

Table 23.2   Cardiovascular Risk Factors.

Hypertension
Cigarette smoking
Obesity (BMI > 30 kg/m^2)
Physicial inactivity
Dyslipidemia
Diabetes mellitus
Age (older than 55 for men, 65 for women)
Microalbuminuria or estimated GFR < 60 ml/min
Family history of premature cardiovascular disease

Table 23.3   Identifiable Causes of Hypertension.

Diagnosis	Diagnostic studies
Sleep apnea	Sleep study
Drug-induced	Medication modification
Chronic renal disease	Urinalysis, serum creatinine, renal ultrasound
Renal artery stenosis	Renal angiogram, ultrasound, magnetic resonance arteriography
Coarctation	Comparison of blood pressure measurements in legs and arms
Cushing syndrome	Plasma cortisol measurements
Primary aldosteronism	Plasma aldosterone level >15 ng/dl in the setting of a low renin level
Pheochromocytoma	Plasma-free metanephrine, urine metanephrines and catecholamines
Thyroid or parathyroid disease	TSH or PTH level

Table 23.4   End Organ Damage Associated with Hypertension.

Organ system	Specific diagnosis
Heart	Left ventricular hypertrophy
	Angina or myocardial infarction
	Congestive heart failure (systolic or diastolic)
	Coronary artery disease
	Cardiac arrhythmias including atrial fibrillation
Neurologic	Stroke
	Transient ischemic attack
	Dementia
Renal	Chronic kidney disease
	End stage renal disease
Vascular	Peripheral arterial disease
	Sexual dysfunction
Ocular	Retinopathy

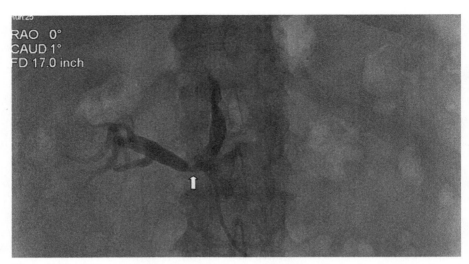

Figure 23.2   80% stenosis of the right renal artery in a patient with refractory hypertension and history of extensive tobacco abuse.

23.6 TREATMENT

For outpatients and long-term risk reduction, treatment of high blood pressure has proven benefits in reducing the progression of hypertension, cerebrovascular accidents, heart failure, and renal dysfunction. Among patients with mild-to-moderate hypertension, antihypertensive therapies have not had as profound an impact on atherosclerotic disease outcomes. The reason for these modest benefits is typically attributed to the choice of antihypertensive therapy and the relatively short duration of the clinical trials. Still, antihypertensive treatments reduce the prevalence of atherosclerotic, cerebrovascular, and renal disease and their associated complications.

Because of the clinical benefits associated with blood pressure regulation, aggressive control in the hypertensive patient is the primary goal. In most patients with hypertension, systolic blood pressure (SBP) control is associated with diastolic blood pressure (DBP) control. Because of this association, clinicians should focus on SBP control. Treating SBP and DBP to targets that are <140/90 mmHg is associated

TAKE HOME POINT #3

For long-term management, current guidelines advocate that thiazide-type diuretics should be used in drug treatment for most patients with uncomplicated hypertension, either alone or combined with drugs from other classes. Certain high-risk conditions are compelling indications for the initial use of other antihypertensive drug classes (angiotensin converting enzyme inhibitors, angiotensin receptor blockers, beta-blockers, calcium channel blockers).

Table 23.5   Lifestyle modifications to manage hypertension*.

Modification	Recommendation	Approximate SBP reduction
Weight reduction	Maintain normal body weight (BMI 18.5–24.9 kg/m²).	5–20 mmHg/10 kg weight loss
Adopt DASH eating plan	Consume a diet rich in fruits, vegetables, and low fat dairy products with a reduced content of saturated and total fat	8–14 mmHg
Dietary sodium reduction	Reduce dietary sodium intake to no more than 100 mmol per day	2–8 mmHg
Physical activity	Engage in regular aerobic physical activity at least 30 min per day, most days of the week	4–9 mmHg
Moderation of alcohol consumption	Limit consumption to no more than 2 drinks per day in most men and to no more than 1 drink per day in women	2–4 mmHg

*The effects of implementing these modifications are dose and time-dependent.
DASH, Dietary Approaches to Stop Hypertension.

with a decrease in CVD complications. In patients with hypertension and diabetes or renal disease, the BP goal is <130/80 mmHg.

Treatment strategies in the outpatient setting can be broadly broken down into nonpharmacologic and pharmacologic therapies. Nonpharmacologic therapies include weight reduction, aerobic exercise, moderation of alcohol intake, elimination of tobacco, and dietary modifications (Table 23.5). Weight reduction has been shown to reduce both systolic and diastolic blood pressure. A 10 lb (4.5 kg) weight reduction may reduce both systolic and diastolic blood pressure by 2–3 mm Hg. Among patients with prehypertension or stage I hypertension, weight reduction may avert the need for pharmacotherapies to reduce blood pressure. Aerobic exercise has been shown to reduce blood pressure independently of its effects on weight reduction. Specifically, exercise can reduce cardiac output and peripheral vascular resistance, both of which contribute to the reduction of blood pressure. The most important element of diet that contributes to hypertension (independently of weight) is the amount of salt consumed. Low salt diets are strongly recommended for patients with hypertension; the benefits are more significant in patients who are older and more sensitive to salt loads.

Pharmacologic therapy should be initiated in patients with stage II hypertension, evidence of target organ damage, cardiac risk factors, or with established cardiovascular disease (Table 23.6). There is a wealth of clinical data on several classes of antihypertensive medications, including angiotensin converting enzyme inhibitors

Table 23.6 Oral Antihypertensive Medications.

Class	Medication	Usual dose range (mg/day)	Usual daily frequency
Thiazide diuretics	Chlorothiazide	125–500	1–2
	Chlorthalidone	12.5–25	1
	Hydrochlorothiazide	12.5–50	1
	Polythiazide	2–4	1
	Indapamide	1.25–2.5	1
	Metolazone	0.5–1.0	1
Loop diuretics	Bumetanide	0.5–2	2
	Furosemide	20–80	2
	Torsemide	2.5–10	1
Potassium sparing diuretics	Amiloride	5–10	1–2
	Triamterene	50–100	1–2
Aldosterone receptor blockers	Eplerenone	50–100	1
	Spironolactone	25–50	1
Beta-blockers	Atenolol	25–100	1–2
	Betaxolol	5–20	1
	Bisoprolol	2.5–10	1
	Metoprolol	50–100	1
	Metoprolol ER	50–100	1
	Nadolol	40–120	1
	Propranolol	40–160	2
	Propranolol LA	60–180	1
	Timolol	20–40	2
Combined alpha and beta-blockers	Carvedilol	12.5–50	2
	Labetalol	200–800	2
ACE inhibitors	Benazepril	10–40	1
	Captopril	25–100	2
	Enalapril	5–40	1–2
	Fosinopril	10–40	1
	Lisinopril	10–40	1
	Moexipril	7.5–30	1
	Perindopril	4–8	1
	Quinapril	10–80	1
	Ramipril	2.5–20	1
	Trandolapril	1–4	1
Angiotensin II antagonists	Candesartan	8–32	1
	Eprosartan	400–800	1–2
	Irbesartan	150–300	1
	Losartan	25–100	1–2
	Olmesartan	20–40	1
	Telmisartan	20–80	1
	Valsartan	80–320	1–2

(Continued)

Table 23.6 (Continued).

Class	Medication	Usual dose range (mg/day)	Usual daily frequency
Calcium channel blockers-nondihydropyridiines	Diltiazem	180–240	1
	Verapamil	80–320	1
Calcium channel blockers-dihydropyridiines	Amlodipine	2.5–10	1
	Felodipine	2.5–20	1
	Isradipine	2.5–10	2
	Nicardipine	60–120	2
	Nifedipine	30–60	1
	Nisoldipine	10–40	1
Alpha-1 blockers	Doxasoin	1–16	1
	Prazosin	2–20	2–3
	Terazosin	1–20	1–2
Central alpha-2 agonists and other central acting drugs	Clonidine	0.1–0.8	2
	Methyldopa	250–1000	2
	Reserpine	0.1–0.25	1
	Guanfacine	0.5–2	1
Direct vasodilators	Hydralazine	25–100	2
	Minoxidil	2.5–80	1–2

(ACEIs), angiotensin receptor blockers (ARBs), beta-blockers (BBs), calcium channel blockers (CCBs), and thiazide-type diuretics. Based on the results of landmark trials including the Antihypertensive and Lipid Lowering Treatment to Prevent Heart Attack Trial (ALLHAT), the most recent JNC VII recommends utilizing thiazide-type diuretics as first-line treatment unless special circumstances dominate. More recently, the Avoiding Cardiovascular Events through Combination Therapy in Patients Living with Systolic Hypertension (ACCOMPLISH) trial has brought into question this recommendation and suggests benefits of ACEIs in combination with CCBs over other regimens, including those utilizing thiazide-type diuretics as first-line agents. Further trials and follow-up will continue to shed light on this controversial topic. However, the overriding theme is that aggressive diagnosis and treatment of high blood pressure is of clinical benefit at both the individual patient level as well as from a public health perspective.

23.7 MANAGING HYPERTENSION IN THE HOSPITAL

Given its high prevalence in the general population, it is likely that patients with hypertension will be admitted for other conditions and that hypertension will have to be managed by hospitalists. Although there are little to no empiric data to guide specific management strategies in these patients, we believe it should be guided by a few general principles. First, the presence of modifying factors that might be associated with transient elevations in blood pressure, particularly pain, must be considered and treated when possible in patients. Second, the hospitalist should understand that the long-term care and management of hypertension in these patients will be provided for in the outpatient setting. While the hospitalist should be actively involved in understanding why certain therapies are prescribed and instituting treatments that she (or he) determines may be more effective (e.g. the use of ACE inhibitors in someone with diabetes), any changes made to a patient's usual regimen should be clearly communicated to the patient and their outpatient physician to avoid confusion. Third, the hospitalist also should recognize that blood pressures will fluctuate at times in hospitalized patients, and avoid the dangers of over-diagnosing or over-treating patients based on an isolated number. Finally, we have found anecdotally that some patients on a large number of antihypertensive therapies who are admitted for other reasons can "bottom-out" their pressures when their home regimen is instituted. Drugs to treat hypertension are ubiquitous in the hospitalized setting and among the most frequently abused in terms of polypharmacy. Always re-institute a home regimen with the cautious understanding that it might be different than what the patient actually takes.

TAKE HOME POINT #4

When substantial changes in home regimens are made to improve blood pressure control in patients with hypertension admitted for other reasons, these changes should be clearly communicated to the patient and outpatient physician.

23.8 HYPERTENSIVE CRISIS

Patients with marked BP elevations and acute target-organ damage (e.g. encephalopathy, myocardial infarction, unstable angina, pulmonary edema, eclampsia, stroke, head trauma, life-threatening arterial bleeding, or aortic dissection) require hospitalization and parenteral drug therapy. Patients with markedly elevated BP but without acute target organ damage usually do not require hospitalization, but they should receive immediate combination oral antihypertensive therapy. They should be carefully evaluated and monitored for hypertension-induced heart and kidney damage and for identifiable causes of hypertension.

The treatment of a hypertensive crisis is dictated by both the level of blood pressure elevation and the presence or absence of acute end-organ damage. The choice of specific pharmacologic agents should be tailored to the situation and the patient. Hypertensive emergency is defined by elevated blood pressure accompanied by acute end-organ damage. Hypertensive urgency is defined by a systolic blood pressure >210 mmHg or diastolic blood pressure >120 mmHg in the absence of end-organ damage. For hypertensive emergency, the short-term objectives to lower mean arterial pressures (MAP) by 25% within 2–3 hours using parenteral drug therapy (Table 23.7). A larger reduction in blood pressure or within a shorter time frame can

Table 23.7 Intravenous Medications for Hypertensive Emergency.

Drug	Dosage
Esmolol	200–500 μg/kg/min for 4 min followed by 50–300 μg/kg/min
Labetalol	20–80 mg IV bolus every 10 minutes; 2 mg/min IV infusion
Nitroprusside	0.25–10 μg/kg/min infusion
Nitroglycerin	5–100 μg/min infusion
Hydralazine	10–20 mg IV push

worsen end-organ damage, particularly neurologic damage. However, if there is evidence of aortic dissection or cardiac failure, blood pressure should be reduced more rapidly. For hypertensive urgency, the objective is to reduce blood pressure within hours using oral agents.

TAKE HOME POINT #5

The management decision in patients with suspected hypertensive crisis revolves around both the blood pressure and evidence of end-organ damage.

KEY REFERENCES

The ALLHAT Collaborative Research Group. Major outcomes in high-risk hypertensive patients randomized to angiotensin-converting enzyme inhibitor or calcium channel blocker vs diuretic: the Antihypertensive and Lipid-Lowering Treatment to Prevent Heart Attach Trial (ALLAT). JAMA 2002; 288:2981–2997.

CHOBANIAN AV, et al. The Seventh Report of the Joint National Committee on Prevention, Detection, Evaluation, and Treatment of High Blood Pressure: the JNC 7 Report. JAMA 2003; 289:2560–2572.

JAMERSON KA, on behalf of the ACCOMPLISH investigators. Benazepril plus amlodipine or hydrochlorothiazide for hypertension in high-risk patients. N Engl J Med 2008;359:2417–2428.

Chapter 24

Valvular Heart Disease

Craig T. Alguire and David S. Bach

24.1 INTRODUCTION

The spectrum of valve disease ranges from a benign murmur to severe hemodynamic instability. Valve surgery accounts for 10–20% of all cardiac surgery in the United States. The causes of valvular dysfunction are broad and can include a primary process directly affecting the leaflets or dysfunction of the adjacent, mechanical supporting structures. It is important to understand the underlying etiology in order for a clinician to effectively diagnose and target medical and surgical therapy.

Acute changes in valvular function usually present with an abrupt onset of symptoms or hemodynamic instability. In contrast, chronic valvular disease typically has an insidious course; symptoms of fatigue, shortness of breath, or decreased functional capacity are seen only late in the progression of disease. When patients have multiple co-morbidities, differentiating nonspecific symptoms of chronic valvular disease and other underlying medical processes can be challenging. When symptoms are difficult to elicit or confounded with co-morbidities, stress exercise testing with evaluation of hemodynamic response can be helpful. Concurrent imaging, usually with echocardiography and Doppler, can assess chamber sizes and function to determine impact of valvular disease on cardiac function.

This chapter reviews valvular disease, focusing on significant regurgitation and stenosis of each valve. It focuses primarily on diagnostic testing and management with the physical examination features associated with valvular heart disease discussed elsewhere. Extensive guidelines are available from the American College of

Inpatient Cardiovascular Medicine, First Edition. Edited by Brahmajee K. Nallamothu and Timir S. Baman.

Cardiology (ACC) and American Heart Association (AHA). However, individual patient characteristics cannot always be captured by algorithms and recommendations are limited by the lack of large randomized trials on valvular disease. In general, consultation with a cardiologist should be considered any time a patient has moderate or severe valve disease.

24.2 AORTIC VALVE

The normal aortic valve has three cusps supported by a fibrous annulus (Figure 24.1). A normal valve opens freely when the left ventricular cavity pressure surpasses aortic pressure allowing unimpeded flow from the left ventricle to aorta. Diseases of the aortic valve can be acquired or congenital and result in stenosis, regurgitation, or both.

24.2.1 Aortic Stenosis

Aortic stenosis is the condition characterized by a significant pressure gradient across the valve. Less commonly, obstruction of the left ventricular outflow tract can occur below (subvalvular) or above (supravalvular) the aortic valve. Dyspnea (or other manifestations of heart failure), angina, and syncope are the classic symptoms of severe aortic stenosis. Aortic valve stenosis occurs primarily from three main etiologies: calcific degeneration of a three leaflet valve (the most common), bicuspid aortic valve, or rheumatic disease. Aortic stenosis is graded as mild, moderate, or severe (Table 24.1), although there is a hemodynamic continuum without absolute cutoffs.

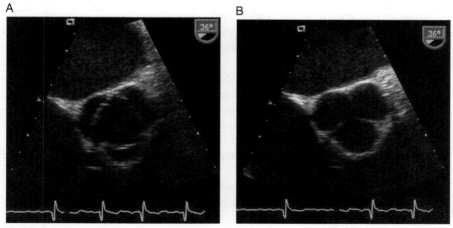

Figure 24.1   Echocardiographic images of a normal tricuspid aortic valve. **A** shows aortic valve in systole; **B** shows closure in diastole.

Table 24.1   Aortic Stenosis Severity.

	Mild	Moderate	Severe
Jet velocity (m/s)	<3	3–4	>4
Mean Gradient (mmHg)	<25	25–40	>40
Valve area (cm²)	1.5–2.0	1.0–1.5	<1.0

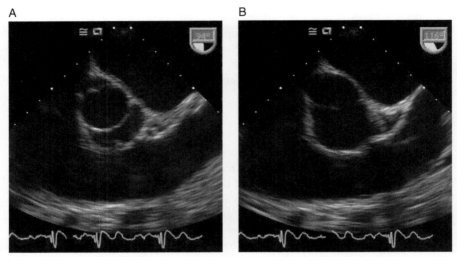

Figure 24.2   Echocardiographic images of a bicuspid aortic valve. **A** shows a bicuspid valve in systole; **B** shows a bicuspid valve in diastole.

The ACC/AHA guidelines recommend transthoracic echocardiography for re-evaluation of asymptomatic patients every year for severe AS; every 1–2 years for moderate AS; and every 3–5 years for mild AS.

Calcific degeneration of an aortic valve (or senile calcification) is the most common cause of aortic stenosis and subsequent valve surgery. The disease tends to be progressive with an average decrease in valve area of 0.1 cm² per year. Although the presence of aortic stenosis is associated with similar risk factors that exist for atherosclerosis (diabetes mellitus, smoking, hypertension, hyperlipidemia, male sex, and age), there is currently no compelling data to support risk factor modification as a treatment for aortic stenosis. When the aortic valve becomes heavily calcified, it can be difficult to differentiate a bicuspid from a tricuspid valve.

Bicuspid aortic valves affect approximately 2% of the population. It is more common in men than women, with a 3:1 ratio. Compared to patients born with a tricuspid valve, patients with a bicuspid aortic valve tend to develop aortic stenosis and insufficiency at an earlier age. In addition, a bicuspid aortic valve is associated with ascending aortic aneurysm and increased risk for dissection. Figure 24.2 demonstrates a short axis of a bicuspid valve. In this view, the valve opens freely without stenosis in an oval shape.

Rheumatic aortic valve stenosis is almost always associated with concurrent rheumatic mitral valve disease. In contrast to senile calcific aortic stenosis, in which calcification extends from the cusp bases, rheumatic disease initially affects the commissural edges and usually progresses gradually over several years.

24.2.2 Low Gradient Aortic Stenosis

Patients with left ventricular dysfunction may have severe aortic stenosis, but measured pressure gradients across the valve can be low due to a "low flow" state. In this situation, the clinician needs to differentiate "true stenosis" from "pseudostenosis." True stenosis refers to an aortic valve with a hemodynamically significant mechanical obstruction with secondary left ventricular dysfunction. Pseudostenosis refers to an aortic valve with limited mobility that is secondary to low cardiac output from the left ventricle, not intrinsic valve disease. Dobutamine stress echocardiography can help distinguish between both conditions. In true stenosis, valve gradients increase with increased cardiac output without a change in aortic valve area. In pseudostenosis, the aortic valve area increases with increased cardiac output and valve gradients are unchanged. Cardiology consultation should be utilized to differentiate patients when low gradient aortic stenosis is suspected, since these patients will benefit from surgery.

24.2.3 Management of Aortic Stenosis

Appropriate patients with severe aortic stenosis and symptoms should undergo aortic valve replacement (Figure 24.3). However, symptom onset can be insidious with slowly progressive disease, and patients often compensate by decreasing activity. Once symptoms develop in the setting of severe aortic stenosis, the prognosis without surgery is very poor. Percutaneous balloon valvuloplasty can be considered as a palliative intervention, but restenosis rates at six months are high and long-term outcomes are inferior to surgery. Early clinical trials have suggested a role for transcatheter aortic valve replacement (TAVR) implanted via percutaneous or transapical access in patients who are poor candidates for sugery.

Medical therapy is limited in aortic stenosis. Diuretics are helpful with fluid overload. Treatment of concurrent cardiac disease should be done with caution as afterload-reducing and preload-reducing medications can precipitate hypotension.

TAKE HOME POINT #1

Severe aortic stenosis with symptoms (dyspnea, angina, syncope) is a class I ACC/AHA indication for aortic valve replacement.

24.2.4 Aortic Regurgitation

Aortic regurgitation is a complex disease that varies broadly in its acuity of presentation, severity, etiology, and management. The most common causes of aortic valve regurgitation are listed in Table 24.2.

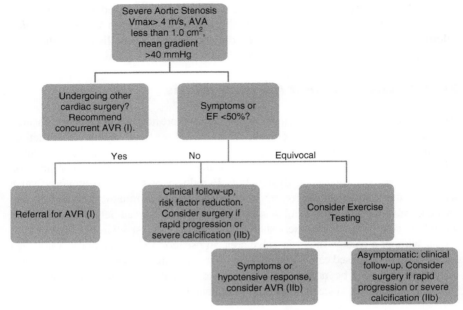

Figure 24.3   Algorithm for appropriate timing of aortic valve replacement (AVR) in aortic stenosis based on 2006 ACC/AHA guidelines. Per these guidelines, Class 1 recommendations "should be done," Class IIa is "reasonable to perform," and Class IIb "should be considered."

Table 24.2   Causes of Aortic Insufficiency.

Dilation of aorta
Congenital valve abnormality (bicuspid)
Calcific degeneration
Rheumatic disease
Infective endocarditis
Aortic dissection

Acute, severe aortic regurgitation can cause cardiovascular collapse due to a rapid increase in end-diastolic volume from regurgitant blood. The diastolic murmur associated with aortic regurgitation is low-pitched and early, and lessens with severity. Echocardiography is the diagnostic test of choice. As a medical emergency, it should be treated in intensive care, with intravenous vasodilators, and with urgent surgical intervention in appropriate patients. An intra-aortic balloon pump is contraindicated and can worsen the severity of aortic regurgitation. It is important to rule out acute aortic pathology (dissection or aneurysm expansion) and endocarditis in acute aortic insufficiency since these are the most common causes.

Chronic aortic regurgitation, in contrast, is a slow and insidious disease process. Patients may frequently remain asymptomatic for several years due to the extensive compensatory mechanisms of the left ventricle that occur over time. Physical findings may be unreliable for grading the severity of chronic aortic regurgitation, but

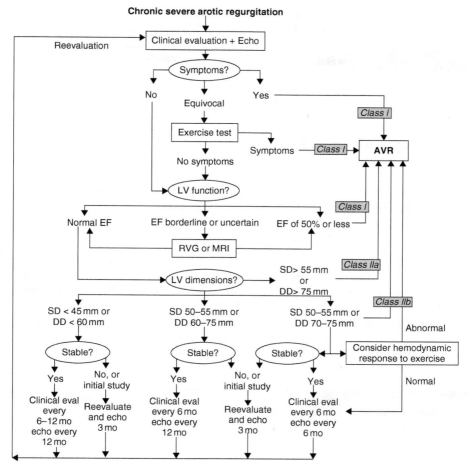

Figure 24.4 Algorithm for appropriate timing of aortic valve replacement (AVR) in aortic regurgitation based on 2006 ACC/AHA guidelines. Per these guidelines, Class 1 recommendations "should be done," Class IIa is "reasonable to perform," and Class IIb "should be considered." (Source: Bonow RO, Carabello BA, Kanu C, et al. 2006. Reproduced with permission of Wolters Kluwer Health).

echocardiography is accurate at grading the severity of regurgitation as well as left ventricular function and size. Patients with symptomatic and severe chronic aortic regurgitation should be evaluated for aortic valve replacement. For asymptomatic patients with severe chronic aortic regurgitation, provoked symptoms on exercise testing, increased left ventricular size, and decreasing ejection fraction all are indications to pursue surgery. Figure 24.4 summarizes the algorithm endorsed by the ACC/AHA for evaluating patients for surgery. If surgery is deferred, timing of follow-up examinations in asymptomatic patients with severe regurgitation on echocardiography depends on left ventricular dimensions and systolic function, as well as the stability of these measurements. Stable patients with normal dimensions should have repeat echocardiograms annually. If cardiac chambers are enlarging, follow-up should be more frequent and referral for surgery should be considered.

TAKE HOME POINT #2

Asymptomatic chronic regurgitation of the aortic valve must be followed carefully to ensure stability of left ventricular size and function.

24.3 MITRAL VALVE

The mitral valve is composed of anterior and posterior leaflets with a support structure including the mitral annulus, chordae tendinae, papillary muscles, and the left ventricle. Dysfunction of any of these elements can lead to stenosis, regurgitation, or both.

24.3.1 Mitral Valve Stenosis

By far the most common cause of mitral valve stenosis in native valves is rheumatic heart disease. This is an autoimmune disorder that occurs after acute pharyngitis from group A *streptococcus*. In developed countries, symptoms of mitral valve stenosis usually occur 15 to 20 years after an episode of rheumatic fever. Due to changing virulence of Group A *streptococcus* and the widespread availability of antibiotic therapy, rheumatic fever prevalence has dramatically decreased in industrialized countries over the last 100 years.

TAKE HOME POINT #3

Mitral stenosis is almost always due to rheumatic heart disease.

The characteristic findings of rheumatic mitral disease are seen in Figure 24.5. The leaflets become thickened and rigid, and the chordae tendinae fuse, thicken, and shorten with a classic "hockey-stick" appearance of the leaflet due to restriction at the commissures. As obstruction worsens, left atrial pressure increases, leading to pulmonary edema and pulmonary hypertension. Patients can present with dyspnea, hemoptysis, chest pain, atrial fibrillation, or embolic events. The transmitral pressure is dependent on flow across the valve; therefore, symptoms can be exacerbated with exercise (or fever, anemia, coexisting mitral regurgitation). As with aortic stenosis, this mechanical obstruction requires invasive intervention for definitive therapy. This may include percutaneous mitral balloon valvuloplasty in select patients with suitable valves based on echocardiographic criteria. Surgical intervention comprises mitral valve repair, which is preferable, or mitral valve replacement. Medical therapy focuses on prevention of recurrence with secondary prophylaxis even into adulthood, aggressive treatment of tachyarrhythmias, and monitoring progression with echocardiography. For prevention of thromboembolism, anticoagulation with warfarin is indicated in

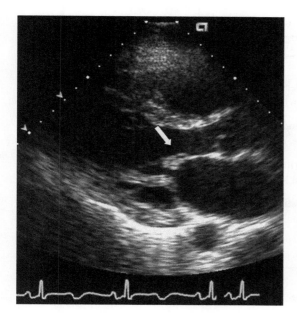

Figure 24.5 Typical echocardiographic features of mitral stenosis secondary to rheumatic heart disease. The image demonstrates thickening of the mitral valve leaflet tips and chordae tendinae with restricted motion or hockey-sticking of the anterior mitral valve leaflet (arrow).

patients with mitral stenosis and atrial fibrillation, prior thromboembolism, or known left atrial thrombus. Cardiology consultation is typically required for patients with significant mitral stenosis to decide between numerous treatment options.

24.3.2 Mitral Regurgitation

Dysfunction of any component of the mitral valve or supporting apparatus can cause acute or chronic regurgitation (Table 24.3). Echocardiographic imaging is the most widely-used tool for the assessment of mitral regurgitation etiology and severity. Organic MR is caused by an anatomic abnormality intrinsic to the mitral valve leaflets or chordae tendinae including myxomatous degeneration (i.e., mitral valve prolapse), rheumatic heart disease, and infectious endocarditis. There is no proven role for medical therapy in the treatment of organic MR when it is severe. Indications for surgical intervention revolve around the presence of symptoms, LV systolic dysfunction (LVEF ≤60%), or significant LV enlargement. In addition, there is an increasingly accepted role for consideration of intervention in an asymptomatic patient with severe MR if there is a high likelihood of successful repair.

In contrast to organic MR, functional MR occurs from failure of normal mitral leaflets to coapt appropriately owing to changes in LV size or shape (typically from dilated cardiomyopathy). Medical therapy for functional MR is aimed at the underlying cardiomyopathy, with afterload-reducing therapy, diuretics, beta-adrenergic antagonists, and biventricular pacing all having been shown to reduce the severity of functional MR. There are no widely-accepted indications for surgical intervention for functional MR, although there may be a role in some

Table 24.3   Causes of Acute and Chronic Mitral Regurgitation.

Mitral leaflet disorders
infection, trauma, tumors (atrial myxoma), myxomatous degeneration

Mitral annulus disorders
infection (endocarditis with abscess), trauma, complication of surgery

Rupture of chordae tendinae
idiopathic, myxomatous, endocarditis

Papillary muscle disorders
coronary disease, global left ventricular dysfunction

Dysfunction of prosthetic valves
perforation, degeneration, or paravalvular leak

Congenital
mitral valve clefts, fenestrations, or parachute valve

patients for mitral valve repair to treat intractable heart failure that persists despite aggressive medical therapy.

TAKE HOME POINT #4

Mitral regurgitation is either secondary to intrinsic abnormalities of the leaflets or chordae tendinae (organic) or secondary to changes in left ventricular size or shape (functional).

Acute severe mitral regurgitation should be treated as a medical and surgical emergency given that its hemodynamic effects can be profound. It is typically due to one of three basic mechanisms: (1) flail leaflet from mitral valve prolapse or infectious endocarditis; (2) chordae tendinae rupture from spontaneous rupture, trauma, or infectious endocarditis; and (3) papillary muscle dysfunction or rupture from acute myocardial infarction or ischemia and trauma. Key components to therapy include afterload reduction, possible intraaortic balloon pump, revascularization, and surgical evaluation. Patients treated with PCI in the setting of acute myocardial infarction or ischemia may demonstrate some improvement in mitral regurgitation.

Mitral valve prolapse syndrome has multiple names, including systolic click-murmur syndrome, Barlow syndrome, billowing mitral cusp syndrome and, more commonly, myxomatous mitral valve syndrome. It can be seen as an isolated process or with connective tissue diseases including Marfan or Ehlers-Danlos syndrome. Mitral valve prolapse is common and seen in up to 2–3% of the population. The most specific echocardiographic finding is superior displacement of one or both mitral valve leaflets at least 2 mm above the plane of the mitral annulus with associated leaflet thickening. Mitral regurgitation can result from leaflet redundancy and excessive motion and elongation or rupture of chordae tendinae.

24.4 RIGHT SIDED VALVE DISEASE

Primary pulmonary and tricuspid valve diseases usually present in childhood as congenital lesions. Ebstein's anomaly is the most common congenital cause of tricuspid disease in which the valve is displaced apically into the right ventricle leading to stenosis or regurgitation. An important acquired cause of triscupid valve disease in adults is the carcinoid syndrome which can lead to thickening and retraction of leaflets resulting in both regurgitation or stenosis. In general, triscupid valve disease typically leads to regurgitation much more commonly than stenosis. Causes of tricuspid regurgitation are listed in Table 24.4.

Because significant tricuspid regurgitation is most commonly due to functional changes, diseases like pulmonary hypertension or right ventricle and atrial dilation must be considered when patients present with isolated tricuspid valve disease. Pulmonary artery systolic pressures can be estimated on echocardiogram using the velocity of the tricuspid regurgitation jet on Doppler interrogation. Management of tricuspid regurgitation usually follows medical therapy with diuretics to control fluid status and to prevent symptoms of hepatosplenomegaly, ascites, and peripheral edema. Surgical repair of the tricuspid valve can be performed but its utility and long-term durability are unknown.

As with tricuspid regurgitation, the most common form of pulmonary regurgitation is pulmonary hypertension of any etiology. Infective endocarditis is another leading etiology. Pulmonary stenosis is usually congenital and often can be treated with balloon valvuloplasty.

24.5 PROSTHETIC VALVES

Prosthetic valves are mechanical or bioprosthetic. Typically encountered mechanical valves are bileaflet or tilting disk, although caged ball valves are still seen. Bioprosthetic valves include heterografts (primarily bovine pericardium or porcine), homograft (human tissue), or autograft (pulmonary valve from same patient). Mechanical valves are more durable than are bioprostheses, but require anticoagulation to reduce the risk of valve thrombosis. Over time, bioprosthetic valves can progressively calcify with subsequent structural degeneration but do not require long-term anticoagulation. Due

Table 24.4 Causes of Tricuspid Regurgitation.

Functional (with an anatomically normal valve)
Pulmonary arterial hypertension
Cor pulmonale
Rheumatic
Endocarditis
Ebstein's anomaly
Myxomatous disease
Carcinoid

to durability, mechanical valves may be preferred in some younger patients although lifestyle considerations also play an important role in valve choice.

The management of oral anticoagulation is problematic for patients with mechanical valves requiring procedures. The risk of valve thrombosis must be weighed against bleeding risk and the need for procedures. In general, anticoagulation can be interrupted for patients with a "low risk" mechanical aortic valve and no other thromboembolic risks, whereas thromboembolic risks or a mechanical mitral valve mandates measures to minimize the interval during which therapeutic anticoagulation is interrupted. At present, low-molecular weight heparin is not approved by the US FDA as an alternative to coumadin or intravenous unfractionated heparin for patients with a mechanical valve. The role of newer agents, such as dabigatran, is also unknown.

TAKE HOME POINT #5

Anticoagulation can be interrupted for short periods of time for patients with a "low risk" mechanical aortic valve and no other thromboembolic risks, whereas thromboembolic risks of a mechanical mitral valve mandates measures to reduce interval in which anticoagulation is interrupted.

The 2006 ACC/AHA guidelines for anticoagulation to prevent thrombosis with prosthetic valves around the time of procedures are summarized in Table 24.5.

Table 24.5   Summary of ACC/AHA Guidelines.

There is evidence and/or general agreement that the following approach to therapy is effective in patients with mechanical valves:

Among patients who are at low risk for thrombosis, which is defined as a bileaflet aortic valve with no risk factors:*

1. Warfarin should be withheld 48 to 72 hours before the procedure to allow the INR to fall below 1.5
2. Warfarin is restarted 24 hours after the procedure
3. Heparin is usually not necessary

Among patients who are at high risk for thrombosis, which is defined as a mechanical aortic valve with any risk factor* or any mechanical mitral valve:

1. Warfarin should be withheld more than 72 hours before the procedure
2. Therapeutic doses of intravenous unfractionated heparin should be started when the INR falls below 2.0 (usually 48 hours before the procedure)
3. Heparin is stopped 4–6 hours before the procedure
4. Heparin and warfarin are restarted as soon after surgery as bleeding stability permits.
5. Heparin is discontinued when the INR reaches therapeutic levels

---

*Risk factors for valve thrombosis: atrial fibrillation, previous thromboembolism, left ventricular dysfunction <30%, a hypercoagulable state, older generation thrombogenic valves (caged ball or tilting disk), a mechanical tricuspid valve, or multiple valves.

Anticoagulation depends on the type of valve and position. Mitral valves, due to lower velocity of flow, are at higher risk for thromboembolic events than aortic valves.

Bridging patients with mechanical valves who require uninterrupted anticoagulation typically involves intravenous heparin. However, the ACC/AHA gives low molecular weight heparin (100 U/Kg every 12 hours) or high dose SC unfractionated heparin (15,000 units every 12 hours) a 2B recommendation (weight of evidence or opinion is less well established for this approach). Decisions should involve patient understanding of risk, preference, and guidance by cardiology consultation as needed.

KEY REFERENCES

BONOW RO, CARABELLO BA, KANU C, et al. ACC/AHA 2006 guidelines for the management of patients with valvular heart disease. Circulation 2006;114(5):e84–231.

CARABELLO B. Aortic stenosis. NEJM 2002;346(9):677–682.

OTTO C. Evaluation and management of chronic mitral regurgitation. NEJM 2001;345(10):740–746.

Chapter 25

Infective Endocarditis

Michael P. Thomas and Preeti N. Malani

25.1 EPIDEMIOLOGY

There are 15,000 new cases of infective endocarditis (IE) per year in the United States with an in-hospital mortality of 15–20% and a one-year mortality that approaches 40%. Native-valve endocarditis compromises approximately three-quarters of all cases with prosthetic-valve endocarditis responsible for one-fifth and the remainder involving pacemakers or intracardiac defibrillators (ICD) (Figure 25.1, Figure 25.2). Three out of every four patients present within one month of the initial signs of illness.

Results from the International Collaboration on Endocarditis-Prospective Cohort Study suggest that infective endocarditis involves the mitral valve and aortic valve equally at rates of approximately 40%. The tricuspid valve is most commonly affected in intravenous drug users. Pulmonic valve endocarditis is rare. Predisposing conditions associated with IE include intravenous drug use, previous IE, invasive procedures within the preceding 60 days, chronic intravenous access, pacemaker or ICD, congenital heart defects, and native valve predisposition including mitral valve prolapse associated with mitral regurgitation and degenerative aortic valve disease (Table 25.1).

> **TAKE HOME POINT #1**
>
> In-hospital mortality for infective endocarditis is 15–20%.

Inpatient Cardiovascular Medicine, First Edition. Edited by Brahmajee K. Nallamothu and Timir S. Baman.
© 2014 John Wiley & Sons, Inc. Published 2014 by John Wiley & Sons, Inc.

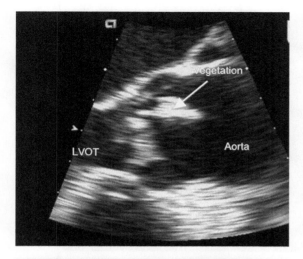

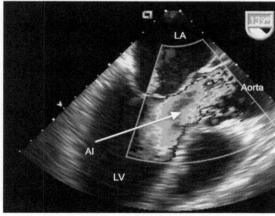

Figure 25.1   TEE of aortic valve endocarditis with aortic regurgitation. AI, aortic regurgitation; LVOT, left ventricular outflow tract. (See Color plate 25.1).

25.2 PATHOPHYSIOLOGY

Developing valvular IE is a complex process involving multiple interacting components. In order for a vegetation to form, the valve surface must first be altered or damaged. Valve surface damage often results in blood flow turbulence and is frequently followed by platelet and fibrin deposition with eventual formation of nonbacterial thrombotic endocarditis (NTE). Bacteria may then colonize the lesion after formation of NTE. The continued proliferation of bacteria and deposition of platelets and fibrin result in a vegetation that can embolize peripherally and result in embolic phenomena. Often, these vegetations create a biofilm, thus making them impermeable to the body's defenses as well as antibiotic therapy.

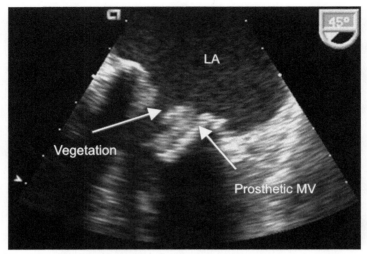

Figure 25.2   TEE of prosthetic mitral valve endocarditis.

Table 25.1   Predisposing Conditions Associated with Infective Endocarditis (IE).

Predisposing conditions
Chronic intravenous access
Congenital heart defects
Intravenous drug use
Invasive procedures within 60 days
Native valve predisposition
Pacemaker/intracardiac defibrillators
Previous IE

The clinical features of IE are a consequence of (1) local cardiac destruction, (2) systemic embolization of the vegetation, and (3) deposition of circulating immune complexes. Intracardiac complications vary from minimal tissue damage to extensive valvular destruction and significant hemodynamic deterioration. Common sites of emboli include the central nervous system, spleen, lung, and skin. Immune complexes can deposit in the glomerular basement membrane, resulting in glomerulonephritis.

TAKE HOME POINT #2

The peripheral manifestations of infective endocarditis are the result of systemic emboli and immune complexes.

Table 25.2 Clinical Findings in Patients with Definite Infective Endocarditis*.

Clinical finding	Percentage of cases (%)
Fever, temperature >38 °C	96
New murmur	48
Hematuria	26
Worsening of old murmur	20
Vascular embolic event	17
Splenomegaly	11
Splinter hemorrhages	7
Conjunctival hemorrhage	5
Janeway lesions	5
Osler nodes	3
Roth spots	2

*Adapted from Murdoch DR, Corey R, Hoen B, et al: Clinical presentation, etiology, and outcome of infective endocarditis in the 21st century: The International Collaboration on Endocarditis – Prospective Cohort Study. Arch Intern Med 2009;169:463.

25.3 CLINICAL FEATURES

The period of time from the onset of bacteremia to symptoms of IE is generally less than two weeks, although this can vary based on the infecting organism. The most common clinical finding of IE is fever observed in more than 95% of patients (Table 25.2). Constitutional symptoms result from cytokine release and include arthralgias, myalgias, anorexia, and malaise. The risk of systemic emboli increases with vegetations greater than 10 mm. Embolization risk decreases shortly after the administration of antibiotics. Stroke occurs in 15–20% of patients and most commonly involves the middle cerebral artery. Congestive heart failure results from valvular destruction, fistula formation, and myocarditis. Renal insufficiency can result from the deposition of circulating immune complexes. Although classically described with IE, peripheral manifestations that can result from either systemic emboli or immune complex deposition are seen in fewer than 10% of IE cases. Such manifestations include petechiae, splinter hemorrhages (linear streaks in the proximal nail bed), Osler nodes (tender subcutaneous nodules in the pulp of digits), Janeway lesions (small erythematous nontender lesions on the palms and soles), and Roth spots (oval retinal hemorrhages with a pale center).

TAKE HOME POINT #3

The most common clinical finding in infective endocarditis is fever. Osler nodes and Janeway lesions are uncommon findings in IE.

Table 25.3   Definition of Infective Endocarditis (IE) According to the Modified Duke Criteria*.

Definite IE

Pathologic criteria

1. Presence of microorganisms by culture or embolized vegetation or an intracardiac abscess

or

2. Vegetation or abscess confirmed by histology showing active endocarditis. Clinical criteria can be confirmed by ANY of the following:
   a. 2 major criteria; or
   b. 1 major criterion and 3 minor criteria; or
   c. 5 minor criteria

Possible IE can be considered by ANY of the following
   a. 1 major criterion and 1 minor criterion; or
   b. 3 minor criteria

Diagnosis of IE can be withdrawn by ANY of the following
1. Alternate diagnosis explaining evidence for IE; or
2. Resolution of IE via antibiotic therapy for ≤4 days; or
3. No evidence of IE at surgery with antibiotic therapy for ≤4 days; or
4. Does not meet criteria for possible IE, as above

*See Table 25.4 for definitions of major and minor criterion.

25.4 DIAGNOSIS

Infective endocarditis can be an imprecise diagnosis as bacteremia often occurs without endocardial involvement and IE can occur with negative blood cultures. There are numerous mimickers of IE including, but not limited to, systemic lupus erythematous, thrombotic thrombocytopenic purpura, carcinoid syndrome, and rheumatic fever. Therefore, clinicians must maintain a high-index of suspicion for IE in any patient with a cardiac murmur, organic valvular disease, congenital heart disease, or a prosthetic valve who presents with fever, anemia, hematuria, or other physical findings suggestive of IE. The Modified Duke Criteria provides a highly sensitive and specific diagnostic strategy to aid in diagnosis (Table 25.3, Table 25.4).

> ### TAKE HOME POINT #4
>
> The Modified Duke Criteria provides a diagnostic strategy to aid in diagnosis of infective endocarditis.

Echocardiography plays an important role in the diagnosis of IE. However, it should not be used indiscriminately as a screening tool in patients with fever and

Table 25.4   Definition of Terms used in the Modified Duke Criteria*.

Major criteria	1. Blood cultures positive for IE from 2 separate cultures
	   a. Microorganisms such as Viridans streptococci, *Streptococcus bovis*, HACEK group, *Staphylococcus aureus*; or community-acquired enterococci with no other source. Blood cultures must be drawn >12 h apart; or all of 3 or a majority of ≥4 separate cultures of blood (with first and last sample drawn at least 1 h apart)
	   b. Single positive blood culture for *Coxiella burnetti* or antiphase IgG antibody titer >1:800
	2. Evidence of endocardial involvement
	3. Echocardiogram which displays ANY of the following
	   a. Evidence of vavular mass or mass noted on supporting structure or on implanted material
	   b. Abscess
	   c. New dehiscence of prosthetic valve
	   d. New valvular regurgitation

Minor criteria	1. Increased risk of IE due to previous heart condition or intravenous drug use 2. Febrile illness >38 °C 3. Embolic phenomenon including Janeway's lesions or embolism to brain, lungs, eyes or peripheral locations 4. Immunologic phenomena including glomerulonephritis, Osler's nodes and Roth's spots 5. Positive blood culture that does not meet a major criterion as noted above

*Adapted from Li JS, Sexton DJ, Mick N, et al. Proposed modifications to the Duke Criteria for the diagnosis of infective endocarditis. Clinical Infectious Diseases 2000;30:633.

positive blood cultures who are unlikely to have IE. Transthoracic echocardiography (TTE) and transesophageal echocardiography (TEE) when applied in the correct clinical setting are helpful in diagnosis. The specificity of TTE in vegetation detection is approximately 98% while the sensitivity is 30–40%. If the pre-test probability for IE is low, TTE offers a cost-effective and clinically appropriate test for evaluation of native valve endocarditis. For concerns of prosthetic valve endocarditis or patients with a high pre-test probability of native valve endocarditis, TEE is an appropriate initial imaging modality. The Modified Duke criteria recommend TEE for patients with prosthetic heart valves, rated at least "possible" IE, or complicated IE (i.e. paravalvular abscess) while a TTE is appropriate for all other patients.

TAKE HOME POINT #5

TTE and TEE are useful tools in the diagnosis and management of infective endocarditis.

In patients with no recent antibiotic use who have IE, 95–100% of initial blood cultures will be positive for bacteremia. At least three sets of cultures from separate

Table 25.5   Laboratory findings in IE.

Anemia, normochromic normocytic
Elevated C reactive protein
Elevated erythrocyte sedimentation rate
False-positive Lyme serologic test
False-positive VDRL
Hypercomplementemia
Leukocytosis
Leukopenia
Low serum iron
Low serum total iron binding capacity
Positive rheumatoid factor
Urinalysis with proteinuria, hematuria RBC casts, pyuria, wbc casts, or bacteria

venipuncture sites should be drawn in both aerobic and anaerobic mediums within the first 24 hours of presentation.

Abnormal laboratory findings associated with IE are displayed in Table 24.5. Three out of every four IE patients have a mild anemia, often normochromic and normocytic. Leukocytosis is seen in one-third of patients while some may exhibit leukopenia. Urinalysis may demonstrate proteinuria and hematuria.

Specialized diagnostic testing can help identify complications associated with IE. An ECG with either a new high-grade atrioventricular or bundle branch block should raise one's concern for valvular abscess. A head CT or MRI should be performed on all patients with IE and neurological symptoms.

25.5 MICROBIOLOGY

The microbial causes of IE vary greatly with patient comorbidities. However, gram-positive infections are the major cause, accounting for approximately 80% of all causes of IE. Of all IE cases, *S. aureus* accounts for one-third and is the most common etiologic agent of IE in drug abusers, native valve endocarditis, and prosthetic valve endocarditis (Table 25.6). In specific instances, special techniques may be necessary for the isolation of certain microorganisms. The microbiology laboratory and Infectious Diseases should be consulted for guidance regarding this evaluation. The microorganism responsible for IE may provide clues to the patient's general condition (Table 25.7).

TAKE HOME POINT #6

S. *aureus* is the most common cause of infective endocarditis. However, some specific microorganisms are associated with particular clinical scenarios.

Table 25.6   Microbiological Etiology of Definite Endocarditis in 2781 Patients*.

Microbiological cause	IVDU (%)	Non-IVDU (%)	PVE (%)
Staphylococcal aureus	68	28	23
Coagulase-negative staphylococcus	3	9	17
Viridans group streptococci	10	21	12
Streptococcus bovis	1	7	5
Other streptococci	2	7	5
Enterococcus species	5	11	12
HACEK	0	2	2
Fungi	1	1	4
Polymicrobial	3	1	0.8
Negative culture findings	5	9	12
Other	3	4	7

IVDU, intravenous drug users; PVE, prosthetic valve endocarditis.

Table 25.7   Microbiological Causes of Infective Endocarditis and their Clinical Associations.

Organism	Clinical associations
Viridans group streptococci	Oral origin
Streptococcus bovis	Gastrointestinal malignancy
Streptococcus pneumoniae	Alcohol abuse, meningitis, rapid valvular destruction (often aortic)
Enterococcus species	Genitourinary tract/manipulation
Staphylococci	
S. aureus	Intravenous drug users, health-care contact, invasive procedures, systemic embolization
Coagulase – *Staphylococci*	Prosthetic valve endocarditis
HACEK*	Fastidious, part of respiratory tract and oropharyngeal flora
Fungal	Immunocompromised, indwelling catheters, intravenous drug users, negative blood cultures
Culture negative	Slow growth of fastidious, fungal, recent antibiotics

*Haemophilus parainfluenzae, Hemophilus aphrophilus, Actinobacillus actinomycetemcomitans,
Cardiobacterium hominis, Eikenella corrodens*, and *Kingella kingae.*

25.6   ANTIMICROBIAL THERAPY

The principles of treatment for IE include eradication of the organism and resolution of the intracardiac and extracardiac manifestations that may result. Successful treatment may require surgical intervention; however, typically, approximately one-half of patients can be treated with antimicrobial therapy alone. There are several considerations when selecting the appropriate regimen for treatment of IE. Selection is generally based on antimicrobial susceptibility, thus emphasizing the need for initial blood cultures to be obtained prior to antibiotic use. Parenteral agents are the overwhelming choice given the erratic absorption and lack of efficacy of oral regimens. Extended durations of parenteral therapy (often 4–6 weeks) are usually necessary. Careful follow-up and monitoring of patients by both Infectious Disease and cardiology are critical.

After initial cultures are drawn, an empiric regimen should be initiated in patients with rapidly progressing acute IE and hemodynamic compromise. Selection of an empiric antimicrobial regimen should take into consideration the most likely pathogens. At a minimum, empiric treatment should provide coverage against staphylococci (including methicillin resistant strains), streptococci, and enterococci. Gram negative and/or antifungal coverage may also be indicated. In patients felt to be medically stable, delaying the initiation of antimicrobial therapy until results of initial blood cultures are obtained is often reasonable. Such an approach allows additional cultures to be drawn without being confounded by the initiation of empiric antibiotics in the event the first cultures are negative.

TAKE HOME POINT #7

For medically stable patients, antimicrobial therapy may be delayed until the results of initial cultures are available.

Practitioners should refer to the ACC/AHA guidelines for the antimicrobial treatment regimens for the management of native valve endocarditis and prosthetic valve endocarditis. For patients suspected of having endocarditis whose cultures remain negative and their clinical course has not been confounded by empiric antimicrobial therapy, fastidious organisms that require special techniques for isolation should be considered. The most common of these include *Bartonella* species and *Coxiella burnetii*.

Outpatient therapy can be considered in patients who have responded to antimicrobials, have not experienced any complications, and have adequate social support to accommodate regular antimicrobial administration as well as frequent follow-up.

25.7 SURGICAL THERAPY

Cardiac surgery plays an important role in the management of IE when there is significant valvular damage, the microorganism is not responsive to antimicrobial therapy and/or when recurrent embolization occurs (Figure 25.3). Other reasons to consider surgical intervention are listed in Table 25.8. Since mortality is directly related to the degree of hemodynamic deterioration, surgery is recommended prior to the development of hemodynamic compromise regardless of the duration of antimicrobial treatment. In patients with Class III–IV heart failure from IE, the reinfection

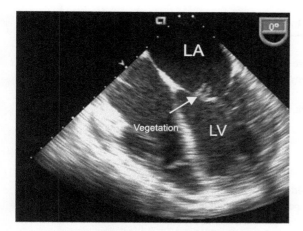

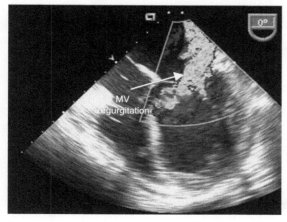

Figure 25.3   TEE of mitral valve endocarditis with leaflet perforation and mitral regurgitation. (See Color plate 25.2).

rate following surgery is less than 5% whereas the mortality rate of congestive heart failure managed with medical therapy alone approaches 50%. Acute mitral or aortic insufficiency due to infective endocarditis requires prompt surgical evaluation.

In patients with prosthetic valve endocarditis, warfarin and aspirin should be discontinued and heparin initiated in the event that urgent surgery is required. Additionally, if neurological symptoms develop, anticoagulation should be stopped until an intracranial process has been excluded with either CT or MRI. The benefit of anticoagulation in patients with native valve endocarditis has not yet been demonstrated. Valve repair, when possible, is favored over valve replacement, which carries a greater risk of infection due to the increased use of prosthetic material. The duration of antimicrobial therapy following surgery is dependent on factors including the previous duration of therapy, the offending microorganism and its susceptibility pattern, type of surgery, and culture status of the vegetation. Infectious Diseases consultation is strongly advised given the complexity of antimicrobial therapy in IE.

Table 25.8   Surgical Indications in Infective Endocarditis.

Indicated
Congestive heart failure caused by valvular dysfunction
New aortic insufficiency or mitral regurgitation
Fungal endocarditis
IE with highly resistant organism
Heart block
Annular or aortic abscess or destructive lesions
Prosthetic dehiscence
Increase in prosthetic valve regurgitation

Strong supportive evidence
Recurrent emboli and persistent vegetation despite antibiotic therapy
Persistent bacteremia with prosthetic valve
Relapse of infection with prosthetic valve

Weak supportive evidence
Vegetation >10 mm

Not indicated
Uncomplicated prosthetic valve endocarditis

TAKE HOME POINT #8

Early surgical referral reduces mortality in select patients with infective endocarditis.

25.8 RESPONSE TO THERAPY

For patients included in the International Collaboration on Endocarditis-Prospective Cohort Study, the in-hospital mortality for IE was 18%. Factors associated with increased risk of death within the cohort included prosthetic valve endocarditis, increased age, presence of pulmonary edema, *S. aureus* infection, coagulase-negative staphylococcus infection, mitral valve vegetations, and paravalvular complications.

Within one week of the initiation of antimicrobial therapy, 70% of the patients will become afebrile while 90% are afebrile at 14 days. For patients whose fever persists greater than 10 days on appropriate therapy, blood cultures should be repeated and an examination for IE complications, such as a paravalvular or intra-abdominal abscess, should be performed. Consideration should also be given to the presence of a drug fever. Many of the laboratory features (Table 25.5) associated with IE are slower to resolve and may not return to baseline until after the completion of therapy. Before or at completion of therapy, a TTE should be obtained to establish a new baseline for the patient. Relapse of IE typically occurs within the first two months following completion of therapy. The most common patient characteristic associated with relapse of infection is ongoing IVDU.

> **TAKE HOME POINT #9**
>
> For patients whose fever persists longer than 10 days following the initiation of antimicrobial therapy, complications of infective endocarditis should be considered.

25.9 PROPHYLAXIS

The ACC/AHA have recently revised the guidelines for prophylaxis against infective endocarditis, greatly decreasing the number of patients for whom prophylaxis is recommended. Only those patients with cardiac conditions who are at highest risk of poor outcomes from IE are now recommended to receive prophylaxis (Table 25.9, Table 25.10). For example, patients with mitral valve prolapse without mitral

Table 25.9 Cardiac Conditions for which Endocarditis Prophylaxis is Recommended.

Prosthetic heart valves or valve repair
Previous infective endocarditis
Congenital heart defects (CHD)
    Unrepaired cyanotic CHD, including palliative shunts and conduits
    Completely repaired CHD repaired with prosthetic material or device during first
    6 months after procedure
    Repaired CHD with residual defects at site or adjacent site to prosthetic material
Cardiac transplant recipients with valve regurgitation due to structurally abnormal valve

Table 25.10 Regimens for Infective Endocarditis Prophylaxis.

Situation	Adult dosing (30–60 minutes before procedure)
Oral	Amoxicillin 2 g
Unable to take oral	Ampicillin 2 g IM or IV
	or
	Cefazolin or ceftriaxone 1 g IM or IV
Allergic to penicillins or ampicillin – oral	Cephalexin 2 g
	or
	Clindamycin 600 mg
	or
	Azithromycin or clarithromycin 500 mg
Allergic to penicillins or ampicillin and unable to take oral	Cefazolin or ceftriaxone 1 g IM or IV
	or
	Clindamycin 600 mg IM or IV

(Source: Adapted from Nishmmura RA, Carabello BA, Faxon DP, et al. 2008. With permission of Elsevier).

regurgitation or leaflet thickening are no longer required to take antibiotics. Prophylaxis is recommended in dental procedures involving manipulation of gingival tissue, periapical region of teeth, or perforation of the oral mucosa. IE prophylaxis is not recommended for transesophageal echocardiography, esophagogastroduodenoscopy, or colonoscopy.

> **TAKE HOME POINT #10**
>
> Patients with cardiac conditions who are at highest risk of poor outcomes from infective endocarditis should receive antibiotic prophylaxis prior to dental procedures.

25.10   CARDIOVASCULAR DEVICE INFECTION

As the number of permanent pacemaker and implantable cardioverter-defibrillator implantations rise, there has been an increase in the rate of device-related infections with generator pocket and device-related endocarditis representing the most common (Figure 25.4). In a single center review by Sohail et al. coagulase-negative staphylocci and *Staphyloccous aureus* accounted for nearly three-fourths of all infections. Nearly all of the patients in the cohort required removal of the device and extended antimicrobial therapy for up to one month. With a combined approach of device removal and antimicrobial therapy, 96% of patients received curative therapy.

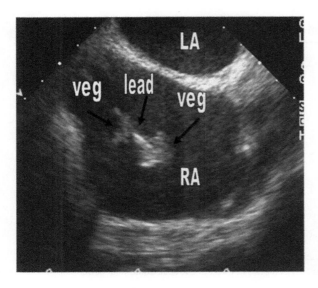

Figure 25.4   TEE of pacemaker endocarditis. LA, left atrium; lead, pacemaker lead; RA, right atrium; veg, vegetation.

KEY REFERENCES

BADDOUR LM, WILSON WR, Bayer AS, et al: Infective endocarditis: diagnosis, antimicrobial therapy, and management of complications. A Statement for Healthcare Professionals from the Committee on Rheumatic Fever, Endocarditis, and Kawasaki Disease, Council on Cardiovascular Disease in the Young, and the Councils on Clinical Cardiology, Stroke, and Cardiovascular Surgery and Anesthesia, American Heart Association: Endorsed by the Infectious Diseases Society of America. Circulation 2005;111:e394.

BAYER AS, BOLGER AF, TAUBERT KA, et al. Diagnosis and management of infective endocarditis and its complications. Circulation 1998;98:2936.

BONOW RO, CARABELLO BA, CHATTERJEE K, et al. 2008 focused update incorporated into the ACC/AHA 2006 guidelines for the management of patients with valvular heart disease: a report of the American College of Cardiology/American Heart Association Task Force on Practice Guidelines (Writing Committee to Revise the 1998 Guidelines for the Management of Patients with Valvular Heart Disease). Endorsed by the Society of Cardiovascular Anesthesiologists, Society for Cardiovascular Angiography and Interventions, and Society of Thoracic Surgeons. J Am Coll Cardiol 2008;52:e1.

LI JS, SEXTON DJ, MICK N, et al. Proposed modifications to the Duke Criteria for the diagnosis of infective endocarditis. Clin Infect Dis 2000;30:633.

MURDOCH DR, COREY R, HOEN B, et al: Clinical presentation, etiology, and outcome of infective endocarditis in the 21st century: The International Collaboration on Endocarditis – Prospective Cohort Study. Arch Intern Med 2009;169:463.

NISHMMURA RA, CARABELLO BA, FAXON DP, et al. ACC/AHA 2008 guideline ipdate on valvular heart disease: focused update on infective endocarditis: a report of the American College of Cardiology/American Heart Association Task Force on Practice Guidelines Endorsed by the Society of Cardiovascular Anesthesiologists, Society for Cardiovascular Angiography and Interventions, and Society of Thoracic Surgeons. J Am Coll Cardiol 2008;52:675.

SOHAIL MR, USLAN DZ, KHAN AH, et al. Management and outcome of permanent pacemaker and implantable cardiovascular-defibrillator infections. J Am Coll Cardiol 2007;49:1851.

Chapter 26

Pericardial Diseases

David C. Lange and Timir S. Baman

26.1 ACUTE PERICARDITIS

26.1.1 Introduction

Acute pericarditis is due to inflammation of the pericardium and accounts for up to 5% of emergency room visits for chest pain without a myocardial infarction (MI). Many electrocardiographic features seen with pericarditis are also witnessed with acute MI, adding great anxiety to those making the final diagnosis. Acute pericarditis can lead to fluid accumulation within the pericardial space known as a pericardial effusion. If the fluid accumulation occurs rapidly, filling of the intracardiac chambers can be impaired during diastole and cardiac tamponade with hemodynamic compromise may result.

26.1.2 Pathophysiology

Pericarditis is due to an inflammatory process affecting the inner visceral layer and outer parietal layer of the pericardium.

26.1.3 Etiologies

As many as 85% of cases of acute pericarditis are due to an unknown etiology. These cases are often preceded by a recent flu-like illness or gastrointestinal symptoms and are

Inpatient Cardiovascular Medicine, First Edition. Edited by Brahmajee K. Nallamothu and Timir S. Baman.

Table 26.1   Causes of Acute Pericarditis.

Etiology	Examples
Infectious	Viral: adenovirus, coxsackievirus, EBV, echovirus, HAV, HBV, HIV/AIDS, VZV, measles virus, mumps virus
	Bacterial: Gram positives (S. pneumo, S. auerus), Gram negatives, *Mycobacterium tuberculosis*
	Fungal: coccidiodomycosis, histoplasmosis, toxoplasmosis, blastomyces dermatitidis, and Candida sp
Autoimmune	Connective tissue disorders: rheumatoid arthritis, sarcoidosis, scleroderma, SLE, Sjögren's, Mixed Connective Tissues Disorder
	Vasculitis: Churg-Strauss, PAN, Wegener's Granulomatosis can cause pericarditis
	Other: Dressler's Syndrome, inflammatory bowel disease, seronegative spondyloarthropathies
Neoplasms	Primary: cardiac neoplasms, mesothelioma
	Metastatic: lung, breast, and renal cell cancers, leukemia, lymphoma
Systemic	Uremia
	Hypothyroidism
	Amyloidosis
Cardiovascular	Acute MI (usually transmural)
	Proximal aortic dissection
Iatrogenic	Irradiation
	Pericardiotomies
	Cardiac catheterization
	Pacemaker implantation
	Myocardial ablation
	Medications: dantrolene, doxorubicin, isoniazid, mesalamine, penicillin, phenytoin, rifampin, procainamide, and hydralazine
Idiopathic	

largely thought to be secondary to the Coxsackie B virus or echovirus. The differential diagnosis for acute pericarditis is extraordinarily broad and includes infectious, autoimmune, neoplastic, systemic, cardiovascular, and iatrogenic causes (Table 26.1).

TAKE HOME POINT #1

Most cases of acute pericarditis are due to an unknown etiology.

Clinical history is imperative for further evaluation of possible etiologies, which can sometimes guide specific treatments. Patients hospitalized for bacterial sepsis or pneumonia may have lymphatic or hematogenous spread to the pericardium. Those who are immunocompromised and present with fever or pericardial effusion should be aggressively evaluated for tuberculosis pericarditis. Pericarditis has been known to afflict up to 20% of individuals with HIV/AIDS. Patients with a recent history of MI are susceptible to post-MI pericarditis (acute phase) or Dressler's syndrome (delayed phase also associated with cardiac surgery). Individuals recently undergoing renal replacement therapy can develop uremic pericarditis with large pericardial effusions. Finally, metastatic carcinomas can lead to acute pericarditis and subsequent pericardial effusion and tamponade.

26.1.4 Clinical Manifestations

Acute pericarditis can present with a variety of signs and symptoms, which tend to vary in accordance with the underlying etiology and the rapidity with which fluid accumulates (as discussed below under Section 26.2, Pericardial Tamponade). Patients with acute pericarditis tend to present with chest pain which is pleuritic, positional (exacerbated by laying supine, alleviated by sitting up and leaning forward), and often retrosternal. The pain of pericarditis often starts substernal and radiates to the trapezius muscle. Chest pain is characteristically not present in rheumatoid pericarditis, and may also be absent in pericarditis due to TB, neoplasm, uremia, and post-irradiation. Patients may also complain of a viral prodrome of fever, nonproductive cough, GI upset, malaise, and myalgias.

Physical exam may reveal a pericardial friction rub. When present, the rub is a leathery, scratchy, high-pitched sound caused by friction between visceral and parietal pericardial surfaces. The friction rub is typically heard best with the diaphragm of the stethoscope along the left sternal border during expiration with the patient sitting upright and leaning forward. Classically, there are three components to the rub, although the rub may be mono- or bi-phasic. The first component is the atrial contraction, followed by ventricular contraction, which is the loudest and most frequently-heard component. Finally, the third component of the rub is ventricular relaxation. While this pericardial friction rub is occasionally detected, it tends to be variable; thus, repeated auscultation is often required.

TAKE HOME POINT #2

Patients with pericarditis often present with chest pain that is worse when lying flat and relieved when sitting upright in a tripod position in addition to the classic tri-phasic pericardial rub heard on auscultation.

26.1.5 Evaluation and Diagnostic Studies

The first step to evaluating acute pericarditis is to perform a complete and thorough history and physical exam. Diagnostic imaging should follow routine laboratory work-up and usually includes an electrocardiogram (ECG), transthoracic echocardiography and chest X-ray. Clinical suspicion for other underlying etiologies such as autoimmune, infectious, neoplastic, etc., should guide additional testing as necessary (e.g. ANA, RF, mycobacterial studies, screen for malignancies, etc.)

Cardiac enzymes such as CK-MB and Troponin I may be mildy increased in as many as 30% of cases of acute pericarditis. Other routine labs that may be abnormal depending upon the etiology include a CBC with leukocytosis, basic chemistry panel revealing the presence of uremia, and elevated inflammatory markers such as CRP and ESR; however, these are nonspecific indicators of inflammation.

The cardiac ECG is helpful in diagnosing acute pericarditis. In acute pericarditis, an ECG classically reveals diffuse ST elevations (concave up) with a down-sloping PR interval (PR depression – very specific finding), and evolving T waves (Figure 26.1). ECG changes transpire in four stages evolving over hours to weeks and any of these manifestations may be present at the time a patient is being examined:

Stage 1:   PR depression with diffuse ST elevations

Stage 2:   ST and PR segments return to isoelectric state, T waves flatten

Stage 3:   T wave inversion

Stage 4:   T waves return to baseline

Numerous electrocardiographic clues distinguish acute pericarditis from acute MI (Table 26.2, Figure 26.2). Diffuse distribution of ST elevations over numerous leads and the presence of PR elevation in lead aVR and PR depression in other leads are common clues to the diagnosis of acute pericarditis. The ratio of ST elevation to T wave amplitude in lead V_6 can also be helpful in distinguishing acute pericarditis from acute MI. If the ST elevation in V_6 to T wave amplitude in V_6 ratio is >0.24, acute pericarditis is highly likely.

Electrical alternans – or beat-to-beat oscillating QRS axes seen on ECG – can signify a large pericardial effusion (Figure 26.3). This is due to the heart rotating in an increased amount of fluid within the pericardial space.

All patients with suspected acute pericarditis should have an echocardiogram performed to rule out significant pericardial effusion, especially in the setting of recent cardiovascular surgery or electrophysiological procedures due to the possibility of postoperative bleeding. Patients with evidence of a pericardial effusion should be assessed for signs of cardiac tamponade both on physical exam and via echocardiography as detailed in later sections. This will require the assistance of cardiology consultation. The vast majority of patients with pericarditis do not have evidence of significant pericardial effusions.

Chest X-rays are routinely normal in patients with acute pericarditis without significant pericardial effusion. If an accompanying pleural effusion is present and there is suspicion for malignancy, a thoracentesis can be analyzed for cell count, total protein, LDH, glucose, gram stain, cultures and cytology.

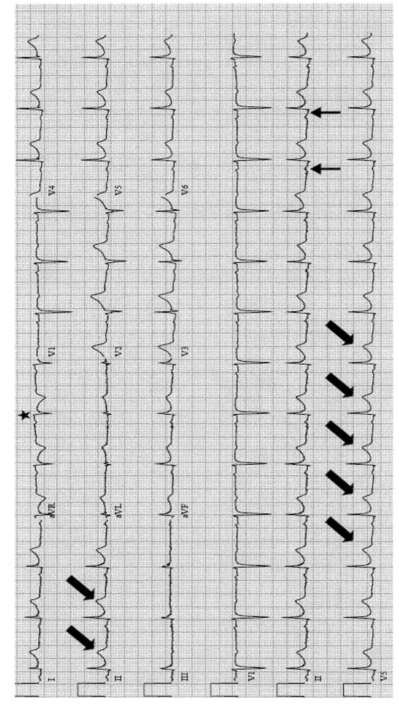

Figure 26.1 Electrocardiogram of a patient with acute pericarditis. Block arrows indicate concave ST elevations; Line arrows indicate PR depression; Star indicates PR elevation in lead aVR.

318

Table 26.2 Electrocardiographic Keys to Differentiate Acute Pericarditis from Acute ST Elevation Myocardial Infarction.

	Acute pericarditis	ST-elevation myocardial infarction
ST Elevation	Usually begins at J point and rarely exceeds 5 mm in height	May be greater than 5 mm in height
	Concave shape	Convex shape
	Distribution over numerous leads	Usually localizes to leads of one coronary territory
	Reciprocal ST segment changes are not seen	Reciprocal ST changes can be seen
	ST changes and T wave inversions are not commonly seen simultaneously	ST changes and T wave inversions are commonly seen simultaneously
PR elevation in aVR	Common	Not common
PR depression	Common	Not common
Q waves	Not common	Common
Hyperacute T waves	Not common	Common
QT prolongation	Not common	Common

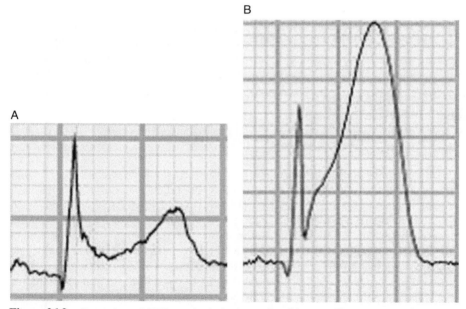

Figure 26.2 Comparison of QRS complex in **A** acute pericarditis versus **B** acute ST elevation myocardial infarction. Notice the PR depression and concave ST elevation in acute pericarditis as to the lack of PR depression and convex ST elevation in acute ST elevation MI.

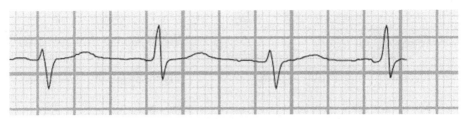

Figure 26.3   Electrocardiogram of a patient with acute pericarditis and subsequent pericardial effusion. Notice the beat-to-beat oscillations in QRS axis

Table 26.3   High-Risk Features of Acute Pericarditis Requiring Hospitalization.

Clinical findings

1. History of trauma, recent surgery or immunosuppressed state
2. Body temperature >100.4° F
3. Large pericardial effusion on echocardiography
4. Cardiac tamponade
5. Anticoagulation therapy
6. Elevated biomarkers

26.1.6   Treatment

The decision to hospitalize patients or to treat medically on an outpatient basis can be a difficult one. Once a diagnosis of acute pericarditis is confirmed, it is reasonable to treat patients without high-risk features on an outpatient basis. Patients with high-risk clinical characteristics should be hospitalized for further evaluation and therapy (Table 26.3).

> **TAKE HOME POINT #3**
>
> Simple acute pericarditis does not require hospitalization for treatment.

Nonsteroidal anti-inflammatory drugs (NSAIDs) are the cornerstone of pharmacologic treatment for acute pericarditis (Figure 26.4). Patients typically require high dose regimens such as ibuprofen 600–800 mg three times a day for 14 days. However, NSAIDs should be avoided if the patient is within 7–10 days post-MI. For those with a recent history of MI, high-dose aspirin is the preferred pharmacologic treatment (e.g. aspirin 800 mg every six hours as needed). If patients have a slow or inadequate response, one can consider the addition of colchicine administered with a 2–3 mg oral loading dose followed 0.5–1 mg per day for 14 days. The addition of colchicine has been shown to decrease duration of symptoms as well as reduce the recurrence rate of acute pericarditis. Glucocorticoids tapered over a two-week period can be used alone, or in combination with NSAIDs for refractory cases; however, there is concern that recurrent relapses may be associated with steroid therapy.

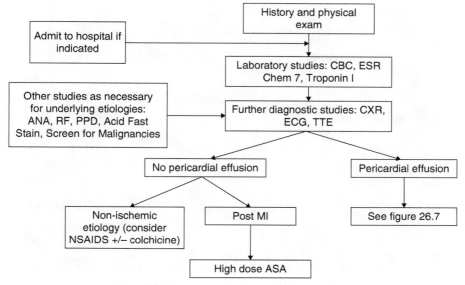

Figure 26.4 Acute pericarditis treatment algorithm.

In addition to pain management with anti-inflammatory drugs as above, the underlying etiology should be treated if known. For example, antibiotics should be given for bacterial causes, steroids for autoimmune etiologies, or dialysis instituted for symptomatic uremia.

26.1.7 Follow-up/Referral

Unfortunately, as many as 30% of patients will have a relapse of acute pericarditis if not treated with colchicine. For the initial relapse, a second course of NSAIDS and/or colchicine has been shown to be moderately effective. A small minority of patients with ongoing recurrent symptoms may need longer courses of prednisone, maintenance therapy with colchicine and/or other immunosuppressive drugs. Pericardiectomy can be considered as a final therapy, although most patients do not experience significant benefit. In cases of relapse, referral to a cardiologist should be considered. Patients with relapses or those with single episodes of acute pericarditis are at risk for developing constrictive pericarditis and this diagnosis should be considered in those who continue to be breathless or show signs of right-sided heart failure.

26.2 PERICARDIAL TAMPONADE

26.2.1 Pathophysiology

Pericardial tamponade results when pericardial fluid impairs diastolic filling of the heart (Figure 26.5). Cardiac tamponade occurs when fluid or blood fills the pericardial

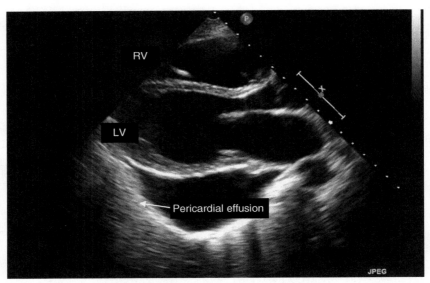

Figure 26.5   Echocardiogram of a patient with acute pericarditis and resultant pericardial effusion.

sac resulting in impaired cardiac filling. Tamponade physiology can occur with minimal amounts of rapid fluid accumulation (<200 ml) due to a lack of stretch in the pericardium. The pericardial space can accommodate up to 1.5 L if the accumulation occurs gradually.

TAKE HOME POINT #4

Clinical manifestations of cardiac tamponade are associated with the *rate* of fluid accumulation in the pericardial sac rather than the *total* amount.

In pericardial tamponade, increased intrapericardial pressure compresses the myocardium throughout the cardiac cycle. This results in a diminished cardiac output due to decreased venous return and stroke volume (Figure 26.6). With continued accumulation of fluid, the pressures in the right atrium, right ventricle, pulmonary artery, left atrium, and left ventricle equalize during diastole. During tamponade physiology, the right atrial diastolic pressure is equal to the right ventricular diastolic pressure which prevents filling during relaxation.

26.2.2   Etiology

Pericardial tamponade can result from any cause of pericarditis, but it is most commonly caused by malignancy, tuberculosis or purulent infection. Other causes of pericardial tamponade include trauma (both penetrating and blunt), proximal aortic

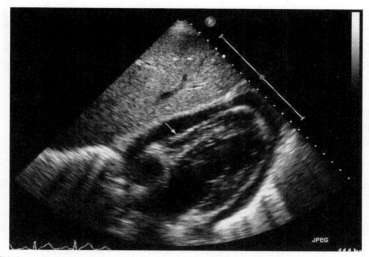

Figure 26.6 Echocardiogram of a patient with acute pericarditis and resultant pericardial effusion causing cardiac tamponade. Arrow indicates right ventricular collapse.

dissection, post-op cardiovascular surgery, myocardial rupture (post-MI), and recent electrophysiology procedures.

26.2.3 Clinical Manifestations

A number of clinical findings can be noted on physical examination indicating cardiac tamponade (Table 26.4). Virtually all patients look uncomfortable and convey an impending "sense of doom." Patients are hypotensive and have evidence of sinus tachycardia unless blunted by pharmacologic therapy. The clinical constellation of distant heart sounds, hypotension, and jugular venous distention (known cumulatively as Beck's triad) is classic for pericardial tamponade. In addition, pulsus paradoxus – defined as a decrease in systolic blood pressure ≥10 mm Hg during inspiration – is often seen. Pulsus paradoxus can be also detected by a decrease in the amplitude of the femoral or carotid pulse during inspiration.

Other exam findings in cardiac tamponade include a narrowed pulse pressure (due to decreased stroke volume), diaphoresis, decreased cognition, and cool extremities caused by hypotension. Finally, patients often complain of tachypnea, but have clear lung fields during auscultation.

26.2.4 Evaluation and Diagnostic Studies

The first step to properly evaluate cardiac tamponade is to perform a complete history and physical exam. Diagnostic studies such as chest X-rays, echocardiograms, and right heart catheterization can also aid in the diagnosis.

Table 26.4 Key Clinical and Diagnostic Findings of Pericardial Tamponade.

Clinical and diagnostic findings
1. Beck's Triad (distant heart sounds, hypotension, and jugular venous distention)
2. Pulsus paradoxus – a decrease in SBP ≥10 mm Hg during inspiration
3. Pericardial effusion on echocardiogram
4. Right atrial or early ventricular diastolic collapse on echocardiogram
5. Respiratory variation of valve velocities on echocardiogram
6. Equalization of pressures on right heart catheterization

Chest X-rays will reveal enlargement of the cardiac silhouette with greater than 250 cc fluid in the setting of clear lung fields. Chest X-rays may also appear normal and thus cannot be used to definitively diagnose or rule out cardiac tamponade.

Similar to acute pericarditis, there are characteristic ECG findings that strongly suggest cardiac tamponade. These include low QRS voltage and electrical alternans described as variations in QRS amplitude due to the pendular swinging of the heart within the pericardial fluid (Figure 25.3). Again, similar to chest X-ray, ECG can neither definitively diagnose nor rule out cardiac tamponade.

Echocardiogram remains the most sensitive and specific noninvasive diagnostic modality and should be performed in all patients suspected of having cardiac tamponade. Characteristic echocardiographic findings include an effusion, septal shift with inspiration, diastolic collapse of right atrium or right ventricle, and changes in transvalvular velocities associated with the respiratory cycle (Figure 26.6).

Clinicians must remember that cardiac tamponade is a clinical diagnosis and cannot be made solely on echocardiographic findings.

TAKE HOME POINT #5

The diagnosis of cardiac tamponade is made clinically and is not based on echocardiographic findings without clinical correlation.

If an echocardiogram is nondiagnostic and clinical suspicion remains high, right heart catheterization can be performed to provide more information. In patients with tamponade physiology, right heart catheterization will reveal elevation and equalization of diastolic pressures in the right atrium, right ventricle, pulmonary artery, left atrium, and left ventricle. As always, other tests should be ordered as necessary in accordance with the underlying etiology (Figure 26.7).

26.2.5 Treatment

The initial step to treating pericardial tamponade is volume resuscitation with intravenous fluid in order to support the patient's preload (increasing venous return)

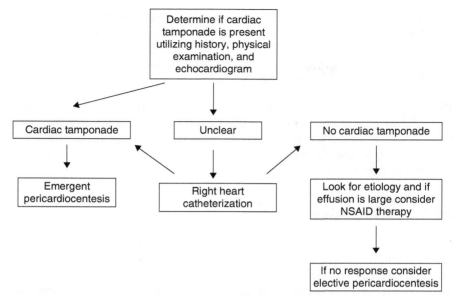

Figure 26.7 Approach to a patient with pericardial effusion.

with hopes of improving cardiac output. If the patient's hemodynamic status does not improve with fluid, or if the patient is severely hemodynamically compromised, use of vasopressors and inotropes to support cardiac function can be considered until a pericardiocentesis is performed. A pericardiocentesis involves placing a needle within the pericardial space to drain the pericardial effusion, which can be performed either in the cardiac catheterization laboratory under fluoroscopy or at the bedside with echocardiography. Drains are usually kept in the pericardial space until the output is <25 cc over 24 hours. This fluid can then be sent for further analysis in order to determine the etiology of tamponade. Typical studies that are sent include cultures, PCR, cytology and adenosine deaminase for tuberculosis screening. Tests to differentiate transudative versus exudative effusion are rarely useful for diagnosis in pericardial fluid. Emergent surgical consultation should be obtained if there is clinical suspicion for hemorrhagic tamponade secondary to trauma, aortic dissection, or myocardial rupture.

26.3 CONSTRICTIVE PERICARDITIS

26.3.1 Introduction

Constrictive pericarditis occurs when adhesions and fibrous scar formation occur in the pericardial layers following an episode of inflammation. It is an uncommon complication of acute pericarditis, but critical to recognize since it is treatable with early recognition and management. Furthermore, constrictive pericarditis often mimics other more common disorders, particularly restrictive cardiomyopathy.

26.3.2 Pathophysiology

The key pathophysiological process in constrictive pericarditis is impaired diastolic filling due to restricted filling from the scarred and adherent pericardium. In diastole, right ventricular filling is impaired and leads to symptoms of systemic venous congestion and right heart failure. Impaired filling of the left ventricle also occurs and leads to low forward cardiac output and hypotension.

26.3.3 Etiologies

The most common cause of constrictive pericarditis is idiopathic, and it typically occurs months to years after an episode of acute pericarditis due to any etiology. In the past, tuberculosis was a common cause of constrictive pericarditis due to the highly inflammatory nature of that disease process in the pericardium. Although this is less seen now in Western countries, it remains an important cause in low-to-middle income countries.

26.3.4 Clinical Manifestations

Constrictive pericarditis is usually characterized by the development of congestive heart failure symptoms and signs over a gradual period of time. These can include fatigue, weakness, hypotension, hepatomegaly, ascites, and peripheral edema. The latter symptoms of hepatomegaly, ascites and peripheral edema are particularly prominent in constrictive pericarditis. For this reason, patients are sometimes mistakenly diagnosed with liver disease early during their course.

Physical exam should start with a careful examination of the neck veins and estimation of the jugular venous pressure. Neck veins will typically become more filled during slow inspiration with an increase in jugular venous pressure. This finding is known as Kussmaul's sign, and differs from what is expected during normal physiology where neck veins collapse and jugular venous pressure falls during inspiration. Examination of the neck veins should be performed with the patient lying at 30 to 45 degrees and also sitting upright. When the jugular venous pressure exceeds 20 cm (equivalent to approximately 15 mm Hg), the pulse may not be visualized at all, since it would be above the angle of the jaw in most patients who are sitting upright. In addition, auscultation of the chest may reveal a pericardial knock. This is an early diastolic sound that represents the sudden cessation of diastolic filling in the left ventricle. It typically occurs earlier than an S3, is higher in pitch, and increases in intensity with inspiration.

TAKE HOME POINT #6

Kussmaul's sign is a classic finding associated with constrictive pericarditis where the normal collapse of neck veins with inspiration is reversed and neck veins increasingly distend with a rise in jugular venous pressure during inspiration.

26.3.5   Evaluation and Diagnostic Studies

Diagnostic studies for constrictive pericarditis can be challenging. A full review of many of the expected findings from different studies are listed in Chapter 14 ("Dilated and restrictive cardiomyopathy"). The EKG is often nonspecific. BNP levels are typically normal even when significant signs of right heart failure are present due to restricted dilation of the atrial and ventricular chambers from the fibrosed pericardium. Chest radiography can show pericardial calcifications.

Echocardiography findings are often subtle. They can demonstrate normal wall thickness (as opposed to restrictive cardiomyopathy), possible pericardial thickening, prominent septal "bounce" due to early diastolic filling, and increased expiratory hepatic vein diastolic flow reversal. Computed tomography and magnetic resonance imaging are more useful in demonstrating pericardial thickening. Final diagnosis frequently requires cardiac catheterization to document hemodynamic effects that differ from restrictive cardiomyopathy. Elevated and equalized diastolic pressures on cardiac catheterization are the rule for constrictive pericarditis. Ventricular filling is rapid early and blunted late by the stiffened pericardial sac, leading to the characteristic steep "y" descent of right atrial pressure and the dip and plateau of ventricular pressure. Although these hemodynamic patterns can be observed in other causes of heart failure such as restrictive cardiomyopathy, discordance between changes in right and left ventricular systolic pressures during respiration (i.e. ventricular interdependence) reliably distinguishes constrictive pericarditis from these other conditions.

26.3.6   Treatment

Most patients with constrictive pericarditis require surgical pericardiectomy. Removal of densely adherent pericardium is usually successful but can be extremely challenging. This is why early diagnosis is crucial as scarring may be less prominent. Moreover, recovery can be delayed for several weeks, and patients in whom the constriction has progressed to the point of abnormal ventricular function, severely reduced cardiac output, cachexia, or end-organ dysfunction derive the least benefit from the procedure. These observations also highlight the importance of early diagnosis and treatment.

TAKE HOME POINT #7

Although it can be challenging, patients with constrictive pericarditis should be referred for surgical pericardiectomy as it represents curative treatment.

KEY REFERENCES

LANGE RA, HILLIS LD. Acute pericarditis. New Engl J Med 2004;351:2195–2202.
TINGLE L, MOLINA D, CALVERT C. Acute pericarditis. Amer Family Physician 2007;76(10):1509–1514.
TROUGHTON RW, ASHER CR, KLEIN AL. Pericarditis. Lancet 2004;363:717–727.

Chapter 27

Pulmonary Hypertension

Scott H. Visovatti and Vallerie V. McLaughlin

27.1 INTRODUCTION

Hospitalists are often faced with patients who present with months of progressive dyspnea on exertion and a systolic murmur on physical examination. A transthoracic echocardiogram (TTE) is often ordered as part of the evaluation and typically shows both tricuspid regurgitation and pulmonary hypertension (PH) with a normal ejection fraction. This chapter is designed to guide hospitalists through the initial evaluation and management of suspected pulmonary hypertension.

Pulmonary hypertension is a broad term used to describe an elevation of pressure in the pulmonary arteries as a consequence of one, or many, diverse disease processes. The strict definition requires a mean pulmonary artery pressure (mPAP) greater than or equal to 25 mm Hg. However, in clinical practice PH is often suggested by a Doppler TTE that reveals tricuspid regurgitation with a right ventricular systolic pressure (RVSP) greater than 40 mm Hg. Normally, the pulmonary circulation and right side of the heart comprise a low-pressure system. Thus, chronically elevated right-sided pressures can have devastating effects, ultimately resulting in overt right heart failure and significant morbidity and mortality if not properly managed.

Pulmonary venous hypertension (PVH) refers to the subset of PH resulting from processes affecting the left side of the heart, resulting in an increased pressure in the pulmonary veins that is transmitted back to the right side of the heart. PVH is the most common form of PH seen by hospitalists due to the high prevalence of systolic and diastolic heart failure seen in the community. It is also important to consider

Inpatient Cardiovascular Medicine, First Edition. Edited by Brahmajee K. Nallamothu and Timir S. Baman.

conditions that raise pulmonary pressure primarily by increasing cardiac output (CO), and thus pulmonary blood flow. Such conditions include fever, anemia, thyrotoxicosis and pregnancy.

Pulmonary arterial hypertension (PAH) is a rare subset of PH and results from restricted flow through the pulmonary arterial system. The diagnosis requires a right heart catheterization (RHC) revealing pressures that meet specific hemodynamic criteria: a mean pulmonary artery pressure (mPAP) greater than or equal to 25 mm Hg, and a pulmonary artery occlusion pressure (PAOP or wedge pressure) less than or equal to 15 mm Hg. The distinction between PVH and PAH is an important one as treatment options and management greatly differ.

TAKE HOME POINT #1

Pulmonary hypertension (PH) is diagnosed by an elevated mean pulmonary artery pressure greater than or equal to 25 mm Hg. Pulmonary arterial hypertension (PAH) is a subset of PH with restricted flow through the pulmonary arterial circulation and must meet specific RHC criteria for diagnosis.

27.2   ETIOLOGIES

The 2008 Dana Point Clinical Classification of Pulmonary Hypertension (Table 27.1) reflects the wide variety of specific disease processes that ultimately lead to PH. The modern groups are based upon similar pathophysiological, clinical and therapeutic characteristics. Scanning the classification list after diagnosing PH may allow for the identification of one or more causes of the elevated right-sided pressure. PH specialists use the classification system when considering treatment options, as the majority of clinical trials involving PH medications have focused on Group 1 diagnoses.

27.3   PATHOPHYSIOLOGY

Though many distinct disease processes may ultimately cause PH, progressive right-sided heart failure is both the final common pathway and the primary cause of death in patients with this condition. For many of the conditions listed above, the mechanism by which a disease process results in an elevated PA pressure may be apparent. For example, occlusion of the pulmonary vasculature due to chronic thromboembolic disease results in elevated right-sided pressures, as blood is impeded from flowing freely towards the left atrium. Likewise, any etiology resulting in elevated left-sided pressure such as systolic or diastolic dysfunction and valvular disorders can lead to elevated right-sided pressures.

The pathogenesis is less clear for those with PAH. Researchers believe affected individuals may have a genetic predisposition towards developing elevated pulmonary pressures. A subsequent "second hit" in the form of an additional genetic factor, a coexisting disease, or an environmental exposure may be necessary before a patient goes on to

Table 27.1   Dana Point Clinical Classification of Pulmonary Hypertension (2008).

1. Pulmonary Arterial Hypertension (PAH)
 1.1 Idiopathic PAH
 1.2 Heritable
  1.2.1 BMPR2
  1.2.2 ALK1, endoglin (with or without herediatary hemorrhagic telangiectasia)
  1.2.3 Unknown
 1.3 Drug- and toxin-induced
 1.4 Associated with
  1.4.1 Connective tissue diseases
  1.4.2 HIV infection
  1.4.3 Portal hypertension
  1.4.4 Congenital heart disease
  1.4.5 Schistosomiasis
  1.4.6 Chronic hemolytic anemia
 1.5 Persistent pulmonary hypertension of the newborn

1'. Pulmonary veno-occlusive disease (PVOD) and/or pulmonary capillary hemangiomatosis (PCH)

 2. Pulmonary hypertension owing to left heart disease
 2.1 Systolic dysfunction
 2.2 Diastolic dysfunction
 2.3 Valvular disease

 3. Pulmonary hypertension owing to lung diseases and/or hypoxia
 3.1 Chronic obstructive pulmonary disease
 3.2 Interstitial lung disease
 3.3 Other pulmonary diseases with mixed restrictive and obstructive pattern
 3.4 Sleep-disordered breathing
 3.5 Alveolar hypoventilation disorders
 3.6 Chronic exposure to high altitude
 3.7 Developmental disorders

 4. Chronic thromboembolic pulmonary hypertension (CTEPH)

 5. Pulmonary hypertension with unclear multifactorial mechanisms
 5.1 Hematologic disorders: myeloproliferative disorders, splenectomy
 5.2 Systemic disorders: sarcoidosis, pulmonary Langerhans cell histiocytosis, lymphangioleiomyomatosis, neurofibromatosis, vasculitis
 5.3 Metabolic disorders: glycogen storage disease, Gaucher disease, thyroid disorders
 5.4 Others: tumoral obstruction, fibrosing mediastinitis, chronic renal failure on dialysis

"Updated Clinical Classification of Pulmonary Hypertension (Dana Point, 2008)" in: Simonneau et al. Updated Clinical Classification of Pulmonary Hypertension. JACC 2009;54(1), Suppl S:S43–54.

develop PAH. Once triggered, the vasoconstrictive, pro-thrombotic phenotype of PAH is likely perpetuated by a complex process involving endothelial cell dysfunction, smooth muscle cell proliferation, inflammation, an underproduction of prostacyclin and nitric oxide with an overabundance of thromboxane A_2 and endothelin-1. These pathophysiological alterations in homeostasis form the basis of pulmonary vasoconstriction and subsequent elevated pressures. Accordingly, many of our therapies are guided towards reversing these alterations with hopes of reducing the vasoconstriction.

27.4 EPIDEMIOLOGY

Given that PH is associated with such a wide variety of underlying diseases, it is helpful to consider the epidemiology of some of the major groups listed in the Dana Point classification scheme. It is important to keep in mind that the majority of patients with PH have elevated right-sided pressures secondary to left heart disease. Table 27.2 shows the prevalence of the major etiologies of PH in a series of 483 patients with pulmonary artery systolic pressures greater than 40 mmHg as measured by transthoracic echocardiogram. "Non-PAH PH," or Groups 2 through 5, are often due to other disease processes resulting in secondary PH. It is estimated that as many as 1% of patients with advanced COPD have severe PH, giving a prevalence of 3–17 per million. However 100–150 per million patients with COPD may have lesser degrees of PH. The finding of PH in the COPD population is important, as mean pulmonary arterial pressure has been shown to be a strong predictor of mortality. Approximately 33% of patients with idiopathic pulmonary fibrosis have been shown to have echocardiographically-defined PH which is also a predictor of mortality in this group. Chronic thromboembolic pulmonary hypertension is an important consideration in any evaluation of PH, as approximately 2,500 new cases are diagnosed each year in the US, many of which occur without any acute symptoms. Sleep-disordered breathing is another common cause of PH, and studies have shown that as many as 70% of patients with obstructive sleep apnea (OSA) have some degree of PH.

PAH (Group 1 of the Dana Classification), and specifically idiopathic PAH, is less common with prevalence estimates of 15 cases per million and 5.9 cases per million, respectively. The incidence rates for IPAH are estimated to be on the order

Table 27.2 Prevalence of PH Groups.

Etiology	Prevalence
Left heart disease (Group 2)	78.7%
Lung disease and hypoxemia (Group 3)	9.7%
PAH (Group 1)	4.2%
CTEPH (Group 4)	0.6%
Unclear diagnosis	6.8%

of 2.4 cases per million, and together with familial and appetite-suppressant-related cases, make up over 50% of PAH cases. Women are twice as likely as men to develop IPAH. The mean age on onset of IPAH is 37 years, though it may occur through the sixth decade. The second most common form of PAH (30% of PAH cases) occurs in patients with the scleroderma spectrum of diseases or mixed connective tissue disease. Studies indicate that between 7% and 12% of patients with limited cutaneous scleroderma develop PAH; this is an especially vulnerable population, as prognosis is poor. PAH associated with congenital heart disease, portopulmonary hypertension, and HIV round out the most common etiologies of this uncommon disease. In endemic regions of the world, schistosomiasis-associated PAH is a significant health problem with an 8% prevalence in Brazilian patients suffering from hepatosplenic schistosomiasis. Given that close to 200 million people worldwide are infected with schistosomiasis, more than 270,000 people could have this form of associated PAH.

27.5   CLINICAL PRESENTATION AND PHYSICAL EXAMINATION

Dyspnea is the most common symptom of PH and forms the basis of the World Health Organization classification system (Table 27.3). At the time of diagnosis, patients with PH typically have experienced progressive dyspnea-on-exertion (DOE) over the course of months to years. Fatigue, light headedness, chest pain, palpitations, orthopnea, edema, paroxysmal nocturnal dyspnea, and cough are other common presenting symptoms. Syncope in a patient with PH is indicative of WHO class IV functional status due to RV failure while PH should always be on the differential diagnosis list of anyone admitted with unexplained syncope.

Exam findings suspicious for the presence of PH include a prominent P2, a parasternal lift, a right ventricular S4, a systolic murmur of tricuspid regurgitation, an early systolic click, and a diastolic murmur of pulmonary regurgitation. Clues to the etiology of PH include central cyanosis, which may be the result of an intracardiac shunt or Eisenmengers syndrome; clubbing of the fingers due to congenital heart disease; sclerodactyly or Raynaud's phenomenon as a result of connective tissue disease; splenomegaly, scleral icterus, and caput medusae from portal hypertension; a left ventricular S3, or mitral and/or aortic valve murmurs as a result of left heart disease; and wheezing or protracted expiration secondary to hypoxic lung disease.

Table 27.3   World Health Organization Classification of Functional Status.

Class	Description
I	No limitation of usual physical activity
II	Mild limitation of physical activity; no discomfort at rest; normal activity causes increased dyspnea, fatigue, chest pain or presyncope
III	Marked limitation of physical activity; no discomfort at rest; less than normal activity causes increased dyspnea, fatigue, chest pain or presyncope
IV	Discomfort at rest; may have signs of RV failure, symptoms increased by almost any physical activity

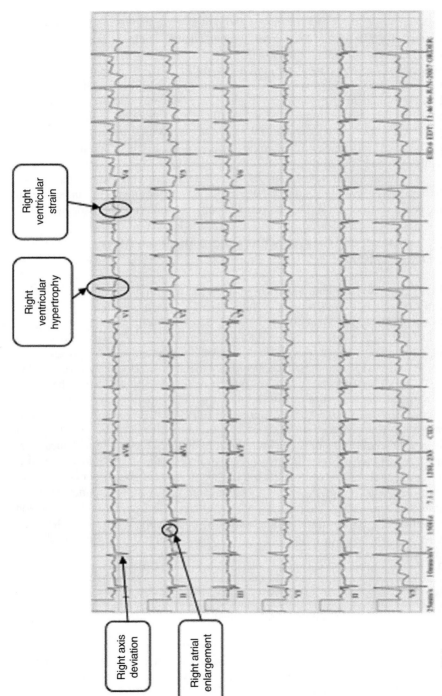

Figure 27.1 This ECG from a patient with pulmonary hypertension shows right axis deviation, right ventricular hypertrophy, and a right ventricular strain pattern. (Source: http://www.cvphysiology.com/Arrhythmias/SAN%20action%20potl.gif, with permission from Dr Richard Klabunde).

Findings in advanced PH with right heart failure may include jugular venous distention, a right ventricular S3, edema, ascites, and hepatomegaly.

27.6 EVALUATION AND DIAGNOSTIC STUDIES

The initial evaluation of any patient with suspected PH should begin with a 12-lead ECG and two-view chest X-ray. PH is supported by ECG findings of right axis deviation, right ventricular hypertrophy, right atrial enlargement, and ST and T wave abnormalities in the precordial leads consistent with right ventricular strain (Figure 27.1). The PA CXR may show prominent central pulmonary arteries and peripheral hypovascularity or "pruning." The lateral view may demonstrate RV obliteration of the retrosternal space due to RV enlargement (Figure 27.2).

If the history, physical examination, ECG and CXR are suggestive of PH, a carefully selected systematic series of diagnostic studies is indicated. Experts endorse the approach in Figure 27.3. Doppler TTE is generally obtained early in the evaluation of patients with suspected PH. The tricuspid regurgitant jet is used to estimate the RVSP, and pressures >40 mm Hg are consistent with PH. However, TTE can both under- and overestimate pulmonary artery pressures, as compared to the gold standard of RHC. In addition to the pressure measurements, TTE is useful in identifying elevated right-sided pressures by showing evidence of right atrial and ventricular enlargement, flattening of the interventricular septum, and an underfilled LV (Figure 27.4).

With the exception of the RHC, most of the pivotal testing can be performed at a patient's local hospital, and prior to referral to an expert. The

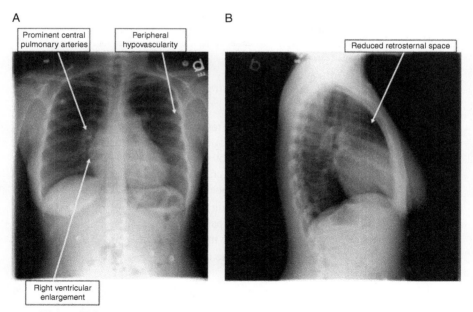

Figure 27.2   **A** The PA and **B** Lateral CXR from a patient with pulmonary hypertension.

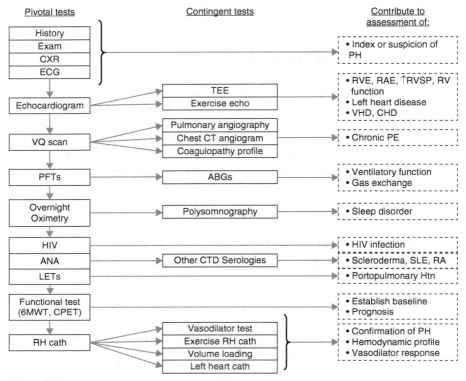

Figure 27.3 The evaluation of suspected pulmonary hypertension. (Source: McLaughlin et al. ACCF/ AHA 2009 expert consensus document on pulmonary hypertension: a report of the American College of Cardiology Foundation Task Force on Expert Consensus Documents. J Am Coll Cardiol 2009;53:1573–619. Reproduced with permission of Elsevier).

following points should be kept in mind when ordering and evaluating tests for PH:

- **Ventilation/perfusion (V/Q) scan**: the test of choice for the initial evaluation of chronic, surgically accessible thromboembolic disease. PE protocol CT is excellent for identifying *acute* PE, but is not sensitive for chronic thromboembolic disease. If indicated, pulmonary angiography can often be scheduled immediately following RHC if chronic thromboembolic disease is highly suspected
- **Pulmonary function tests** (PFTs): may show only mild restrictive disease and a mildly decreased diffusing capacity for carbon monoxide (DLCO); scleroderma patients may have a more marked decrease in DLCO
- **Polysomnogram**: should be performed if a patient endorses symptoms of sleep-disordered breathing
- **Serological testing**: given the association between PH and both connective tissue disorders and chronic liver disease, antinuclear antibody (ANA) and liver function tests (LFTs) are routinely performed. HIV testing should be performed if a patient endorses risk factors

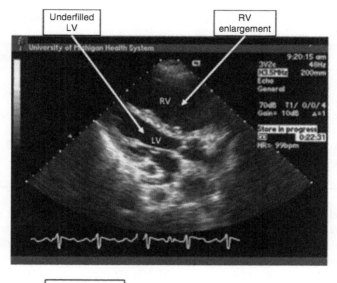

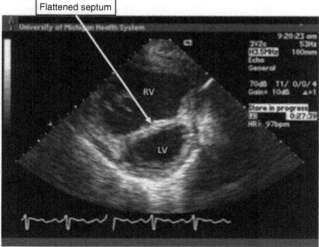

Figure 27.4   The transthoracic echocardiogram in pulmonary hypertension.

- **Six-minute hall walk (6MWT):** commonly used to objectively assess functional capacity. This test is often performed at baseline and repeated periodically to assess response to treatment; it is frequently used as an end-point in clinical PAH trials.

A diagnosis of PAH requires RHC in order to provide evidence of elevated pulmonary pressures in the setting of normal left-sided pressures. A complete set of pressure measurements should be performed (right atrium, right ventricle, pulmonary artery, pulmonary artery occlusion pressure, cardiac output, cardiac index, systemic

Table 27.4   Right Heart Catheterization Pressures in Patients with Pulmonary Arterial Hypertension.

	Normal (mm Hg)	PAH (mm Hg)
RA (mm Hg)	≤6	normal or ↑
RV (mm Hg)	15–30	↑
PA (mm Hg, systolic/diastolic/mean)	15–30/8–15/6–19	mPAP >25, typically 30–60
PAOP (mm Hg)	≤12	≤15 mm Hg
PVR (Wood units)	1–3 (increases with age)	>3
CO (L/min)	4–8	normal or ↓
CI	2.2–4.4	normal or ↓

BP, and calculated pulmonary vascular resistance) as well as oxygen saturations (superior vena cave, inferior vena cava, pulmonary artery, and systemic artery) in order to rule out shunts. Typical RHC pressure measurements for the diagnosis of PAH are included in Table 27.4. It is recommended that the RHC be performed at a high-volume center that is familiar with PH. Vasodilator testing can be performed by comparing RHC pressure measurements before and after the administration of inhaled nitric oxide (NO), intravenous epoprostenol or intravenous adenosine. A positive response requires a decrease in mean pulmonary artery pressure (mPAP) greater than or equal to10 mmHg, a final mPAP less than or equal to 40 mmHg, and an unchanged or increased cardiac output. Patients who exhibit a response to vasodilator testing may respond to calcium channel blockers (CCBs), though such patients must be followed closely, and may not maintain a long-term clinical response. The initiation of a CCB without vasodilator testing during a RHC could cause significant deterioration.

After heart catheterization, it is important to localize the disease process responsible for the PH (Figure 27.5) in order to determine the appropriate therapy

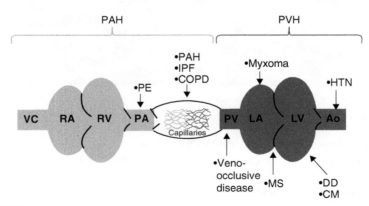

Figure 27.5   Locations of disease processes resulting in PH. Ao, aorta; CM, cardiomyopathy; COPD, chronic obstructive pulmonary disease; DD, diastolic dysfunction; HTN, hypertension; IPF, interstitial pulmonary fibrosis; LA, left atrium; LV, left ventricle; MS, mitral stenosis; PA, pulmonary artery; PAH, pulmonary arterial hypertension; PE, pulmonary artery; PV, pulmonary vein; RA, right atrium; RV, right ventricle; VC, vena cava. (See Color plate 27.1).

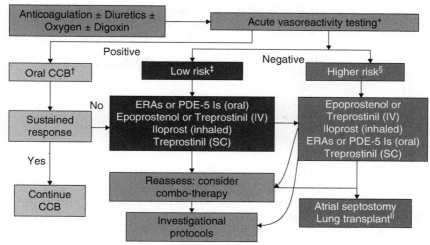

Figure 27.6 Treatment Algorithm for PAH. Background therapies include warfarin anticoagulation, which is recommended in all patients with IPAH without contraindication. Diuretics are used for management of right heart failure. Oxygen is recommended to maintain oxygen saturation greater than 90%. *Acute vasodilator testing should be performed in all IPAH patients who may be potential candidates for long-term therapy with calcium channel blockers (CCBs). †CCBs are indicated only for patients who have a positive acute vasodilator response, and such patients need to be followed closely both for safety and efficacy. ‡For patients who did not have a positive acute vasodilator testing and are considered lower risk based on clinical assessment, oral therapy with ERA or PDE-5I would be the first line of therapy recommended. If an oral regimen is not appropriate, the other treatments would need to be considered based on patient's profile and side effects and risk of each therapy. §For patients who are considered high risk based on clinical assessment, continuous treatment with intravenous (IV) prostacyclin (epoprostenol or treprostinil) would be the first line of therapy recommended. Treprostinil may be delivered via either continuous IV or subcutaneous (SC) infusion. Combination therapy should be considered when patients are not responding adequately to initial monotherapy. ‖Timing for lung transplantation and/or atrial septostomy is challenging and is reserved for patients who progress despite optimal medical treatment. (Source: McLaughlin et al. ACCF/AHA 2009 expert consensus document on pulmonary hypertension: a report of the American College of Cardiology Foundation Task Force on Expert Consensus Documents. J Am Coll Cardiol 2009;53:1573–619. Reproduced with permission of Elsevier).

(Figure 27.6). If a patient has PVH (i.e. a "lesion" distal to the pulmonary capillary bed), medications that dilate the pulmonary vasculature (CCBs or any PAH vasodilator) could lead to life-threatening pulmonary edema.

TAKE HOME POINT #2

The diagnosis of PH, and especially PAH, requires confirmation beyond a TTE; such confirmation (including a RHC) must take place before treatment options are considered.

If pre-RHC testing supports the diagnosis of PAH, it is reasonable to refer the patient to a PAH center for an initial evaluation, RHC with vasodilator testing, and interpretation of all results within the context of the patient's specific presentation.

TAKE HOME POINT #3

Given the complexity of PAH, its treatments, and the need for close monitoring, patients with this condition should be followed by a PH specialist.

27.7 TREATMENT

General treatment recommendations for PH include sodium restriction, limited aerobic exercise, and consideration of birth control for women (Table 27.5). Non-PAH PH is further treated by addressing the underlying cause, and by adding supplemental oxygen and diuretics as needed. As the vast majority of patients with PH have either diastolic or systolic heart failure, treatment of volume status can often alleviate the PH, resulting in increased functional capacity.

PAH-specific therapies should be utilized under the direction of a PAH specialist. These therapies may include warfarin, diuretics, calcium channel blocker (for those with a positive vasodilator response during RHC), prostacyclin, endothelin receptor antagonist, and phosphodiesterase-5 inhibitor (Table 27.6). Expert consensus regarding the selection of therapy in PAH is outlined in Figure 6. Invasive therapies are considered for those with certain etiologies of PH (Table 27.7).

Intravenous epoprostenol is a prostacyclin that causes vasodilation, inhibition of platelet aggregation and inhibition of vascular smooth muscle cell proliferation. Epoprostenol has been shown to improve survival, functional class, hemodynamics, and exercise endurance in patients with IPAH. Patients with the scleroderma spectrum of diseases have also shown improved hemodynamics and exercise tolerance as a result of intravenous epoprostenol therapy. Epoprostenol is delivered using continuous

Table 27.5   General Treatment Measures.

Diet	
Sodium restricted diet	<2400 mg per day
Exercise	
Aerobic exercise	Encouraged (low level)
Isometric exercise	Discouraged (exertional syncope)
Travel	
Advise caution when flying	May require supplemental O_2
Pregnancy	
Advise use of birth control	Hemodynamics of pregnancy/delivery result in a maternal mortality rate of up to 50%
	Medication contraindications with pregnancy

Table 27.6   Medications.

Supplemental oxygen	As needed to treat symptoms (may be needed for air travel)
Anticoagulation	
warfarin	Improved survival in observational studies involving patients with IPAH
	Also recommended in advanced associated PAH
	INR 1.5 to 2.5
Diuretics	
furosemide	As needed to treat symptoms
Calcium channel blockers	
diltiazem	Mechanism: reduces intracellular calcium
nifedipine	Indicated only in patients with positive vasodilator response during RHC; empiric administration without hemodynamic guidance may result in rapid deterioration
amlodipine	Avoid verapamil (decreased inotropy)
	Administration: oral
	Side effects: hypotension, headache, dizziness, flushing
IV Epoprostenol	
Flolan, Veletri	Mechanism: replenishes PGI_2 resulting in vasodilation, inhibition of platelet aggregation and inhibition of vascular SMCs
	Indication: WHO class III to IV symptoms (IPAH or scleroderma spectrum of PAH)
	Randomized trials: improved functional class, exercise tolerance, hemodynamics and survival in IPAH
	Observational studies: improved exercise tolerance and hemodynamics in associated PAH
	Administration: continuous infusion requires a central venous catheter (should quickly switch to peripheral IV in an emergency, as half-life is 4 to 6 *minutes*)
	Side effects: flushing, jaw pain, nausea, diarrhea, rash, musculoskeletal pain
	Overdose can result in high-output heart failure
Treprostinil	Mechanism: same as epoprostenol
Remodulin	Indication: WHO class II to IV symptoms (PAH)
Tyvaso	Open label trials: improved exercise tolerance
	Administration: continuous infusion via central venous catheter or subcutaneous sites (Remodulin), intermittent inhalation (Tyvaso)
	Switch to peripheral IV in an emergency (Remodulin)
	Half-life: 4.5 *hours*
	Side effects: flushing, jaw pain, nausea, diarrhea, rash, musculoskeletal pain, site pain (subcutaneous infusions)

(continued)

Table 27.6   (Continued).

Iloprost Ventavis	Mechanism: same as epoprostenol Indication: WHO class III to IV symptoms (PAH) Randomized trial: improved exercise tolerance Administration, inhaled 6 to 9 times per day Side effects: cough, headache, flushing, jaw pain

**Endothelin receptor
antagonist**
bosentan (Tracleer)
	Mechanism: non-selectively blocks vasoconstrictive and SMC
	   mitogenic effects of endothelin-1 (ET_A and ET_B)
	Indication: WHO class II to IV symptoms (PAH)
	Randomized trial: increased exercise tolerance, decreased
	  clinical worsening, improved hemodynamics
	Administration: oral, 125 mg po BID
	Side effects: peripheral edema, nasal congestion, sinusitis,
	   flushing
	Considerations: must monitor LFTs and hemoglobin,
	   potential teratogen, may reduce sperm count

**Endothelin receptor
antagonist**
ambrisentan (Letairis)
	Mechanism: blocks vasoconstrictive and SMC mitogenic
	   effects of endothelin-1 by selectively antagonizing ETA
	   receptor (allows NO production via ETB receptor
	   activation)
	Indication: WHO class II to III symptoms (PAH)
	Randomized trial: increased exercise tolerance, improved
	   time to clinical worsening
	Administration: oral, 5 mg or 10 mg once daily
	Side effects: peripheral edema, nasal congestion, sinusitis,
	   flushing
	Considerations: must monitor LFTs and hemoglobin,
	   potential teratogen, may reduce sperm count

**Phosphodiesterase-5
inhibitor**
sildenafil (Revatio)
	Mechanism: prevents degradation of cGMP, resulting in
	   vasorelaxation
	Indication: (WHO group I PAH)
	Randomized trial: increased exercise tolerance, delay clinical
	   worsening, improve hemodynamics
	Administration: oral, 20 mg po TID
	Side effects: headache, flushing, dyspepsia, epistaxis
	Considerations: contraindicated in patients taking nitrates,
	   may be used in conjunction with IV epoprostenol

Table 27.6 (Continued).

Phosphodiesterase-5 inhibitor	
Tadalafil (Adcirca)	Mechanism: prevents degradation of cGMP, resulting in vasorelaxation
	Indication: (WHO group I PAH)
	Randomized trial: increased exercise tolerance, delay clinical worsening
	Administration: oral, 40 mg po daily
	Side effects: headache, flushing, dyspepsia, epistaxis
	Considerations: contraindicated in patients taking nitrates

Table 27.7 Invasive Therapies.

Pulmonary thromboendarterectomy	Treatment of choice for surgically accessible chronic thromboembolic pulmonary hypertension in appropriate patients, should be performed at high-volume centers
Atrial septostomy	Creates $R \rightarrow L$ interatrial shunt
	Results in improved CO but increased hypoxemia
	Reserved for carefully selected, critically ill patients (15% procedural mortality)
Right ventricular assist device	Not yet tested in patients with PAH
Lung and combined heart/lung transplantation	Indicated in selected patients with an inadequate response to aggressive medical therapy
	Increased operative mortality; long-term survival rates comparable to patients with other indications for transplantation

intravenous infusion. Doses range from 25 to 40 ng/kg/min depending on the symptoms and toleration of side effects. Common side effects include jaw pain, headache, flushing, nausea, diarrhea, skin rash and musculoskeletal pain. The initiation of IV prostacyclin analogs requires admission to an inpatient service familiar with this medication, the placement of a central venous catheter, comprehensive education for the patient and family members, and close monitoring as the medication is started.

TAKE HOME POINT #4

Once initiated, prostacyclin analogs should not interrupted, even for short periods of time. It is important to make sure that patients who are admitted on these medications have an adequate supply of the drug and a functional infusion pump, as interruption of therapy for even a few minutes can lead to hemodynamic collapse. The patient's PH specialist should be contacted immediately.

Treprostinil is less potent than epoprostenol, and its effects are limited to improved exercise tolerance. Delivery options include continuous infusion through intravenous or subcutaneous routes, or through an inhaled formulation. Side effects of treprostinil are similar to epoprostenol, but include the possibility of pain and erythema (subcutaneous treprostinil), and cough (inhaled treprostinil).

Endothelin receptor antagonists block the vasoconstrictive and smooth muscle cell mitogenic effects of endothelin-1. Boesentan (initiated orally at 62.5 mg twice daily and titrated up to 125 mg twice daily after one month) and ambrisentan (administered orally at doses of either 5 mg or 10 mg once daily) improve hemodynamics, exercise capacity and the clinical course of PAH. Side effects of these medications include lower extremity edema, headache, nasal congestion, liver injury (monthly liver function tests must be performed), and anemia (monthly hemogloblin monitoring must be performed).

The phosphodiesterase type-5 antagonists sildenafil (20 mg orally three times daily) and tadalafil (40 mg orally once daily) prevent degradation of cGMP resulting in vasorelaxation. Common side effects include headache, flushing, dyspepsia, and epistaxis.

27.8 CARE OF THE CRITICALLY ILL PAH PATIENT

Though beyond the scope of the current discussion, some key concepts to consider when treating critically ill PAH patients are included in Tables 27.8 and 27.9. Acute hypoxemia in patients with PAH is a true medical emergency, and can be secondary to decreased cardiac output due to progression of their disease, interruption of medication administration due to pump or central line malfunction, sepsis, or pulmonary embolism. Given the tenuous hemodynamics of patients with PAH, any one of these events may be enough to cause cardiovascular collapse. Initial interventions may include the re-establishment of intravenous

Table 27.8 Causes of Acute Worsening of Hypoxemia in PAH.

1. RV failure and decreased cardiac output
2. Pump or catheter malfunction in patients who are on continuous therapy
3. In-situ thrombosis
4. Pulmonary embolism (unlikely for patients who are therapeutic on warfarin and/or who are on prostacyclin analogues)
5. Pneumonia/atelectasis
6. Sepsis
7. Right to left shunt via a patent patent foramen ovale (PFO) or atrial septal defect (ASD)
8. Large pleural effusion
9. Pneumothorax

Source: Rubenfire M, Bayram M, Hector-Word Z 2007. Reproduced with permission of Elsevier.

Table 27.9   Causes of Rapid Deterioration in PAH.

1. Natural history of the disease
2. Catheter occlusion or pump malfunction (prostacyclin)
3. Pneumonia
4. Indwelling catheter infection
5. RV ischemia, stunning, infarction
6. Pulmonary embolism
7. In-situ pulmonary thrombus
8. Gastrointestinal (GI) bleeding
9. Anemia
10. Ischemic bowel
11. Pancreatitis
12. Acute renal failure
13. Hypothyroidism
14. Hyperthyroidism
15. Arrhythmias (atrial fibrillation/flutter)
16. Subdural hematoma (confusion/central nervous system (CNS) symptoms)
17. Hyponatremia
18. Hypokalemia

Source: Rubenfire M, Bayram M, Hector-Word Z 2007. Reproduced with permission of Elsevier.

PAH medication administration through a peripheral IV, initiation of antibiotics, and hemodynamic support. The patient's PH specialist should be contacted immediately for further advice, or to initiate transfer to a PH center.

KEY REFERENCES

ACCF/AHA 2009 Expert consensus document on pulmonary hypertension. Circulation 2009; 119;2250–2294.

McLaughlin VV, Shillington A, Rich S. Survival in primary pulmonary hypertension: the impact of epoprostenol therapy. Circulation 2002;106:1477–1482.

Pulmonary Hypertension Association. www.PHAssociation.org

Rubenfire M, Bayram M, Hector-Word Z. Pulmonary hypertension in the critical care setting: classification, pathophysiology, diagnosis, and management. Critical Care Clinics 2007;23:801–834.

Chapter 28

Cardiac Tumors

Auroa Badin and Timir S. Baman

28.1 INTRODUCTION

Cardiac tumors are rarely primary in origin (<0.01%), with metastatic involvement 40 times more prevalent than primary cardiac tumors. Metastases to the heart are present in up to 20% of patients with terminal cancer, although the majority of these affect the pericardium. Most cardiac tumors are found incidentally on routine echocardiography during evaluation of unrelated conditions. For hospitalists, cardiology consultation is always recommended when cardiac tumors are suspected as treatment decisions can often be challenging even when a diagnosis is confirmed.

TAKE HOME POINT #1

Most cardiac tumors are found incidentally on echocardiography.

28.2 EPIDEMIOLOGY

Benign myxomas are the most common type of cardiac neoplasm accounting for up to 50% of all primary cardiac tumors (Table 28.1). Myxomas can manifest in all

Inpatient Cardiovascular Medicine, First Edition. Edited by Brahmajee K. Nallamothu and Timir S. Baman.

Table 28.1 Differential Diagnosis of Cardiac Tumors.

Cardiac tumor	Epidemiology	Gross description	Histology	Clinical description
Myxoma	Most common primary cardiac tumor Mean age of presentation in sporadic cases was 56 years 70% predominance for females 86% occurrence in left atrium	90% are solitary intra-atrial masses Pedunculated and gelatinous Sizes are range from 1 to 15 cm in diameter Usually smooth, but in 35% can be friable which increases risk for embolization	Scattered germ-like cells within mucopolysaccharide stroma Produces vascular endothelial growth factor (VEGF) which aids the early angiogenesis in tumor growth IL-6 production may cause fever, weight loss, anemia or elevated ESR	Classical triad includes: obstructive cardiac symptoms (67%); embolic phenomena (30%); constitutional symptoms (35%) Pulmonary congestion, split S1, and mitral regurgitation murmur can be common 5–10% associated with the Carney Complex (an inherited, autosomal dominant disorder with multiple cardiac and extracardiac tumors, including myxomas, schwannomas, and various endocrine tumors)
Papillary fibroelastoma	Second most common primary cardiac tumor in adults 80% of are found on heart valves Usually on the left side of the heart with the rest being intraventricular	Resemble sea anemones, with frond-like arms emanating from a stalked central core Size can vary from 2–70 mm	Characteristic avascular branching papillae	First manifestation is usually a stroke or transient ischemic attack due to embolization, either of the tumor itself or thrombus 30% are asymptomatic and diagnosed incidentally

347

Table 28.2   Clinical Presentation of Metastatic Cardiac Tumors.

Clinical symptomology
Hemorrhagic effusion
Precordial pain
Right-sided location
Combined intramural and intracavitary location
Extension into pulmonary veins

age groups; however, they are most common in the third to sixth decades of life. Most are located in the left atrium, but they can be found elsewhere. Women have a higher predominance of myxomas compared to men. Other less common etiologies of benign tumors include papillary fibroelastomas, rhabdomyomas, and fibromas.

Metastatic involvement of the heart is relatively common (Table 28.2), most often with involvement of the pericardium. Cardiac metastases can be due to direct invasion, distal metastases, or intravascular extension into the right side of the heart. Malignant melanomas, lung cancer, breast cancer, renal cell carcinomas, and soft tissue sarcomas are among the most common tumors to metastasize to the heart.

TAKE HOME POINT #2

Benign myxomas account for the vast majority of primary cardiac tumors.

28.3 CLINICAL MANIFESTATIONS

Although the majority of patients with cardiac tumors are asymptomatic, those neoplasms that present clinically can have varied presentations (Table 28.3). The degree of patient symptomology often depends on tumor size and location rather than the histopathology. Approximately 80% of cardiac myxomas manifest in the left atrium (Figure 28.1). If the size of the tumor is significant, patients can present with congestive heart failure, dyspnea, or syncope due to mitral valve obstruction (Figure 28.2, Figure 28.3). Tumors that occur in the right atrium or ventricle may be associated with signs of right heart failure. Smaller size tumors can lead to electrophysiologic abnormalities such as atrial tachyarrhythmias or conduction abnormalities. Systemic embolization is the most common cause of complications and occurs due to thrombus formation on the tumor with subsequent dislodgement or embolization of the tumor cells themselves.

Table 28.3 Clinical Manifestations Associated with Cardiac Tumors.

Mechanism	Clinical manifestation
Mechanical Obstruction of circulation	Symptoms of heart failure, syncope, sudden death
Interference with heart valves	Valvular regurgitation
Invasion	
Myocardium	Impaired contractility, arrhythmias, heart block, pericardial effusion
Lung	Respiratory symptoms
Embolization	Stroke, pulmonary embolism
Cytokines (IL-6)	Constitutional symptoms such as fever, fatigue, and lethargy

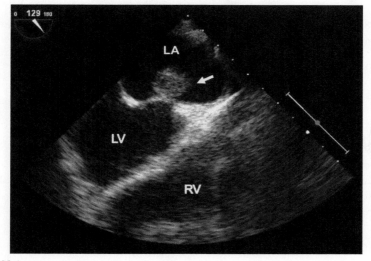

Figure 28.1 Transesophageal echocardiography with white arrow depicting left atrial myxoma. LA, left atrium; LV, left ventricle; RV, right ventricle.

Finally, malignant tumors can invade the pericardial sac causing pericardial effusion, cardiac tamponade, or constrictive pericarditis.

TAKE HOME POINT #3

Clinical presentation of cardiac tumors is determined by the size and location of the tumor in the heart rather than by its histopathology.

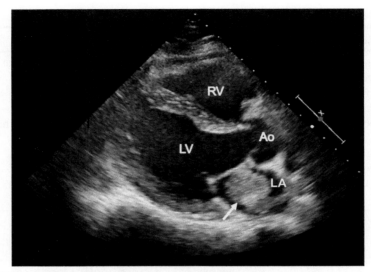

Figure 28.2 Transthoracic echocardiography depicting left atrial myxoma causing mitral valve obstruction (white arrow). Ao, aortic outflow; LA, left atrium; LV, left ventricle; RV, right ventricle.

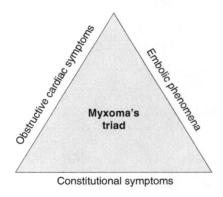

Figure 28.3 Triad of clinical symptoms for atrial myxomas.

28.4 DIAGNOSTIC EVALUATION

Cardiac tumors are extraordinarily difficult to diagnose due to their low incidence and highly varied clinical presentation. Some key physical examination findings that can indicate the presence of a cardiac tumor and necessitate further evaluation with an imaging study are summarized in Table 28.4.

The primary purpose of diagnostic evaluation is visualizing the size and location of the cardiac tumor, and its association with other structures such as heart valves or the pericardium. The etiology of a cardiac tumor is never determined by an imaging study, and histological analysis is always required. Echocardiography is a simple, widely available, and noninvasive diagnostic tool with a sensitivity and

Table 28.4   Key Physical Exam Findings Based on Tumor Location.

Location of tumor	Key finding
Left atrium	"Tumor plop", mitral regurgitation murmur, diastolic murmur, S4, delayed or split S1
Right atrium	Tricuspid stenosis (TS) murmur, diastolic murmur, and possible "tumor plop"
Left ventricle	Systolic ejection murmur can be heard
Right ventricle	Signs of right ventricular failure (jugular venous distention, peripheral edema, hepatomegaly)

specificity of >90% for cardiac mass detection. Moreover, utilization of Doppler echocardiography can ascertain if valvular obstruction is present. Transthoracic echocardiography (TTE) is usually the initial evaluation technique of choice when cardiac tumors are suspected. However, transesophageal echocardiography (TEE) may provide superior spatial resolution depending on location of the tumor (e.g. smaller tumors and those located on the posterior wall). TEE is also utilized to aid in planning for and intraoperative surgical resection of cardiac tumors (Figure 28.4).

TAKE HOME POINT #4

Echocardiography is the initial test of choice for cardiac tumors as the specificity and sensitivity of diagnosis is >90%.

Cardiac magnetic resonance (CMR) and cardiac computed tomography (CT) both provide higher resolution than echocardiography and can further characterize the lesion and extent of neoplasm involvement. CMR, if available, is preferred over cardiac CT for evaluation of cardiac tumors (Table 28.5) due to increased spatial resolution (Figure 28.5). This can be particularly useful when differentiating thrombus or hypertrophic papillary muscle from intracavitary tumor.

TAKE HOME POINT #5

Cardiac MR can provide detailed information regarding the surrounding environment of the tumor as well as provide clues to the etiology of the tumor.

Although CMR can help elucidate the type of cardiac tumor (Figure 28.6), histological evaluation with surgical biopsy continues to be recommended. Obtaining fluid for cytology examinations is possible when pericardial effusion is present. Percutaneous or transvenous biopsy can be considered but is frequently challenging to perform. If these modalities are not successful, thoracoscopy or thoracotomy may need to be performed.

A

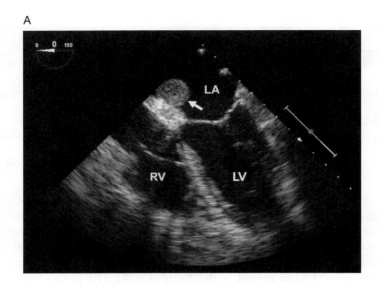

B

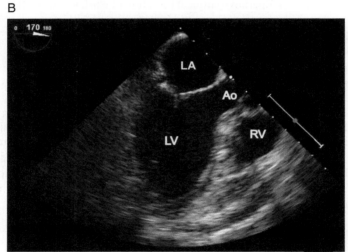

Figure 28.4   Transesophageal echocardiography **A** pre-resection of left atrial myxoma (white arrow), **B** post resection. Ao, aortic outflow; LA, left atrium; LV, left ventricle; RV, right ventricle.

Table 28.5   Comparison of Transthoracic Echocardiography (TTE) and Cardiac Magnetic Resonance (CMR).

Technology	Advantages	Disadvantages
TTE	Availability; relatively inexpensive	Limited tissue differentiation
CMR	High resolution; can differentiate tumors from thrombus	Expensive; not always available; use of gadolinium contrast

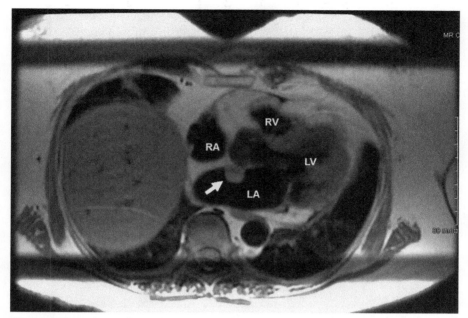

Figure 28.5 Cardiac magnetic resonance imaging of left atrial myxoma (white arrow). LA, left atrium; LV, left ventricle; RA, right atrium; RV, right ventricle.

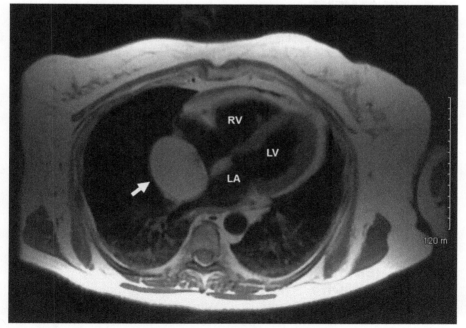

Figure 28.6 Cardiac magnetic resonance imaging showing a large right atrial lipoma (white arrow). The lipoma appears bright on a fat enhancing sequence. LA, left atrium; LV, left ventricle; RV, right ventricle.

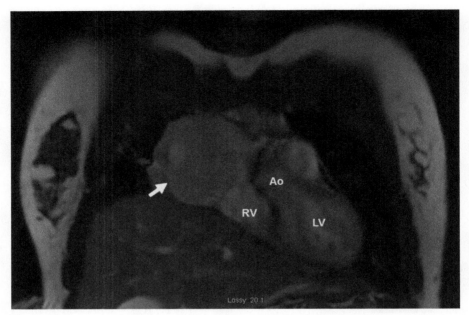

Figure 28.7   Large right atrial polymorphic sarcomas seen with cardiac magnetic resonance imaging (white arrow). Ao, aortic outflow; LV, left ventricle; RV, right ventricle.

28.5 TREATMENT

Surgical excision is the gold standard therapy for cardiac tumors with urgency to intervene based on type of tumor that is suspected as well as patient symptomology and clinical presentation. For asymptomatic patients with atrial myxomas, surgical intervention is recommended due to the high risk of embolic and cardiac complications. Surgical mortality for tumor excision is ~5% with a 3% recurrence rate up to 10 years. Recurrences can also occur in the heart, brain, lung, skeletal muscle, kidney, or gastrointestinal tract due to growth of embolized tissue. Patients who undergo myxoma resection should be followed by a cardiologist long term.

Treatment for other tumors is often individualized according to patient, tumor histology, and size. Malignant cardiac tumors, such as sarcomas (Figure 28.7), often are associated with a high mortality and morbidity as these tumors metastasize quickly and infiltrate the myocardium, thus causing cardiac obstruction. Surgical resection with or without chemotherapy can be considered but is associated with poor results and high rates of relapse.

28.6 OTHER UNCOMMON PRIMARY CARDIAC TUMORS

Rhabdomyomas: These tumors develop mostly before the age of one year, and are
   usually associated with tuberous sclerosis. They are usually found in the ventricular

walls or on the atrioventricular valves. Rarely resection will be needed, since most rhabdomyomas regress spontaneously.

Fibromas: These are the second most common cardiac tumor in children, occurring more commonly in the left ventricle causing heart failure or valvular dysfunction. If of significant size, cardiac transplantation may be indicated at time of resection.

Teratoma: These tumors can arise within the pericardium and can be associated with acute tamponade. These neoplasms carry a high risk of death *in utero* or immediately after birth.

KEY REFERENCES

McManus BE, Lee CH. Primary tumors of the heart. In: Libby, Bonow, Mann, Zipes (eds) Braunwald's Heart Disease, 8th ed, WB Saunders, 2007.

Reynen KL. Cardiac myxomas. N Engl J Med 1995;333:1610–1617.

Salcedo EE, Cohen GI, White RD, Davison MB. Cardiac tumors: diagnosis and management. Curr Probl Cardiol 1992;17:73.

Index

Inpatient Cardiovascular Medicine, First Edition. Edited by Brahmajee K Nallamothu and
Timir S Baman.
© 2014 John Wiley & Sons, Inc. Published 2014 by John Wiley & Sons, Inc.